This book is dedicated
to the next generation of doctors

Dunn's Surgical Diagnosis and Management

A GUIDE TO

GENERAL SURGICAL CARE

David C. Dunn MB, MChir, FRCS
Formerly Consultant Surgeon
Addenbrooke's Hospital
Hills Road
Cambridge CB2 2QQ

Nigel Rawlinson MB, MChir,
FRCS (Ed), FFAEM
Consultant in A & E Medicine
Bristol Royal Infirmary
Bristol BS2 8HW

THIRD EDITION

Blackwell
Science

© 1985, 1991, 1999 by
Blackwell Science Ltd
Editorial Offices:
Osney Mead, Oxford OX2 0EL
25 John Street, London WC1N 2BL
23 Ainslie Place, Edinburgh EH3 6AJ
350 Main Street, Malden
  MA 02148 5018, USA
54 University Street, Carlton
  Victoria 3053, Australia
10, rue Casimir Delavigne
  75006 Paris, France

Other Editorial Offices:
Blackwell Wissenschafts-Verlag
  GmbH
Kurfürstendamm 57
10707 Berlin, Germany

Blackwell Science KK
MG Kodenmacho Building
7–10 Kodenmacho Nihombashi
Chuo-ku, Tokyo 104, Japan

The right of the Authors to be
identified as the Authors of this
Work has been asserted in
accordance with the Copyright,
Designs and Patents Act 1988.

First published 1985
Reprinted 1989
Second edition 1991
Reprinted 1992, 1993, 1994, 1995,
1996
Four Dragons edition 1991
Reprinted 1992, 1994, 1996
Third edition 1999

Set by Semantic Graphics, Singapore
Printed and bound in Great Britain
at the University Press, Cambridge

For further information on
Blackwell Science, visit our Website:
www.blackwell-science.com

DISTRIBUTORS
Marston Book Services Ltd
PO Box 269
Abingdon, Oxon OX14 4YN
(Orders: Tel: 01235 465500
         Fax: 01235 465555)

USA
Blackwell Science, Inc.
Commerce Place
350 Main Street
Malden, MA 02148 5018
(Orders: Tel: 800 759 6102
              781 388 8250
         Fax: 781 388 8255)

Canada
Login Brothers Book Company
324 Saulteaux Crescent
Winnipeg, Manitoba R3J 3T2
(Orders: Tel: 204 837-2987)

Australia
Blackwell Science Pty Ltd
54 University Street
Carlton, Victoria 3053
(Orders: Tel: 3 9347 0300
         Fax: 3 9347 5001)

A catalogue record for this title
is available from the British Library

ISBN 0-86542-718-6

Library of Congress
Cataloging-in-publication Data

Dunn, David C. (David Christy)
    Surgical diagnosis and
management: a guide to general
surgical care/David C. Dunn,
Nigel Rawlinson. — 3rd ed.
        p.   cm.
    Includes index.
    ISBN 0-86542-718-6
    1. Diagnosis, Surgical.
    2. Surgery. I. Rawlinson,
Nigel.
II. Title. III. Title: Guide to
general surgical care.
    [DNLM: 1. Diagnostic
Techniques, Surgical.
    2. Surgical Procedures,
Operative. WO 141 D923s 1998]
RD35.D75 1998
617'.075 — DC21
DNLM/DLC
for Library of Congress
                        98-14103
                             CIP

David Dunn

David Dunn died whilst in the process of creating this third edition of *Dunn's Surgical Diagnosis and Management*. He was an outstanding teacher of surgery. His logical mind saw many ways of providing essential information in an easily digestible format — a great benefit to generations of students at the Cambridge Clinical Medical School and the original basis for this book.

His initial training was at Cambridge and St. Bartholomew's Hospital and he returned to Cambridge, firstly as Assistant Director of Research to the Academic Surgical Unit and subsequently to the NHS Consultant staff, to which he was appointed in 1974 and on which he remained until his premature retirement through ill health in 1997.

During his twenty-three years as a Consultant he displayed a keen interest in many of the emerging areas of surgical practice; these included transplantation, vascular and paediatric surgery, surgical audit and latterly, and with tremendous success, minimally invasive techniques. His ability to identify likely areas of surgical expansion was uncanny, and few surgeons in modern times have been able to achieve such success in so many different fields.

His overall surgical ability stemmed from a very secure basic knowledge. His concise analysis of surgical principles form the cornerstone of this highly successful book, written with Nigel Rawlinson, his former House Surgeon, and now into its third edition. This book will continue to be deservedly popular at Cambridge and at many other Clinical Schools for years to come, and will remain a lasting tribute to its senior author.

W A B Smellie
September 1998

Contents

15 Trauma Surgery, 627

List of Operations, 685

Index, 689

The Contributors

M. Drake Registrar in Urology, Paediatric Urology, Churchill Hospital, Old Road, Headington, Oxford OX3 7LJ

D. Griffith Consultant Surgeon, Rotorua Hospital, Private Bag 3023, Rotorua, North Island, New Zealand

J. Harper Professor of Orthopaedic Surgery, Glenfield University Hospital, 134 Groby Road, Leicester LE3 9QP

P. Kent Consultant Vascular Surgeon, Department of Vascular Surgery, St James' University Hospital, Beckett Street, Leeds LS9 7TF

C.L. Lawrence Consultant Dermatologist, Department of Dermatology, Royal Victoria Infirmary, Queen Victoria Road, Newcastle-upon-Tyne NE1 4LP

I.W. Mills Urology Research Fellow, Department of Pharmacology, University of Oxford, Mansfield Road, Oxford OX1 3QT

N.J.M. Mortenson Clinical Reader, Colorectal Surgery, Department of Surgery, John Radcliffe Hospital, Headley Way, Oxford OX3 9DU

R.E. Mountain Consultant ENT Surgeon, Department of Otolaryngology, Ninewells Hospital, Dundee DD1 9SY

D.A. Rew Senior Lecturer and Honorary Consultant, Department of Surgery, University Surgical Unit, Glenfield Hospital, 134 Groby Road, Leicester LE3 9PQ

R.A. Walker Reader in Pathology, Breast Cancer Research Unit, Glenfield Hospital, 134 Groby Road, Leicester LE3 9QP

F.C. Wells Consultant Cardiothoracic Surgeon, Papworth Hospital, Papworth Everard, Cambridge CB3 8RE

Preface to the Third Edition

The death of David Dunn, on August 19th 1998, was a great loss to many colleagues and friends in the surgical world. He had spent much of the previous year preparing this edition. He asked specialists in various fields to review the relevant sections, and then since the spring of this year he and I have been collating this, and checking a revised layout. This edition has been re-styled in a taller and thinner size. At the time of his last illness we were set to complete the final draft.

All the text has been revised. The structure of the first two chapters describing general management of patients in surgical wards has remained largely unchanged. The rest of the book has been re-organized to reflect the increased specialization within surgery, with new chapters such as Chapter 4 (Endocrine Surgery), including thyroid, parathyroid, adrenal, and pancreatic surgical management. Many of these sections have been carefully revised in an attempt to reflect the changing practice of surgery. When we set out to produce a concise, readable text, clearly laying out the principles of general surgery, we recognized that this clarity would not allow full justice to the areas where management is controversial or developing. We ask that this is understood and hope that other surgeons will be tolerant if the practice laid out in this book is widely different from their own. There is space for personal notes.

The layout of each condition has remained essentially unchanged, particularly the division into the headings 'Recognizing the pattern', 'Proving the diagnosis' and 'Management'. In an attempt to break up the text we have shaded the paragraphs that deal with management and operative notes. The popular surgical codes remain unchanged and are intended to be a general guide to a house surgeon gaining informed consent. We fully accept that such details of practice may vary between different surgeons and it is important that a house surgeon checks this information when there is doubt.

At the beginning of the book there is a tribute written by Mr W.A.B. Smellie, Consultant Surgeon at Addenbrooke's Hospital, Cambridge, and David's senior colleague for many years. Following this preface is a personal note from Anne Dunn, David's wife.

I hope that this third edition of *Dunn's Surgical Diagnosis and Management* will remain a popular and valid contribution to the training of clinical students, house surgeons and SHOs. I know that David would be very concerned to feel that this book was still relevant and able to instil knowledge and enthusiasm to those who use it, encouraging them to work to the highest professional standards. He would also hope that these same junior doctors recognized that behind every surgical condition there is a person, who is often afraid, vulnerable, and in need of individual and sensitive care.

Nigel Rawlinson

Personal Note

Before David died on August 19th 1998, he was going to finish this edition. As it turned out time ran out and it was not to be. I am so grateful to Nigel Rawlinson for picking up where David left off and I am sure that he will finish this edition in the style that David would approve of. I am particularly indebted to Michael Stein at Blackwell Science for extending the publishing deadline, giving Nigel time to get everything sorted out. I would also like to thank the reviewers, Ros Clipper and of course Anna Woodford for their assistance in producing this edition.

Anne Dunn

Preface to the First Edition

The stimulus to the production of this book has been the repeated demands of our medical students and housemen for a concise practical text which lists the methods of diagnosis and management of the main general surgical conditions they will have to deal with. It has been derived from a popular series of seminars in surgery given in Cambridge.

The combinations of authors is unusual. One (D.C.D.) has been a consultant since 1974 and the other (N.R.) was his houseman when the work started. We hope that this combination has helped us to concentrate on a layout which answers the needs of the houseman and medical student, needs which have often become obscure to senior doctors. Most surgical texts, for instance, fail to deal with questions which regularly confront the houseman, such as how much blood should be cross-matched for an operation, and how long patients will be in hospital and off work.

The book is designed to be easy to use for rapid reference and a similar layout is used for each subject, with headings suggested by the questions our students ask, such as:

What is that condition?

What makes you think that the diagnosis is likely?

How will you prove whether you are right or not?

What is the management, before, during, and after the operation?

What do I tell the patient when I'm obtaining his consent?

We have tried hard to make sure that the facts in the book are as accurate as possible and are grateful to our many colleagues who have checked the text. Inevitably, however, some errors may have crept in and we hope that our readers will write to us about these so that they may be corrected later.

The housesurgeon and patient have generally been described as 'he' in this book, a choice which is merely convenient and one which we hope will not upset our many excellent female junior staff.

Both authors have found the exercise of coorperating on this book to be interesting and illuminating. We hope our readers will also benefit from what we have produced.

David C. Dunn
Nigel Rawlinson

Acknowledgements

The following contributors are very gratefully acknowledged:
M. Drake, Registrar in Urology; D. Griffith, Consultant Surgeon; J. Harper, Professor of Orthopaedics; P. Kent, Consultant
Vascular Surgeon; C.L. Lawrence, Consultant Dermatologist;
I.W. Mills, Urological Research Fellow; N.J.M. Mortenson,
Clinical Reader in Colorectal Surgery; R. Mountain, Consultant ENT Surgeon; D.A. Rew, Senior Lecturer and Honorary
Consultant (breast surgery); R.A. Walker, Reader in Pathology,
and F.C. Wells, Consultant Cardiothoracic Surgeon.

The Layout of this Book

The first two chapters deal with the routine of patient management before and after any operation. In the subsequent chapters individual surgical conditions and their management are described. Each is presented under the following headings.

The condition
This section gives a brief descriptive outline of the disorder being dealt with.

Recognizing the pattern
When an experienced clinician is faced with a patient complaining of a symptom, he makes a diagnosis by taking an accurate history and by a careful examination. As he does this, however, he is constantly comparing the findings in the patient with a 'typical' picture he associates with various disease states. When he recognizes one of several familiar patterns of symptoms, he will ask subsidiary questions to strengthen or weaken his developing hypothesis as to the cause of the symptom. This process depends on a background knowledge of the typical pattern of each disease. In this section such typical patterns are presented.

Proving the diagnosis
The usual investigations necessary to prove the diagnosis are given.

Management
The general management of each condition is discussed and, after Chapter 2, highlighted using a grey background tint. Because this is a surgical textbook, this will usually involve an operative procedure. A brief description of the preoperative preparation is given, followed by a short account of the operation itself. All operation texts are highlighted with a vertical rule in the margin, and are (in most cases) general, rather than very detailed. In a few cases, however, where it is considered that a junior doctor might be called upon to do the procedure himself, more details are included.

Codes
The 'Codes' given at the end of each operative procedure are

an attempt to provide the houseman with some guidelines for answering those questions which frequently arise at the time of any operation. Notes on their use are given below and should be read before drawing any conclusions.

We are sensitive to the fact that these figures may prove controversial and there is considerable variation between the practices of individual consultants. Where the junior doctor finds that the figures for his unit are markedly different, we suggest that he alters them in the text for his own future reference.

The figures do not represent the *personal* experience of the senior author (D.C.D.) but are the sort of statistics he would give to a patient asking for them, regardless of which surgeon was operating. We hope that other surgeons will be tolerant if they feel they are an inaccurate representation of their own experience.

Notes on the use of 'codes'

Please read this carefully before drawing any conclusions from the figures given for each operation.

Blood. Refers to the amount of blood it is advisable to have available for the operation. It does not represent the amount usually lost.

GA/LA. GA, general anaesthetic; LA, spinal or local infiltration anaesthetic.

Opn time. Refers to the amount of time that might be allowed for this operation during an operating list. The actual time taken varies very widely according to the pathology encountered and the individual surgeon's operative technique.

Stay. Refers to the approximate time a patient can be told to expect to be in hospital. The length of stay will be prolonged if there are complications. It also varies with individual surgeons and hospitals and with the pressure on available beds.

Drains out and sutures out. Different surgeons vary widely in their practices but the figures given are thought to be reasonable to the authors and may help when no other information is available. Further general information is given in Section 2.3.

Off work. The figure for this is necessarily very approximate.

Nevertheless, such information is usually difficult to find so an attempt has been made to provide it. It must be emphasized that the figure given is only an estimate suitable to give the patient as a prediction. It should not be used in any legal arguments about whether or not a particular patient should be back at work.

1 The Daily Management of Patients in Surgical Wards

1

Pulmonary collapse and bronchopneumonia
Inhalation of vomit
Pneumothorax

1.7 Cardiovascular complications
Haemorrhage
Blood transfusion reactions
Myocardial infarction
Left ventricular failure
Stroke
Deep venous thrombosis
Pulmonary embolus

1.8 Urinary complications
Urinary tract infection
Postoperative retention of urine
Postoperative renal failure
Urinary fistula
Urinoma

1.9 Infections, abscesses and fistulae
Wound infection
Wound dehiscence
Infected intravenous drip site
Subphrenic abscess
Hepatic abscess
Pelvic abscess
External intestinal fistula
Bed sores
Septicaemia

1.10 Laparoscopic and endoscopic surgery
General points about laparoscopic surgery

1.11 The intensive care unit
The houseman's role in the intensive care unit
The intensive care unit chart
Daily management of patients on the intensive care unit

1.1 Admitting the Surgical Patient

The first two chapters of this book deal with the daily tasks a surgical houseman has to perform. They should be useful to those who are starting a surgical housejob. They will also help medical students to understand what is going on in a surgical ward and to prepare themselves for the task of being a surgical houseman after qualification. In the subsequent chapters the diagnosis and management of individual general surgical conditions are dealt with, the layout being as described in the preface (p. xvii).

Managing people who need operations

Many people tend to assume that young doctors are trained to regard the human body as a collection of mechanical tubes and pipes and that they overlook the importance of the 'individual'. In fact, most doctors find their work fascinating because they are dealing with a human body enclosing a mind and a spirit as well as complex, delicate biological systems.

The management of patients in surgery is dominated by this difference between the mechanical and the human, the difference between a technician and a surgeon. To obtain good results in surgery the mechanics must, of course, be correct. The anastomosis must not leak, the electrolytes must be kept in the correct range. Over and above this, however, the patient has to believe in their management and obtain confidence from their medical helper. Efforts spent on developing a trusting, friendly and honest relationship can pay huge dividends during the patient's illness. Every practising doctor knows this and has experience of patients surviving by their own will or dying because they have just given up. Maintaining the patient's morale can be just as important as maintaining his blood pressure.

During this book, we have not dwelt too much on this important and overriding principle in medicine, mainly because the relationship of one human being with another cannot be satisfactorily dealt with in a book of this type. It is, however, of supreme importance, and the ability to develop good relationships with patients will transform the knowledgeable bad doctor into the excellent and successful practitioner whom most students aspire to be.

The houseman plays a central role in the organization of a surgical firm. While the more senior members of the firm have to split their time between the ward, the outpatient department and theatre, the houseman's main priority is the ward. He or she is privileged to be the link between the patient, the surgical staff, the nurses and the paramedical staff and must coordinate all aspects of patient care.

The daily ward work

The routine ward work can be split into five parts:

1 Admitting the patient
2 Preoperative management
3 Organizing the operating list
4 The housesurgeon in theatre
5 The daily postoperative ward round.

Admitting the patient

Make sure that you have seen the outpatient notes and the consultant's letter before you start the routine clerking. Check that any X-rays, scans or investigations taken previously are available on the ward. Note which diagnosis the patient has been labelled with, but make your assessment critically and avoid blindly following a predetermined diagnostic pathway. By keeping an open mind you will be able to spot things which may have been missed in the often hurried outpatient assessment.

A full clerking is then carried out on all patients. Some points require special attention when an operation is being planned and these are listed below.

Detecting future problems

History

You are looking for any indication that the patient may not be fit for surgery or may be liable to develop problems postoperatively. Particular points are listed below.

Systems

Chest

Look for the following:

1 Pre-existing chest disease
2 Shortness of breath on minor exertion or at rest
3 Cough, and is it productive?

4 A history of asthma
5 Smoking habit.

Cardiovascular system
Is there a history of the following:
1 Chest pain or angina?
2 Symptoms of cardiac failure (such as oedema, nocturnal dyspnoea, orthopnoea or palpitations)?

Alimentary system
Ask about the following:
1 Anorexia and weight loss. This may indicate poor nutrition resulting in slow healing. In such patients check the serum proteins. The operation may need to be delayed until a protein deficit has been restored (see p. 96).
2 Bowel habit. Any patient prone to constipation who will be restricted to bed may well require suppositories to keep the bowels moving.
3 Heartburn and reflux. A patient with reflux may aspirate under anaesthesia and the anaesthetist should be warned.

Micturition
Ask about micturition. Poor stream, nocturia or hesitancy may be a clue to postoperative retention or infection. Bladder distension may be difficult to detect in the presence of a fresh lower abdominal incision.

Periods
Heavy periods are a common cause of anaemia in women.

Locomotor system
Does the patient suffer from arthritis? Are there any particularly stiff joints? Intubation may be difficult in the presence of cervical joint disease. It may be difficult or impossible to put patients in the lithotomy position on the table when they have stiff hips, knees or back.

Past history
Find out about the following:
1 Previous operations, and whether they were followed by any complications such as deep venous thrombosis or infection.
2 Previous anaesthetics. Were there any problems such as drug reaction, excessive vomiting, scoline sensitivity or malignant hyperpyrexia?

3 Previous history of rheumatic fever which may have damaged the heart valves. With such a history you must examine the heart carefully. Prophylactic antibiotics may be needed for a significant valvular lesion.

4 Previous history of jaundice.

Medical conditions

Does the patient suffer from any other diseases which will influence your management? These are dealt with in section 1.3 and include diabetes, heart disease and chest disease.

Drug history

Many drugs interfere with anaesthetic agents. Some may lead to electrolyte abnormalities (e.g. diuretics). Care must be taken with those on anticoagulants. The antiplatelet effect of aspirin lasts up to 7 days and is not reversible by platelet transfusion.

There is controversy regarding the oral contraceptive in the perioperative period. We advise offering deep venous thrombosis prophylaxis to all young women on the pill.

Allergies

Ask about allergies to:

1 Anaesthetics

2 Antibiotics

3 Applications (e.g. iodine or Elastoplast).

Check whether the allergy is genuine by determining what sort of reaction the patient had when he was exposed to the agent. Many patients say they are allergic to antibiotics because they felt ill or nauseated at the time they took them. Where there is any possibility of allergy, however, the patient's record should be marked and that drug avoided.

Family history

Is there a family history of reaction to an anaesthetic? A patient with a relative who developed anaesthetic problems will be anxious. Inform the anaesthetist as completely as possible about the reaction. Malignant hyperthermia and pseudocholinesterase deficiency can be inherited and reactions avoided by preoperative testing or avoiding certain anaesthetic agents.

Social history

Important points are as follows:

1 The patient's job. This will determine when the patient can go back to work.

2 Support. What sort of support is available from the family or friends postoperatively?

3 Habits. Check how much the patient drinks and smokes. A heavy drinker may be resistant to the normal doses of anaesthetic agents. A heavy smoker will be very liable to develop a chest infection postoperatively and preoperative physiotherapy may be indicated to minimize this risk.

The examination

Always try to improve on the findings made during the rapid outpatient assessment. Finding a supraclavicular lymph node, for instance, may save a patient with cancer from an unnecessary abdominal operation.

Details in the general examination which may be important are as follows.

General condition

Look for signs of dehydration, anaemia or cachexia. These may require correction before the operation is undertaken.

Mental state

Any patient will be anxious about the operation and in some this anxiety is extreme. Careful explanation and reassurance is required. A mild hypnotic or tranquillizer given on the night before the operation is sometimes helpful.

Cardiovascular system

Perform a full examination and inform the anaesthetist of any significant abnormalities. Pay particular attention to the blood pressure. If it is high come back and check it later as it often normalizes once the patient settles into their new environment.

Chest

Assess the shape of the chest looking for signs of emphysema. Check that there are no signs of pleural fluid, lung consolidation or bronchospasm.

Abdomen

The presence of abdominal scars provides a useful check on the patient's history. They may also indicate that a routine operation will be more difficult than usual and require more operative time because of adhesions.

All patients should have a rectal examination before abdominal surgery. Make a note of the amount and hardness of the faeces. Constipation should be relieved before the operation is undertaken. In males note the size of the lobes of the prostate. This information will be of value if the patient develops urinary problems postoperatively. Once in retention, the size of the prostate is much more difficult to assess.

Joints and teeth
The presence of false teeth or crowns, limitation of movement of the neck and micrognathia will make intubation more hazardous. These features should be brought to the attention of the anaesthetist.

Investigations
The following five investigations should be considered preoperatively.

1 Urea and electrolytes. These should be performed if:
   (a) the patient is on intravenous fluid therapy
   (b) the patient is on diuretics or steroids
   (c) the patient is over 70 years of age
   (d) the patient has acute or chronic renal disease
   (e) the patient is diabetic
   (f) there is a history of heart disease or hypertension
   (g) there has been recent significant fluid loss
   (h) you anticipate postoperative fluid therapy to continue for more than 24 h.

2 Full blood count. This should be performed if:
   (a) anaemia is suspected
   (b) the patient is over 70 years of age
   (c) there is a history of malignancy
   (d) there is a history of cardiac or vascular disease
   (e) there is haematological disorder or a coagulopathy
   (f) there is a potential for major blood loss.

3 Chest X-ray. This is indicated in:
   (a) suspected malignancy
   (b) major upper abdominal or thoracic surgery
   (c) patients over 50 years of age
   (d) those with signs or symptoms of significant cardiac or pulmonary disease (excluding asthma).

4 Electrocardiogram (ECG). This should be performed:
   (a) in known cardiovascular disease (including hypertension)
   (b) in males over 50 and females over 60 years
   (c) in those with diabetes or hyperlipidaemia.

5 Liver function tests. The serum albumin gives a good indication of the state of nutrition of the patient and should be

undertaken where this is in doubt. Other liver function tests may form part of the work-up for general liver disease such as hepatic metastases or cirrhosis.

Other investigations can be considered depending on the operation intended, or findings from the history and examination.

Some common pitfalls in surgical management

Diagnosis

Avoid accepting the diagnosis with which the patient has been labelled, until you have confirmed or altered this as a result of your own history and examination.

When taking the history do not blindly accept non-specific terms used by the patient. Define the symptoms they are trying to describe. While a patient might tell you they have had pleurisy, they may mean haemoptysis, shortness of breath and pleuritic chest pain more indicative of a pulmonary embolus and this will affect your management.

Management

Be aware of the patient's previous medications. Find out which can be stopped, which must continue (using alternative forms if appropriate) and which may have affected the patient's electrolyte balance (such as diuretics).

Avoid the temptation to treat postoperative fever with antibiotics. The causes of fever are myriad and should be investigated prior to introduction of antibiotics.

1.2 Preparing for the Operation

Preoperative management
The following is a useful checklist to run through for each patient on the next day's operating schedule.

Identification
Check that the correct patient is having the correct operation on the correct side. Mark such things as hernias, lumps in the breast, varicose veins and small lumps and bumps, using a permanent skin marker.

The As, Bs and Cs

Anaesthetist
The anaesthetist needs to be told a number of facts on the afternoon of the day before surgery.
1 A brief summary of the patient's general health, outlining any relevant problems, past medical history, drugs and examination findings.
2 The proposed surgery.
3 The position of the patient on the list.
4 When the patient last ate or drank (in emergency cases).
The anaesthetist also needs to be asked a number of questions.
1 If he will be writing up the premedication.
2 If he requires any further preparation.
3 If any extra monitoring needs to be arranged for theatre.

Antibiotics
Is cover required? See p. 110.

Anticoagulation
Does the surgeon require the patient to have prophylactic anticoagulation? For indications, see p. 53.

Blood
Is the haemoglobin available?

Biochemistry
Are the electrolytes available and within the normal range? A blood sugar series should be available in diabetics.

Bacteriology
Make sure the result of a culture swab is available on any patients who have preoperative sepsis.

Cross-match
Check that this has been arranged and that the blood will be ready on time (see individual operations).

Chest X-ray
If required.

Cardiogram
If required.

Consent
This is not simply a signature. Time must be spent explaining simply and concisely what the operation will involve. Use the opportunity to tell the patient something about what to expect in the postoperative period. Mention such things as drains and nasogastric tubes, explaining why they are needed. Tell him how long he will be in bed and unable to eat or drink, and how long he is likely to stay in hospital. This information is given in the relevant section later in the book and summarized in the Codes (see p. xvii).

Investigations
Make sure that the results of all the investigations that have been asked for preoperatively are available before the operation starts. These often contain some surprises that affect what should be done.

Organizing the operating list
Having admitted each individual patient, it is the housesurgeon's job to organize the operating list and to coordinate the various personnel in the departments involved.

The following headings summarize the main steps and may be used as a checklist. This should be done on the day before the operations are scheduled.

Surgeon
Be sure you know the following from him:
1 All the patients on the list.
2 What operations he intends to perform. Check you know the precise description and the most complicated alternative

procedure likely to be performed. Find out whether any special instruments or preoperative investigations will be needed.

3 The order of the list.

4 What time the surgeon wants to start.

5 In cases where you are uncertain, check with him whether or not blood is required.

Anaesthetist

Is he/she fully informed as on p. 10?

Assistant

One assistant of adequate experience should be available (some procedures will require more).

Theatre

All the information collected needs to be passed on to the theatre staff. This is done by providing an operating list (Fig. 1). They need to know:

1 The surgeon's name.

2 The anaesthetist's name.

3 The place and time at which the list will take place.

4 The name and age of the patients (children require special instruments).

5 The order of the list.

Please note: when making up the list of operations write clearly with no abbreviations. Always indicate the side of the operation in capital letters.

6 The operation intended, and any alternatives thought likely.

7 Any special equipment needed, e.g. nerve stimulator in parotid surgery, staple gun for bowel anastomosis, monitoring equipment, etc.

LIST OF OPERATIONS

DATE 24. 12. 91   SURGEON: Mr Cutfaster   ANAESTHETIST: Dr Snooze

TIME 8.30 a.m.   THEATRE 8

Number	Patient's Name	Number	Age	Ward	Operation
1	Andrew SMITH	54321	6 months	D2	LEFT inguinal hernia (baby)
2	Jane BLOGGS	68624	55	D8	Cholecystectomy and exploration of common bile duct. Operative cholangiogram.
3	Susan McARTHUR	72643	60	D8	Laparotomy for abdominal mass. ?RIGHT hemicolectomy ? oophorectomy.
4	Henry SMITH	629953	39	D8	RIGHT nephrectomy for hypernephroma ? Exploration of inferior vena cava.

Fig. 1 Specimen operating list.

Wards

A copy of this list is sent to all the wards involved.

Peroperative investigation

The relevant departments need to be informed of any special investigations that will be undertaken during an operation, e.g. histopathology for frozen section, radiology for operative cholangiogram.

Blood

Blood should be considered a potentially hazardous item, and should be transfused only if absolutely necessary.

Certain operations have a predictable blood loss. For this reason a cross-match is often performed preoperatively to ensure adequate amounts of blood are available when needed. Other operations may occasionally be associated with rapid haemorrhage and in these cases it is wise to have cross-matched blood available. If blood is less likely to be required, most blood banks can group and save the patient's serum so that blood can be rapidly cross-matched, if needed, during the following 7 days.

Autologous blood transfusion (that given by the patient to themselves) is likely to become more popular in the future.

A rough guide to the amount of blood many surgeons would wish to have available is set out in Table 1. Further details are given under each individual procedure.

Table 1 Quantities of blood that should be available for operations.

Cholecystectomy	
Amputation–lower leg	Group and
Thyroidectomy	save serum
Parathyroid exploration	
Vagotomy	
Mastectomy	
Staging laparotomy	
Transurethral prostatectomy	
Nephrectomy	
Gastrectomy	2 units
Colectomy	
Anterior resection	
Vascular surgery distal to common iliac vessels	
Whipple's procedure	4 units
Abdominoperineal resection	
Aortic surgery	6 units

1.3 The Management of Patients with Pre-existing Medical Diseases

It is important to identify any patients with an illness that could influence the postoperative course, and to do so in time to allow adequate treatment before the operation. The procedure may have to be delayed until the patient is made as fit as possible. The following medical conditions will be considered in this chapter.

1 Respiratory disease: acute and chronic
2 Cardiovascular disease
3 Diabetes
4 Patients on steroids
5 Patients on anticoagulants
6 Haemophilia
7 Patients with blood-borne diseases
8 Patients with acquired immune deficiency syndrome (AIDS).

Respiratory disease

Acute

Coughs, colds, sore throats and acute infections are all contraindications to elective surgery. Recovery usually takes place very quickly, especially in children, and unless the operation is urgent it should be delayed until the patient is fit. This usually means a delay of 2–4 weeks. The final decision as to whether a patient is fit for anaesthetic is left to the anaesthetist.

Chronic

Any patient with chronic respiratory disease has an increased risk of developing problems after an operation. Factors adversely affecting the chest include immobility, abdominal distension, an inability to cough due to pain and suppression of the cough reflex by analgesics.

The risks are increased by certain factors.
1 The nature and extent of the disease. Chronic airways obstruction is more of a problem than restrictive chest disease.
2 The severity of the operation. A prolonged anaesthetic or postoperative recovery enhances the risk of chest infection.
3 The site of the operation. Chest problems are more common after thoracic or abdominal operations, where coughing is very painful.

14

4 Type of anaesthetic. General anaesthetics potentially cause more problems than local anaesthetics.

5 Continued smoking. Increased secretions occur if smoking continues up to the time of surgery. Postoperative atelectasis is therefore more likely to occur.

In certain patients preoperative physiotherapy to the chest may reduce the risk of chest infection.

Assessment
Patients at risk should be recognized and the severity of their condition assessed.

Investigations
1 Full blood count. The haemoglobin may be elevated reflecting secondary polycythaemia due to chronic hypoxia. This indicates severe respiratory impairment.
2 Blood gases. Both hypoxia and hypercarbia in a blood gas sample reflect severe respiratory impairment.
3 Chest X-ray. This is an important preoperative baseline investigation for comparison with later postoperative X-rays, especially for patients with pre-existing lung disease.
4 Respiratory function tests.

Vitalography
The vitalograph measures the rate at which a patient can exhale. The patient is instructed to take a full inspiration and then blow as hard and for as long as possible into the mouthpiece. The instrument plots the volume exhaled against time. From the best plot obtained one can determine the volume of air exhaled in the first second (FEV_1 = forced expiratory volume in 1 s) and the total volume exhaled (FVC = forced vital capacity). The peak expiratory flow rate (PEFR) is another simpler measurement and is related to the FEV_1. Normal values depend on age, weight, sex, etc., and nomograms are available.

Airways obstruction or volume restriction affects the shape of the graph in a characteristic way (Fig. 2). A useful measure from the graph is the ratio of FEV_1 to FVC. (Normal value is above 75%.)

Airways obstruction reduces the rate at which air can be expelled more than the total volume. Thus the ratio of FEV_1 to FVC is less than 75%. If it is less than 50% significant obstruction is present and an attempt should be made to improve the situation before anaesthesia. Previous vitalographs may also be useful for comparison.

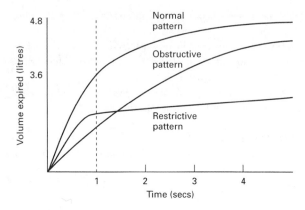

Fig. 2 The vitalograph plots the volume exhaled against time.

Restrictive airways disease (e.g. fibrosing alveolitis). The vital capacity is decreased more than the FEV_1 and the ratio may therefore be above 75%.

Management

Preoperative
1 The patient should stop smoking at least 1 month before surgery. The attempt to stop must therefore be made from the outpatient appointment. Explain that they are likely to develop pneumonia after their anaesthetic if they continues smoking. Most patients understand this and try to do something about it.
2 Try to admit the patient a couple of days before the operation for assessment and preoperative treatment. This consists of the following:
(a) physiotherapy — this may be both active (breathing exercises and loosening of secretions) and passive (postural drainage)
(b) bronchodilators — there is usually an element of reversible airways obstruction and bronchodilators are therefore used. Nebulized salbutamol (2.5 mls 0.1% solution 4-hourly by inspiration) is effective and the commonest in current use. Aminophylline suppositories at night help nocturnal dyspnoea and bronchospasm
(c) perioperative steroid use could be considered
(d) antibiotics — these may be given if surgery is performed despite a chest infection, but in general should be avoided as they encourage emergence of resistant strains.

3 If possible perform procedure under local rather than general anaesthetic.

4 The operative time should be kept to a minimum.

Postoperative care

1 Encourage early mobilization as this will improve chest expansion and decrease ileus.

2 Continue active physiotherapy.

3 Good analgesia enables an effective cough to clear secretions. Various excellent postoperative systems are available including epidurals and patient-controlled analgesia. In some hospitals a pain team may be available to help monitor postoperative pain.

4 Bronchodilators.

5 Prompt treatment of infection. Watch for signs of infection such as increased respiratory rate, pyrexia, purulent sputum and shortness of breath. Give broad-spectrum antibiotics after taking appropriate cultures. Change if necessary once sensitivities are known.

Asthma

Asthma is characterized by reversible airways obstruction. It may be precipitated by an allergen, exercise or cold. There may be no obvious precipitating factors.

Assessment

Find out about the following:

1 Any known precipitating factors.

2 The frequency and severity of attacks and the treatment needed to reverse them.

3 What normal maintenance treatment is required to prevent attacks?

Management

1 A mild well-controlled asthmatic is rarely a problem.

2 Severe asthmatics should be admitted early to allow time for assessment and for the patient to settle on the ward.

3 Reassurance and good premedication are important as anxiety may well precipitate an attack.

4 Discuss the case with the anaesthetist and ask if he/she wants any particular preoperative medication, such as nebulized salbutamol or steroid cover.

5 Listen for bronchospasm postoperatively and treat it early. Similarly, treat any developing chest infection quickly.

Cardiovascular disease

The following problems will be considered:

1 Myocardial ischaemia:
    (a) history of infarction
    (b) angina.
2 Hypertension
3 Left ventricular failure
4 Cardiac dysrhythmias, e.g. atrial fibrillation
5 Heart murmurs.

These pre-existing conditions should be spotted in the general assessment of the patient during the history and examination. If present, a full cardiovascular assessment is required.

Assessment

All patients with a cardiovascular abnormality should have the following investigations:

1 Haemoglobin: to exclude anaemia
2 Chest X-ray:
    (a) assess heart size and shape
    (b) look for pulmonary congestion
    (c) look for unfolding of the thoracic aorta (seen in long-standing hypertension)
    (d) look for calcification in the cardiac valves or aorta.
3 ECG:
    (a) look for evidence of dysrhythmia
    (b) look for changes of ischaemia
    (c) look for conduction defects.

The management of each condition is discussed below.

Myocardial ischaemia

Myocardial infarction

An elective operation should not be undertaken in the first 6 months after a myocardial infarct, as there is a substantial risk of perioperative reinfarction and death during this time. The risk is increased if the patient is hypertensive, if the operation is likely to be prolonged or if the operation involves thoracic or abdominal surgery. Patients who have had a myocardial infarction more than 6 months previously have a small risk of reinfarction.

Angina

If the patient has a history of angina, assess its severity using the following parameters:

1 The frequency of attacks
2 The duration of attacks
3 The state of improvement with rest or glyceryl trinitrate
4 How severe the circumstances were which brought on the attack.

Management of patients with myocardial ischaemia

1 Inform anaesthetist and surgeon. If appropriate, refer to a cardiologist for consideration of investigation, and delay operation.
2 Intraoperatively severe swings of blood pressure should be avoided.
3 Postoperatively give adequate analgesia and avoid fluid overload.

Hypertension

Drugs
Patients receiving treatment for hypertension usually stay on this treatment while in hospital. It is important that the anaesthetist knows which drug is being used as it will influence his management (e.g. β-blockers may mask any sympathetic response to hypotension). He will also have to decide whether any alternative therapy should be given when the patient is taken off oral drugs just before operation. Sudden cessation of certain drugs can lead to rebound hypertension.

Control
Check the blood pressure is well controlled. It may need to be taken on at least two occasions preoperatively.

Electrolytes
If the patient is on long-term diuretics check the electrolytes. Such patients are often sodium- or potassium-depleted.

Secondary effects
Look for left ventricular hypertrophy, myocardial ischaemia, ECG changes and impaired renal function.

Left ventricular failure
If this is acute it should be brought under control with diuretics

and angiotensin-converting enzyme (ACE) inhibitors prior to surgery. The help of medical colleagues should be sought.

If it is chronic, the following must be done:

1 Assess the present degree of failure. An ECG may be helpful to determine left ventricular function.

2 Note the treatment the patient is receiving.

3 Check the urea and electrolytes and relay this information to the anaesthetist.

4 Postoperative fluid management is difficult. It may be an advantage to run the patient rather more dehydrated than usual.

Dysrhythmia (e.g. atrial fibrillation)

Acute dysrhythmias are often precipitated by surgical emergencies and the treatment of these is best discussed with the anaesthetist. Chronic dysrhythmias are usually stable but the anaesthetist should be informed of current treatment.

Heart murmurs

Define the murmur by clinical assessment and evaluation of the ECG, chest X-ray and echocardiogram. If you are in any doubt about the interpretation of the murmur seek expert advice.

Assess the physiological significance of the murmur by looking for secondary effects such as dilatation of the chambers of the heart, or left or right ventricular failure. Check the patient's notes for evidence of previous problems.

Management of patients with valvular disease and septal defects

1 Treat any cardiac failure or dysrhythmia.

2 Antibiotics. Any diseased valve may act as a site for subacute bacterial endocarditis. Its surface may be colonized by organisms during a transient bacteraemia. Therefore prophylactic antibiotics are given to those patients with a murmur who are having the following procedures:

    (a) oral or dental surgery (*Streptococcus viridans*)

    (b) large bowel surgery

    (c) cystoscopy, prostatectomy, genitourinary surgery (*Streptococcus faecalis*)

    (d) biliary surgery

    (e) abortion (*Streptococcus faecalis*).

The drugs used are those indicated by the possible infecting organism. They should be given intravenously with the premedication. Amoxycillin and gentamicin is a popular combination. Vancomycin can be used if *S. aureus* is a possible infecting organism.

3 As in all cardiac disease, avoid any hypovolaemia or fluid overload.

Diabetes

Diabetic treatment is normally planned and adjusted for the individual patient to follow his usual lifestyle, while maintaining a normal blood sugar. Admission for a surgical operation disturbs this balance of 'treatment versus lifestyle', due to the catabolic response to surgery. Diabetics also have an increased risk of developing problems at the time of surgery due to the following factors:

1 Infection.

2 Cardiovascular disease.

3 Renal disease: diabetic nephropathy may affect the elimination of drugs by the kidney.

4 Autonomic neuropathy: this causes postural hypotension, affects the bladder causing retention, and has been implicated in sudden cardiorespiratory arrest in diabetics undergoing surgery.

Assessment

Determine how severe and how unstable the particular patient's diabetes has been. In addition look for evidence of diabetic complications. Assess the following:

1 Cardiac function (by history, examination, chest X-ray and ECG).

2 Renal function (by measurement of the blood pressure, looking for the presence of oedema, testing the urine for protein and checking the serum urea and electrolytes).

3 The neurological system (look for autonomic neuropathy by taking blood pressure supine and upright).

Ideally, diabetic patients needing major surgery should be admitted 24 h before the operation for assessment and stabilization. More time will be needed if their method of diabetic treatment is to be changed (see below).

Monitoring sugar levels

Urinalysis

This method is unreliable as it is retrospective. The urine reflects the blood sugar content some hours previously. It is inferior to blood sugar estimations.

Blood sugar estimation

All patients should have a blood sugar specimen analysed to provide a baseline. However, for serial monitoring, the sugar level in the blood can be tested either by the visual 'sticks' (Dextrostix or BMstix) or a reflectance meter (glucometer). The latter is more commonly used.

Management

The aim of management is to maintain good control and prevent hypoglycaemia and ketoacidosis. Ketoacidosis is prevented by supplying adequate calories and insulin, and hypoglycaemia is prevented by ensuring that the insulin given is covered by sufficient glucose input. Hypoglycaemia is to be strenuously avoided. If it occurs under anaesthetic and is not picked up, brain damage may occur.

Patients can be divided into three main groups:

1 Diabetics controlled by diet
2 Diabetics controlled by oral hypoglycaemics
3 Insulin-dependent diabetics.

Procedures can be divided into:

1 Small operations, where the patient may eat as soon as he wakes up.
2 Large operations, where the patient may have no oral intake for a variable length of time postoperatively.

The precise management will depend on which combination of these factors is present.

Diabetics controlled by diet

Small operations
No specific measures.

Large operations
1 Measure the blood sugar just before anaesthetic.
2 Regular 3–4-hourly blood sugar measurements postoperatively for 24 h.
3 Usually there is no problem, but the combination of stress and bed rest may cause a rise in blood sugar and make the patient temporarily insulin-dependent (see section 1.3, p. 23).

For patients withdrawn from oral feeding, a standard intravenous regime (e.g. 1 L of normal saline, 2 L of 5% dextrose, each with 20 mmol potassium) will give the patient 100 g of carbohydrate. Insulin may or may not be added to this.

Diabetics controlled on oral hypoglycaemics

Small operations
1 No hypoglycaemic on the day of operation.
2 Measure blood sugar just before anaesthetic, postoperatively and 4 h later.
3 Restart oral hypoglycaemics as soon as oral intake is established.

Large operations
Patients must be stabilized and managed on short-acting insulin. Ideally they should be admitted 24–48 h before the operation for conversion to a short-acting soluble insulin. Further management is then as for patients on insulin.

The effects of oral hypoglycaemics may last many hours and insulin requirements will vary. Therefore use a sliding scale of insulin.

Insulin-dependent diabetics
Discuss the preoperative management with the anaesthetist. There are different ways of managing such diabetics and the anaesthetist may well have a preference.

Small operations
If possible plan the operation early in the list.
1 Omit any long-acting insulin the night before the operation.
2 Low insulin requirement: omit the morning dose of insulin. Set up an intravenous infusion for the pre- and perioperative period of 1 L of 5% dextrose with 16 units Actrapid and 20 mmol KCl, infused at 100 mL/h. Patients having small operations later in the day can have a light breakfast covered by half the normal dose of insulin in the morning. They are then starved and an infusion is set up as above.
3 Check the blood sugar before operation, immediately after operation and 4-hourly until eating normally.
4 As soon as oral intake is re-established after the operation, restart the insulin.

Large operations
There are many possible regimes one may use for intravenous insulin administration. One regime is listed below, but your anaesthetist may prefer to use a different one.

Plan the operation early in the list.

Table 2 Sliding scale for insulin infusion rate according to hourly blood sugar measurement.

Ward glucometer test (mmol/L)	Insulin i.v. (units/h)
< 2	Give 50 ml 50% glucose i.v
2–5.9	None
6–8.9	0.5
9–10.9	1.0
11–16.9	2.0
17–28	4.0

1 The day before the operation give the patient his normal dose of insulin in short-acting form.

2 On the morning of the operation start an intravenous infusion of 5% dextrose with 16 units Actrapid and 20 mmol KCl, infused at 100 mL/h.

3 Postoperatively, the insulin is given by continuous infusion from an insulin pump 'piggy-backed' into the side of the drip (strength: soluble insulin 1 unit/mL in saline). The infusion is governed as in Table 2. This system needs good nursing care as the glucose and insulin are given independently and there is a risk that they may get out of phase (in particular, there is a danger of hypoglycaemia).

An insulin infusion is ideal, especially for a long period of care when the patient is going to have no fluid or restricted fluid by mouth. Once the patient begins to drink and becomes re-established on a diet, a twice- or thrice-daily soluble insulin regime can be restarted and adjusted according to blood sugar levels. The initial total daily insulin should roughly equal the patient's preoperative dose. It should be increased by about 20% in the presence of infection or when the patient is taking high-dose steroids. Fifty units Actrapid plus 50 mL 0.9% saline via intravenous infusion pump are administered according to the scale shown in Table 2. One litre 5% dextrose is infused intravenously concurrently over 8–10 h. The saline requirement is given through a second line. Potassium requirements can be added as usual.

NB. The dose may need doubling or quadrupling if the patient is severely ill, shocked or taking steroids or sympatho-mimetic drugs.

Measure the blood sugar hourly postoperatively until stable, adjusting the infusion rate according to the above chart. Once stable, measure it 2–4-hourly. Monitor the potassium levels.

Emergency surgery in diabetics

Diet-controlled diabetics and those on oral hypoglycaemics can usually be managed by putting up a 5% dextrose infusion and administering subcutaneous Actrapid, according to a gentle sliding scale.

Insulin-dependent diabetics and those who are extremely ill should have an insulin dextrose infusion as outlined. It is usually better to run the blood sugar a little too high, rather than a little too low. Ketoacidosis can mimic the acute abdomen, therefore patients should be stabilized and reassessed prior to operation.

Patients on steroids

If the patient has been on regular steroids in the 6 weeks preceding the operation he may have adrenal suppression and be unable to respond to stress and trauma in the usual way. Additional steroid cover is then required.

The dose given is influenced by the severity of the operation and the length of the previous steroid treatment. A commonly used regime for a major operation is listed below.

1 Hydrocortisone 100 mg i.m. with premedication.

2 Hydrocortisone 100 mg 8-hourly over the day of the operation.

3 Hydrocortisone 50 mg 8-hourly on the second postoperative day.

4 Hydrocortisone 50 mg 12-hourly on the third postoperative day.

5 Then 25 mg 12-hourly gradually decreasing to the patient's normal dose over a further week. It is useful to remember that 5 mg of prednisolone is equivalent to 20 mg of hydrocortisone.

6 If the patient's blood pressure falls postoperatively and other causes have been excluded, suspect adrenal insufficiency and give extra hydrocortisone (e.g. 100 mg hydrocortisone i.v.) until the blood pressure is restored.

Patients on anticoagulants

The precise management depends on the policy of the local surgical unit, anaesthetists and haematologists. Patients are usually on anticoagulants as prophylaxis against venous or arterial thrombosis. This is discussed fully on pp. 112–113. In each case a fine balance needs to be kept between effective anticoagulation and minimal risk of haemorrhage during surgery.

The anticoagulant effect of both heparin and warfarin can be reversed. The action of heparin is reversed with protamine sulphate. The action of warfarin is reversed with fresh frozen plasma (FFP) and vitamin K.

The management of a patient on warfarin will depend on the reason for warfarinization. Those with prosthetic heart valves should be managed more precisely than those on warfarin for atrial fibrillation.

In some patients it may be suitable to omit warfarin for 2–3 days and operate when the international normalized ratio (INR) falls to approximately 1.6. In others, the patient may need to be fully stabilized on heparin prior to elective surgery. In the emergency setting use FFP and small doses of intravenous vitamin K (in consultation with the haematologist) to achieve an INR of less than 2.

Haemophilia

Classical haemophilia is due to a deficiency of factor VIII. Christmas disease is due to a deficiency of factor IX. The severity of the condition varies between different patients, but all need special management when surgery has to be undertaken. Capillary bleeding initially ceases due to platelet aggregation (primary haemostasis). Because of the factor deficiency, the clotting cascade is inadequately activated and insufficient fibrin is produced to stabilize the clot. Continued bleeding therefore occurs in the postoperative period unless replacement therapy is given.

Management

Any patient with a history suggestive of a bleeding diathesis, or a family history of haemophilia, should have a full clotting screen undertaken before an operation is contemplated. Patients with proven haemophilia are managed in close cooperation with the haematology department, which must be given as much advance warning as possible. They will usually arrange for the defective factor to be replaced. This may be done using concentrates of factor VIII or IX. Some patients develop antibodies to the missing factors, making management much more difficult. The patient is screened for such antibodies before operation, and if present elective surgery is usually contraindicated.

Patients with mild haemophilia can have their own factor VIII levels stimulated by giving a non-vasoactive vasopressin analogue deamino-D-arginine vasopressin (DDAVP).

If the clotting factor deficiency is corrected, the care of haemophiliacs is similar to that of other patients. However, after major surgery, factor VIII levels may need to be measured and factor VIII given twice daily. Factor IX may need to be given once a day. The morning dose should be given first thing before the patient is bathed and the wound dressed. Intramuscular injections should be avoided. Sutures should be left in longer than usual (10 days) as there is a tendency to bleed around the eighth or 10th day and this may be precipitated by removal of the sutures. Similarly, bleeding may occur after the removal of drains. If effective anti-haemophilic therapy is assured, drains should only be used where they would otherwise be indicated and not inserted specially because of the haemophilia.

Other bleeding disorders and prothrombotic states

A number of other bleeding disorders may require careful preoperative management. They are rare and include:

1 Disorders of the clotting cascade (e.g. factor X or XI deficiency).

2 Disturbances of platelet vessel wall interaction (e.g. von Willebrand's disease).

3 Abnormalities of platelet function (e.g. thrombasthenia).

A careful personal and family history of excess bleeding, especially after tooth extraction or tonsillectomy, will often raise suspicion of the presence of one of these disorders. A basic clotting screen (bleeding time, prothrombin time, partial thromboplastin time (PTT) and fibrinogen) will frequently produce initial confirmation of clinical suspicions.

It is increasingly recognized that congenital and acquired disorders of coagulation are common causes of postoperative thrombosis. Such conditions, frequently due to a reduction of the level of naturally occurring anticoagulants (such as protein C, protein S and antithrombin III) will require careful pre- and postoperative management. Once again a personal or family history of deep venous thrombosis or pulmonary embolism, especially before the age of 40 years, will give a clue as to whether further detailed investigations are required.

Blood-borne diseases

Health-care professionals have quite rightly become concerned about the transmission of certain diseases from patients to those dealing with them or their specimens. Contamination with human immunodeficiency virus (HIV) and hepatitis B most commonly require consideration. As doctors we are at particular risk of transmission from patients' blood; from needle-stick injuries during cannulation, to major contamination in theatre.

For some diseases all those at risk can be immunized (e.g. hepatitis B), and occupational health departments are active in ensuring this. Others, while detectable, have no known vaccine, and new diseases may be discovered by the time you read this book.

The only practical solution therefore, is to minimize the risk of exposure by adopting certain precautions.

1 Cover all open wounds with appropriate dressings.

2 Wear gloves when coming into contact with patient body fluids.

3 Avoid contact with sharps. Avoid resheathing needles, use sharps bins for needles, syringes and scalpel blades, use other instruments when manipulating sharps (no-touch technique).

4 In theatre use a sharps receiver to pass scalpels and needles to one another.

5 In theatre wear eye protection to avoid contamination via the conjunctiva.

6 Double glove.

Occupational exposure to HIV

Report needle-stick injuries immediately to the relevant authority. Recent evidence suggests that the risk of acquiring HIV after a contamination incident is reduced by post-exposure prophylaxis with Indinavir, Lamivudine and Zidovudine. You and the patient may then be tested after relevant counselling. If you do have the misfortune to acquire a disease, testing will enable you to prove your seroconversion was occupationally related. This could be important in future compensation or insurance claims.

AIDS

AIDS, caused by HIV, is a major new disease which has profound implications for both patients and staff. Infection can be acquired by drug abuse, through homosexual or heterosexual intercourse or due to treatment with blood products contaminated with HIV. Quite apart from the effects of the disease, the consequences of diagnosis on an individual's mortgage, insurance, compensation and family can be devastating.

Transmission of the disease occurs with difficulty and requires intimate contact with infected human blood, serum or semen. Once infection has occurred, the virus may remain dormant for many years. Eventually, most, if not all, carriers develop the full-blown immune deficiency syndrome in which there is an absence of T-cell helper activity. This syndrome can present in a wide variety of ways due to lowered resistance to other infections. These may involve any of the surgical specialties. Among the common presentations are atypical pneumonia (pneumocystis), orogenital candidiasis, progressive lympha-denopathy and Kaposi's sarcoma. Although at the time of writing there is no cure for this infection, active treatment can improve the patient's length and quality of life. Patients have a right to confidentiality particularly as there is still intolerance by society to this diagnosis.

Recognizing the pattern
The diagnosis should be considered in any patient presenting with an unusual condition who might be in a high-risk group for infection. The main high-risk groups are listed below.
1 Homosexual males
2 Bisexual males
3 Intravenous drug users
4 Haemophiliacs
5 Recipients of blood products before HIV testing started
6 Residents of African countries south of the Sahara
7 Sexual partners of any of the above
8 Children of infected mothers
9 Prison inmates, past or present.
Heterosexual transmission is now increasingly recognized.

Proving the diagnosis
The patient's informed consent must be obtained prior to HIV testing. Occasionally the virus can be isolated from the host tissues, but this is unreliable.

HIV antibodies appear in serum up to 3 months after infection. The patient can transmit infection during the seron-egative phase. HIV antigen can also be detected in serum, but this test is less widely available than that based on the antibody.

Management
It is unethical for a doctor to refuse treatment to a patient infected with HIV on the grounds that there is a risk of the doctor becoming infected (General Medical Council 1988). Therefore adequate precautions must be taken to prevent cross-infection from any patient by the means listed under Blood-borne diseases (p. 28).

1.4 The Operation and Afterwards

The housesurgeon in theatre

The housesurgeon should ensure that the operating list runs as smoothly as possible. A bleep can be very distracting to the surgeon and should not be worn in theatre.

Before scrubbing up:

1 Check whether the patient requires a bladder catheter.

2 Check that any necessary preoperative antibiotics have been given.

3 Fill in a histology form for frozen section if this is required. If the operating list is running late, inform any other department that might be affected, e.g. those providing peroperative radiology or frozen section histology.

Assisting at operation

The principle of assisting is to make the operation as easy as possible for the surgeon. If you are the first assistant try and follow the operation, imagining you were having to do it yourself, and thus anticipating what is required.

When sutures are being tied have a pair of scissors ready to cut the ends when asked to do so. Always use the tips of the scissors. If you use the blade higher up there is a danger of inadvertently cutting neighbouring structures. Skin sutures should be cut so that the ends are as long as the distance between each suture. In this way they can be seen easily for removal, but are not in the way of the next knot. For internal sutures ask how long the surgeon would like the ends cut, as this will vary with the type of material used.

Ensure that the area the surgeon is operating on is as well exposed as possible, using suitable retractors or forceps to display the structures. Keep the field clear of blood using swabs or suction.

Never try and 'dictate' what the surgeon should do next; simply make it as easy as possible for him to achieve what he has decided to do.

There is usually less to do as a second assistant and you may find yourself holding on to a retractor for hours. This is an important role, as a good demonstration of the operative field may make all the difference between a successful or unsuccessful operation for your patient. Do it willingly and cheerfully.

The immediate postoperative period

The houseman should check the following things after each operation.

1 Laboratory specimens. Have they been labelled and the forms signed? Make sure any microbiology specimens have gone to the laboratory.

2 Operation note. Has it been written?

3 Prescription chart. Check this in order to be certain of the following:

    (a) adequate analgesia and night sedation are written up

    (b) an intravenous fluid regime is written up if the patient requires it.

4 Intravenous lines, arterial lines, drains and catheters. After a large operation make a mental note of the position of these. Are they all necessary in the postoperative period and how long will the surgeon require them to be left in?

5 Nursing observations. Note which observations are required postoperatively and inform the nurses of any particular problems such as the presence of a chest drain or drains requiring measurement of output.

The daily postoperative ward round

The houseman should see every patient under his care at least once a day. This enables him to keep in touch with the patient's progress, and to pick up any postoperative problems as they arise.

The following is a basic plan for such a round, designed to check quickly on every aspect of patient care. If you find something positive the methods of management can be followed up in sections 1.5–1.9.

History

Ask about pain and vital functions.

1 Pain: if the patient has any new or unexpected pain, diagnose the cause. Ask particularly about pain in the legs or chest (thromboembolism), or increasing pain in the wound (wound infection). Has adequate analgesia been prescribed?

2 Breathing: shortness of breath, cough, haemoptysis.

3 Eating: appetite, nausea, vomiting.

4 Bowels: passage of flatus, motions.

5 Urine: has the patient passed urine? Has the patient had any dysuria or difficulty?

Examination

Check the following:

1 Temperature charts for pyrexia, change in pulse rate, blood pressure and respiratory rate.
2 Chest: examine for signs of infection, collapse or oedema.
3 Wound: check for developing localized tenderness.
4 Bowel sounds (after abdominal surgery).
5 Legs: check for localized tenderness over the soleal muscles.
6 Mental state.

Fluid balance

Examine the fluid chart and check the input (oral, i.v.) against the output (urine, nasogastric tube, drains and insensible loss). Is the patient in positive or negative fluid balance?

Drains and tubes

Check the position of intravenous lines, drains and any urinary catheter. Are they all draining? Can any be removed? Have any become infected?

Drugs

Check the prescription sheet for any unnecessary drugs which can be deleted.

Investigations

Order any tests which may be necessary (e.g. haemoglobin, urea and electrolytes, serum proteins).

1.5 Postoperative Complications: Presenting Symptoms

Some of the common problems you will be called upon to deal with in the postoperative period are dealt with in this section. They are listed in Table 3. Further notes on subsequent management are given in sections 1.6–1.9.

Table 3 Common postoperative problems.

Common presentations	Causes	Page reference
Pyrexia	Pulmonary collapse or bronchopneumonia	44
	Wound infection	66
	Intra-abdominal abscess (pelvic or subphrenic)	70–74
	Urinary tract infection	59
	Inflamed drip site	70
	Thromboembolism	52
	Blood transfusion reaction	49
	Septicaemia	76
Postoperative pain	Wound haematoma or infection	66
	Chest	36
	Heart	36, 50
	Abdomen	36
	Legs	36
	Deep venous thrombosis	52
Discharging wound	Abscess	66
	Fistula	64, 74
	Dehiscence	68
Nausea and vomiting	Drugs	36
	Intestinal obstruction	320
	Acute dilatation of the stomach	43
Constipation	Paralytic ileus	42
	Drugs	37
Breathlessness	Pulmonary collapse	44
	Bronchopneumonia	44
	Pulmonary embolism	54
	Left ventricular failure	51
	Inhalation of vomit	45

Continued on p. 34

Table 3 *Continued.*

Common presentations	Causes	Page reference
Confusion	Hypoxia	⎫
	Toxaemia	⎬ 38
	Drugs, alcohol withdrawal	⎭
	Electrolyte disturbances	
Collapse	Inhalation of vomit	45
	Haemorrhage	48
	Septicaemia	76
	Pulmonary embolus	54
	Myocardial infarction	50
	Stroke	51
Oliguria/anuria	Postrenal, renal and prerenal failure	61
	Retention of urine	60

Postoperative pyrexia

The temperature chart is a very good indicator of developing postoperative problems and should be inspected every day. The time of onset of the fever will help you decide the cause.

Early postoperative fever, days 0–2

A mild pyrexia in the first 24 h after operation is commonly due to tissue damage and necrosis, or haematoma formation at the operative site. A higher and more persistent pyrexia may be due to pulmonary collapse, or specific infections related to the surgery, e.g. urinary infection after bladder surgery or biliary infection after a cholecystectomy. A fever due to blood transfusion may also appear in this early period.

Fever, days 3–5

A pyrexia developing in this period is likely to be due to either developing sepsis (e.g. wound infection or pelvic or subphrenic abscess formation) or bronchopneumonia.

Fever, days 5–7

Problems presenting at this time include those associated with failure of a bowel anastomosis, e.g. leakage and fistula formation, and a fever due to venous thrombosis either in the limbs or in the pelvic veins.

Fever after the first week

This is less likely to be due to a problem directly related to the operation, although the development of wound or deep sepsis can be delayed if the patient has received prophylactic antibiotics. Other causes include the development of distant sepsis such as a hepatic abscess or cerebral abscess. Thrombotic disease may also be delayed in onset and appear at this time.

Making the diagnosis

Carry out the following routine.

1 Ask about symptoms of cough, sputum, dysuria, urinary frequency or calf pain.

2 Examine:

    (a) the respiratory and pulse rates

    (b) the chest

    (c) the wound

    (d) the drip site and drain sites

    (e) the calves for tenderness localized over the soleus muscle

    (f) the abdomen if an abdominal operation has been performed.

3 Consider performing these investigations: culture specimens of sputum, urine, blood (if temperature above 38°C), a wound swab and a chest X-ray.

Management of the underlying condition

Some common causes of postoperative pyrexia are shown in Table 3. Further details of these conditions are given in subsequent chapters.

Postoperative pain

Pain relief is almost always required in the postoperative period and analgesic therapy is discussed on p. 104.

The cause of any pain must be determined in the same way as in other circumstances but there are important causes in a postoperative patient.

Wound pain

Pain in the wound is worse on movement and is usually maximal in the first 72 h. Thereafter it usually settles. If the pain is getting worse after this, check for signs of a wound infection, either superficial or deep. Occasionally, patients suffer quite severe 'spasms' of pain in an abdominal wound. This is more common in those who are excessively tense.

Treatment

Appropriate analgesia for wound pain: small doses of tranquillizers (e.g. diazepam 2–5 mg 8-hourly) are helpful for muscle spasms.

Chest pain

Excluding any pain due to a thoracic wound, two other significant types of chest pain occur postoperatively.

1 Pleuritic. Sharp, localized and severe pain increased by inspiration. This may be due to infection involving the pleura or pulmonary infarction after an embolus (see pp. 44 and 54).

2 Cardiac pain (due to myocardial infarction). The patient may complain of a retrosternal tight pain with or without radiation into the arm (see p. 50).

Abdominal pain

Possible causes of increasing abdominal pain include:

1 Intra-abdominal sepsis (see pp. 70–74)

2 Anastomotic leakage (p. 74)

3 Retention of urine (p. 60)

4 Constipation (p. 37)

5 New intra-abdominal pathology, e.g. ischaemic bowel (p. 324), intussusception (p. 325), intestinal obstruction (p. 320).

Legs

1 Deep or superficial venous thrombosis (p. 53)

2 Sciatica

3 Postoperative arterial thrombosis or embolism.

Discharging wound

A copious discharge from the wound may be due to the release of a wound abscess. You should also consider the possibility of the development of an intestinal fistula (p. 74), a urinary fistula (p. 64) or a deep wound dehiscence (p. 68).

Nausea and vomiting

The common causes of postoperative vomiting are as follows:

1 Drugs:
   (a) analgesics (opiates)
   (b) anaesthetic agents
   (c) other drug therapy, e.g. digoxin toxicity.

2 Intestinal obstruction:
   (a) paralytic ileus
   (b) mechanical.

Making the diagnosis

1 Note which drugs the patient has received.

2 Check possible drug interactions. For example, an elderly

patient may be on digoxin and develop hypokalaemia with in-travenous fluid and diuretics. This may precipitate digoxin toxicity.

3 Assess the oral input and listen for bowel sounds. Nausea and vomiting when the patient has just started drinking after ab-dominal surgery may be due to a persistent paralytic ileus. In that case the abdomen will be distended and bowel sounds absent.

4 If nausea and vomiting occur after the patient has been tol-erating oral fluids, consider the possibility of a mechanical obstruction. Here there is usually colicky pain with active bowel sounds. An abdominal X-ray will show distended loops and fluid levels with paucity of distal gas on the erect film.

Treatment

1 Pass a nasogastric tube to drain the stomach.
2 Paralytic ileus (p. 42).
3 Mechanical obstruction (p. 321).
4 Drug-induced vomiting. Treat with an antiemetic (e.g. prochlorperazine 12.5 mg i.m. 4–6-hourly, or metoclopramide 10 mg i.m. 4–6-hourly). Cyclizine and ondansetron could be considered in resistant cases.

Constipation

Constipation occurs frequently after an operation and can cause great discomfort to the patient. A rectal examination is essential. Faecal impaction causes considerable distress and the cause is not always apparent to the patient. The early use of supposi-tories while the patient is still immobile often avoids the need for enemas or manual evacuation later on.

Opiate analgesics are a major cause of such constipation.

Breathlessness

Breathlessness in a postoperative patient is usually due to one of the following factors:

1 Pulmonary collapse (p. 44).
2 Bronchopneumonia (p. 44).
3 Pulmonary embolism (p. 54).
4 Left ventricular failure either due to fluid overload or myo-cardial infarction (p. 51).
5 Pneumothorax (p. 46). This occasionally complicates the in-sertion of a central venous pressure (CVP) line or intercostal anaesthetic blocks, or may even occur spontaneously.

Confusion

It is quite common for a surgical patient, often elderly, to become confused after an operation. This is distressing both for the patient and the relatives. There is usually a cause which may well be amenable to treatment.

Causes

1 Hypoxia (bronchopneumonia, pulmonary embolus)
2 Toxaemia (sepsis, urinary tract infection, chest infection)
3 Drugs (analgesics, sedatives, steroids)
4 Withdrawal (alcohol or drug)
5 Electrolyte imbalance
6 Uraemia
7 Pain (wound, retention of urine).

Making a diagnosis

The symptoms of confusion are disorientation and agitation. Review with the above causes in mind. Always examine the chest. Bronchopneumonia is a frequent cause of confusion in the elderly. Check for a past history of alcohol abuse and see what drugs have been given. Remember that more than one of the causative factors may be operating.

Proving the diagnosis

The investigations may include:
1 Haemoglobin and haematocrit
2 Urea and electrolytes
3 Blood sugar
4 Blood gases
5 Microbiology where appropriate, e.g. blood cultures, samples of sputum and urine
6 Appropriate X-rays.

Management

1 Talk to the patient. Gentle reassurance is required. A confused, elderly patient is usually aware of his own strange behaviour and terrified he is going to be permanently insane. Reassure the patient, and also the relatives, as they are usually more upset than the patient (who will not remember the events when he recovers).
2 Check the drug chart for anything which may be causing the confusion and, if possible, stop the drug concerned.
3 Treat any organic cause found.

4 If the patient is still agitated or potentially hostile despite the above measures, then sedation may be required. There is no ideal drug to recommend; however, small incremental doses of chlorpromazine or diazepam may be used. Watch for respiratory depression in this situation.

Collapse

When a patient suddenly collapses after an operation there is often a degree of panic and it is important to take charge and make a careful assessment.

The collapse is usually associated with cerebral impairment, either due to cerebral depression by anoxia, toxaemia or drugs, or due to a fall in the cerebral blood supply. Whatever the initial cause, the final picture tends to be similar as one system failure results in failure of another (Fig. 3).

Common primary causes to think of include the following conditions.

1 Hypoxia:
   (a) inhalation of vomit (p. 45)
   (b) bronchopneumonia (p. 44).
2 Central circulatory failure:
   (a) myocardial infarction (p. 50)
   (b) pulmonary embolism (p. 54).
3 Peripheral circulatory failure:
   (a) haemorrhage (reactionary or secondary) (p. 48)
   (b) oligaemia (e.g. pancreatitis, mesenteric infarction).
4 Toxaemia:
   (a) septicaemia (p. 77)
   (b) drug overdose (e.g. opiates, digoxin).
5 Cerebral causes:
   (a) stroke (p. 51)
   (b) epilepsy.

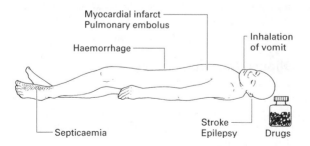

Fig. 3 Postoperative collapse.

Making the diagnosis

Make a quick appraisal of the following:

1 Circulation. Blood pressure, pulse rate and character. Listen to the heart. Jugular venous pulse (JVP).

2 Peripheral resistance. Are the extremities warm (vasodilated) or cold (vasoconstricted)?

3 Respiration. Rate and character. Quiet or dyspnoeic? Laboured? Tracheal tug? Are there any physical signs in the chest?

4 Oxygenation. Pink or cyanosed?

5 Cerebral function. Level of consciousness.

If the blood pressure and pulse are adequate then the cause is anoxia, toxaemia or a cerebral problem such as a stroke.

If there is circulatory collapse (low blood pressure and tachycardia), then you have to decide whether this is due to central (cardiac) failure or peripheral failure (oligaemia or vasodilatation).

In central failure there is venous hypertension (raised JVP, peripheral oedema, pulmonary oedema).

Peripheral failure may be due to inadequate blood volume (in which case the patient is cold and sweating and the peripheries are vasoconstricted), or due to toxic vasodilatation (in which case the blood pressure is low but the peripheries are warm and well perfused).

The following investigations may help in making further progress:

1 ECG

2 Chest X-ray

3 Electrolytes

4 Haemoglobin and white cell count.

While arranging these remember to cross-match blood if this is likely to be needed.

Management

Initial management involves attention to the airway and setting up an intravenous infusion as necessary. The further management depends on the cause of the collapse.

Oliguria/anuria

It is not uncommon for a patient to have a diminished urine output after a major operation, due to the effects of fluid and blood loss and the physiological response of the adrenal cortex to stress (see intravenous fluid therapy, p. 87). This temporary oliguria should recover after 12–24 h. An output of less than 500 mL in 24 h is not satisfactory and should be investigated.

There are three possible causes to consider for poor post-operative urine output.

1 Retention of urine
2 Prerenal failure
3 Acute renal failure.

These are dealt with in section 1.8. Retention of urine is diagnosed by finding a full bladder on examination and confirming this by catheterization. If no evidence of retention is found then renal failure must be suspected and appropriate steps taken.

1.6 Gastrointestinal and Respiratory Complications

Paralytic ileus

Paralytic ileus ('ileus') is atony of the intestine causing intestinal obstruction. It has a complex aetiology and is common after any operation when the stomach or bowel have been handled, or where there has been peritonitis. The condition is exacerbated by chemical derangement (hypokalaemia, uraemia, diabetes), by reflex sympathetic inhibition (e.g. after retroperitoneal haematoma or injury) or by anticholinergic drugs. It is rare after a laparoscopic procedure.

There may be an ileus for a variable period after open abdominal surgery. Oral feeding can only be restarted once bowel function has returned and you will be called upon to make a decision about this.

Management

Surgeons differ widely in their attitudes towards reintroducing fluids after abdominal operations. Immediately after the operation, unless a nasogastric tube is present, the patient is either kept 'nil by mouth', or only allowed small volumes of water to drink (e.g. 15 mL/h) or ice to suck, occasionally. The fluid requirements are given intravenously. If a nasogastric tube is in place, the patient may drink more and this keeps the mouth and pharynx comfortable. The tube should be aspirated before each drink is given. You should check that it is draining freely and not blocked. If in doubt, test by giving fluid to drink and then reaspirating it up the tube.

Recovery from ileus

The end of the ileus is demonstrated by:
1 The return of bowel sounds
2 Passage of flatus
3 The patient beginning to feel hungry
4 A decrease in the nasogastric aspirate
5 An increase in the urinary output as fluid is absorbed from the bowel.

Listen to the abdomen daily. When bowel sounds return, oral fluids may be increased slowly. The nasogastric tube can be removed once the oral intake exceeds the nasogastric drainage over a few hours. Large volumes of aspirate may persist if the tip of the tube has passed into the duodenum, or if a pyloric bypass operation such as a pyloroplasty or gastroenterostomy has been performed.

As the ileus recovers the patient frequently has some abdominal distension and 'wind' pains, and will require reassurance about these. They are relieved when flatus is passed.

Prolonged ileus
If the ileus persists for more than 4 days, there may be some other cause operating such as continuing peritonitis, intra-abdominal abscess formation, anastomotic leakage or mechanical intestinal obstruction. A prolonged ileus is also common where a truncal vagotomy has been performed or large amounts of narcotic agents have been given.

Providing none of the above causes are apparent, encourage the patient to mobilize, pushing his drip stand before him. Rectal suppositories may help. Metoclopramide (10 mg i.m.) is a good antiemetic, as it not only has central action but also helps gastric emptying. A prolonged ileus may eventually necessitate the introduction of intravenous feeding.

Simple constipation
This is dealt with on p. 37.

Acute dilatation of the stomach
This is a rare complication of any laparotomy in which there is overdistension of the stomach. It contains several litres of fluid, mucus and air. As distension progresses the duodenum becomes kinked causing mechanical obstruction to outflow. The stomach wall becomes thinned out and congested, with occasional mucosal erosions. Eventually there is circulatory collapse and a risk of aspiration pneumonitis.

Acute dilatation is seen occasionally after splenectomy, vagotomy or operations on the biliary tree, but can occur after any abdominal procedure. It may rarely also occur after trauma, childbirth, the application of plaster of Paris, during acute infection or in diabetic coma.

Recognizing the pattern
The most important factor is to think of the possibility. The condition can occur any time in the first week after an operation and can be rapid in onset. Do not be misled by the presence of a nasogastric tube as this may not have been aspirated efficiently. The patient complains of progressive distension, hiccups

and vomiting. The vomiting becomes effortless, and is of dark brown fluid. On examination the upper abdomen is distended. The patient may be dehydrated with a tachycardia and hypotension.

Proving the diagnosis

The diagnosis is proved by passing a nasogastric tube and aspirating large volumes of dark-coloured fluid.

An abdominal X-ray shows a very large gastric air bubble. A chest X-ray may show a raised left hemi-diaphragm and some basal collapse.

The following investigations are important:

1 Urea and electrolytes to check the potassium
2 Haematocrit to assess the degree of hypovolaemia.

Management

1 The nasogastric tube is left in place and aspirated regularly to keep the stomach empty. The patient immediately feels better. No fluids should be given orally for 24 h. Clear fluids can then be gradually reintroduced. The gastric ileus recovers rapidly once the stomach is decompressed.
2 Intravenous fluid is given to provide both the body requirement and to replace that lost by vomiting and aspiration. This should correct the hypovolaemia. Watch the potassium level.

Pulmonary collapse and bronchopneumonia

Pulmonary collapse, or atelectasis (Fig. 4) is due to the blockage of bronchi with retained secretions and absorption of air from the distal segment. It usually happens within 48 h of operation. If the sputum plug persists then secondary bronchopneumonia ensues.

Recognizing the pattern

The most constant feature is an early postoperative pyrexia which may be quite high (e.g. 39°C). If initial treatment fails to dislodge this blockage, the pyrexia remains high and eventually purulent sputum is produced.

The patient may complain of shortness of breath and a dry cough. He may feel there is something he wants to cough up but is unable to. On examination the patient has a raised respiratory rate and a tachycardia. Examination of the chest usually fails to show anything very significant in the early stages.

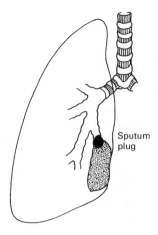

Fig. 4 Pulmonary collapse.

Proving the diagnosis

The collapsed segment may be visible on chest X-ray after a few days. As soon as a sample of sputum is produced it should be sent off to the microbiologists for culture in case antibiotics are required later.

Management

The condition may be prevented by adequate analgesia and encouraging coughing in the first few hours after operation. If it occurs however, physiotherapy is used to help the patient cough. This is both active (chest percussion and breathing exercises) and passive (postural drainage). Adequate analgesia is essential if this is to be successful. Nebulized saline can make the mucus less tenacious.

In severe cases bronchoscopy and suction may be indicated.

If the pyrexia persists for more than 48 h then antibiotic therapy should be instituted to treat secondary infection. In those with no previous chest disease, *Pneumococcus* is the most likely organism and penicillin is a suitable drug (benzyl penicillin 600 mg i.v. or i.m. 6-hourly). In those with chronic chest disease there could be a number of bacteria responsible and broad-spectrum antibiotics are suitable.

Inhalation of vomit

This usually occurs in the early postoperative period and may be associated with acute gastric dilatation or a pre-existing hiatus hernia with reflux. Inhalation of vomit causes an aspiration pneumonitis (Mendelson's syndrome). The chemical inflammation causes bronchospasm, pulmonary oedema, and respiratory and circulatory collapse, the extent of which depends on the volume and the acidity of the aspirate.

Recognizing the pattern

There is often a history of unconsciousness, vomiting or difficult intubation. There is progressive deterioration in respiratory function with cyanosis, tachycardia and dyspnoea. There are generalized bronchospasm, poor air entry and diffuse crepitations in the chest. The blood pressure is low and the peripheral vessels are vasoconstricted.

Proving the diagnosis

A chest X-ray shows widespread pulmonary infiltrates.

Management

1 Clear the airway
2 Give oxygen
3 Notify the anaesthetist or intensive care team
4 Commence broad-spectrum antibiotics
5 Consider using hydrocortisone and bronchodilators
6 Monitor oxygenation with a pulse oximeter or serial blood gases. If the oxygen saturation deteriorates, consider mechanical ventilation.

Pneumothorax

Pneumothorax can occur during or after an operation. It can arise:

1 Spontaneously.
2 Due to rupture of the lung occurring during positive pressure ventilation.
3 Following insertion of a CVP line.
4 If the pleura has been opened accidentally (e.g. in nephrectomy or cervical sympathectomy).

Tension pneumothorax is described on p. 650.

Recognizing the pattern

The chest on the affected side is immobile and hyperresonant with decreased breath sounds.

Proving the diagnosis

The air in the pleural space is visible on a chest X-ray.

Management

A pneumothorax large enough to impair breathing is treated by chest drainage. The insertion and management of a chest drain is discussed in section 6.1. Where the pneumothorax is not complicated by the presence of blood or fluid in the chest, a small tube placed anteriorly in the second intercostal space provides a satisfactory method of management. The tube is connected to an underwater seal drain.

1.7 Cardiovascular Complications

Haemorrhage

The condition of postoperative haemorrhage may be:

1 Primary — bleeding at the time of operation from uncontrolled vessels.

2 Reactionary — occurs within 24 h of operation. This is from uncontrolled vessels after vasospasm relaxes. Such haemorrhage also occurs as the blood pressure rises after recovery from anaesthesia, and with increases in venous pressure on moving and coughing.

3 Secondary — occurs 7–14 days after operation and is due to reopening of a vessel by separation of the thrombus or to erosion due to infection. Such haemorrhage is often preceded by a 'warning' minor bleed.

Making the diagnosis

The pattern of presentation depends on the rate of bleeding.

Minor bleed

With a slow haemorrhage there will be a tachycardia with mild hypotension made worse by an upright posture. The patient often notices blood in the bed or a blood-soaked dressing.

Major bleed

Acute severe haemorrhage presents as collapse. The patient becomes semiconscious, appearing restless, pale, cold and sweaty. The pulse is weak and there is tachycardia with a low blood pressure and low JVP/CVP.

Look for external bleeding (e.g. from the wound) or increasing abdominal distension suggesting intra-abdominal haemorrhage. Check whether there is blood issuing from any drains.

Early detection of haemorrhage is important as it significantly reduces morbidity and mortality. Regular reliable observations should be carried out on any patient at risk, half- to one-hourly, for at least 12 h after an operation.

Management

1 Stop the bleeding. Pressure dressings may help. If the loss is rapid the patient may need to go back to theatre for laparotomy

or exploration of the wound. Wound dressings must be changed regularly as blood-soaked dressings are a good medium for infection.

2 Replace the lost blood volume. Insert two large-bore cannulae (14 or 16 gauge). Cross-match some blood urgently. Initial fluid replacement should be with plasma expanders or blood as discussed on p. 90. Give oxygen and ideally catheterize the patient to monitor the urine output.

3 A chronic slower bleed may require blood transfusion over the next 24 h.

Blood transfusion reactions

A reaction to blood transfusion is quite common and occurs for a number of reasons. The most serious, though rarest, reaction is that following transfusion of incompatible blood due to an error of identification. This causes intravascular haemolysis with haemoglobinaemia and haemoglobinuria and later circulatory collapse, acute renal failure and jaundice. Disseminated intravascular coagulation and a bleeding tendency can develop.

More commonly, milder reactions occur due to the presence of pyrogens in the donor blood, or recipient antibodies to donor white cells. This results in a mild febrile reaction. Atopic individuals may have antibodies to exogenous antigen, e.g. milk or egg protein present in the donor plasma, which may cause an urticarial reaction. This very occasionally causes acute anaphylactic shock.

Making the diagnosis

A mild pyrexia (37.5–38.0°C) commonly occurs during or within 2 h of blood transfusion. It is usually harmless, lasting a few hours, and the patient is otherwise well. Sometimes, an itchy urticarial rash may develop. There may be a past history of allergy.

The symptoms and signs of a haemolytic reaction include pain in the transfused limb, constricting pain in the chest and pain in the loins. On examination there is flushing, pyrexia, rigors, hypotension and bronchospasm. There may be persistent bleeding, and this can be the first indication of incompatible blood transfusion during operation.

Management

The following guidelines may be helpful:

1 Mild pyrexia with no other symptom or signs:
  (a) leave the blood transfusion running

(b) watch for any deterioration in the routine observations

(c) reassure the patient.

2 Pyrexia with an itchy urticarial rash, no other abnormalities:

(a) slow the transfusion down

(b) the itching and rash may be relieved by antihistamine drugs. Chlorpheniramine (10 mg i.m.) can be used. If the patient has a past history of repeated urticarial reactions to blood he may be started before transfusion on chlorpheniramine (4 mg orally 8-hourly)

(c) if the rash persists, remove the unit of blood.

3 Patients with more serious symptoms which suggest either a haemolytic reaction or anaphylactic shock:

(a) take the blood and the giving set down. Send it with a fresh sample of the patient's blood and urine to the laboratory for analysis

(b) give hydrocortisone (200 mg i.v.), adrenaline (1 : 1000 0.5–1.0 mL (i.m.), and oxygen

(c) watch the pulse, blood pressure, clotting time and urine output very carefully and treat accordingly.

Overall, if you are in doubt, change the unit being transfused.

Myocardial infarction

Myocardial infarction may occur after operation. People who have a past history of infarction or angina are particularly at risk, as are those undergoing vascular surgery.

Recognizing the pattern

The history is of central crushing chest pain which may radiate down the arms or into the neck.

Usually the patient is pale, cold, clammy and tachycardic. Postoperative infarction may be silent, or simply present as an unexplained hypotensive episode.

Proving the diagnosis

The ECG shows:

1 ST elevation

2 T-wave inversion

3 Q waves.

Cardiac enzymes are elevated over the next 2 or 3 days as follows:

1 Creatine phosphokinase, Marsh–Bender factor (CPK MB): up 2–4 h, maximum 36 h

2 Lactate dehydrogenase (LDH): up 10 h, maximum 92 h.

Management
Initial management is analgesia with diamorphine, oxygen and bed rest. Further management is beyond the scope of this book and a textbook of medicine or cardiology should be consulted.

Left ventricular failure
Left ventricular failure occurs in surgical patients who have been overloaded with fluid, particularly where there is a past history of heart failure or myocardial ischaemia. When the left ventricle fails the lungs become oedematous and the patient dyspnoeic.

Recognizing the pattern
The patient, who is often elderly, complains of shortness of breath. This may come on acutely or slowly, and is worse on lying flat. Urine output may be poor.

On examination the patient is dyspnoeic, often very distressed and cyanosed. There is a tachycardia with a triple rhythm, and bilateral fine basal crepitations with or without bronchospasm in the lungs. In the absence of chronic obstructive airways disease, acute bronchospasm in the elderly is often due to pulmonary oedema.

There may also be associated signs of right heart failure, such as a raised JVP, hepatomegaly and peripheral oedema.

Proving the diagnosis
A chest X-ray shows hilar congestion. An ECG must be performed. In severe cases blood gas measurements are helpful.

Management
Sit the patient up and give oxygen. Intravenous diuretics (e.g. frusemide 80–120 mg) and diamorphine (5–10 mg i.v.) are effective in the acute attack.

Preventative measures are important. The elderly need less fluid and this must be remembered during the administration of intravenous fluid therapy (see section 2.1). Blood transfusion should be undertaken with caution. At night the patient should be propped up in bed.

Stroke
A stroke is due to intracerebral haemorrhage, thrombosis or embolism with subsequent ischaemia or infarction of cerebral tissue. Preoperative predisposing factors include hypertension

and vascular disease. During or after operation severe hypovol-aemia may result in intracerebral thrombosis. Emboli may arise from the myocardium, heart valves, great vessels, or carotid and basilar arteries.

Recognizing the pattern

The patient usually suffers a sudden collapse and becomes unconscious.

On examination there may be neurological signs of hemiple-gia (e.g. paralysis on one side, up-going plantar responses, difficulties with speech). There may also be evidence of raised intracranial pressure such as a progressively slowing pulse, rising blood pressure and the appearance of papilloedema and pupil dilation.

Proving the diagnosis

This is usually made obvious by the neurological deficit. It may be necessary to order a CT scan to help with the diagnosis and aid in prognostication.

Management

1 The initial management is conservative, comprising nursing care, catheterization, attention to fluid balance and regular observations.

2 Treat any excessive hypertension.

3 The patient may be referred acutely to the neurologists for further management. They may decide to treat raised intra-cranial pressure.

4 Most patients who have had a stroke have long-term prob-lems and are going to be dependent on others for some time. A team consisting of occupational therapist, physiotherapist, social worker and physician for the elderly will be available to help with ongoing issues of mobilization, rehabilitation and placement.

Deep venous thrombosis

Virchow's triad describes three predisposing factors for throm-bosis:

1 Increased coagulability of the blood

2 Decreased flow in the vessel

3 Local injury to the intima.

Once a localized thrombus has formed in a vein it may extend proximally and there is a danger that fragments of the clot will break off as emboli.

Thromboembolism is particularly common after any surgical procedure since the criteria of the triad are all likely to be fulfilled. There is an increase in blood viscosity after an operation, associated with dehydration and alteration in the serum proteins. The patient is immobile and there may be local injury to vessels while lying on the operating table or during abdominal and pelvic surgery. In addition, there is an increase in blood coagulability following the physiological response to trauma.

The risks are particularly increased by long operations in the pelvic or hip regions. Other risk factors include a past history of deep venous thrombosis or pulmonary embolus, obesity, smoking, carcinomatosis and taking the contraceptive pill.

Common sites of postoperative phlebothrombosis are in the pelvis and in the venous plexus in the soleal muscles of the calf.

Recognizing the pattern

A characteristic sign of venous thrombosis is a persistent tachycardia and a mild 'rumbling' fever. Other signs depend on the site of the thrombus formation.

Pelvic phlebothrombosis is difficult to diagnose. Apart from the systemic signs, there is little to find.

Acute thrombosis of the iliac veins or femoral veins leads to a grossly swollen painful leg. There is localized tenderness over the involved vein. Axillary vein thrombosis similarly presents with a marked swelling of the arm.

When thrombosis occurs in the soleal plexus there is tenderness in the soleal muscle, which is swollen and turgid compared with the other side. The enlargement can be measured accurately with a tape measure.

Proving the diagnosis

The best non-invasive investigation is a duplex scan of the femoral veins. Although iliac and calf veins are difficult to see, calf venous thrombosis is unlikely to lead to embolization and a normal femoral vein usually excludes iliac vein disease.

A venogram can still be performed where duplex is not available, to detect clot in iliac or inferior vena cava and for placement of caval filter.

Management

Prevention
This is very important. Identify any patient who is at risk (see above). During the operation avoid prolonged calf compression

(rest the heels on a pad to elevate the calves; do not lean on the calves). It is also possible to aid venous return by compression stockings or intermittent calf compression with inflatable stockings. Subcutaneous low molecular weight heparin should be given to 'at-risk' patients (5000 units subcutaneously 8-hourly). This is started with the premedication and continued until the patient is fully mobile. Passive leg exercises should be encouraged whilst the patient is in bed, and the foot of the bed should be elevated to increase the venous return. Early mobilization should be the rule for all surgical patients.

In certain procedures the surgeon may not wish to give subcutaneous heparin because of the risk of bleeding and you should always check with him before starting therapy.

Treatment

If deep venous thrombosis is proven, full anticoagulation with intravenous heparin is the treatment of choice, followed by oral warfarinization. There is speculation that deep venous thrombosis may be treated in the community effectively with low molecular weight heparin in the future. Suitable regimes for treatment are described on p. 112.

Compression stockings, analgesia and mobilization when comfortable, are important factors in treatment.

Pulmonary embolus

Pulmonary embolism occurs when a thrombus from the peripheral venous system becomes detached, passes through the right side of the heart, and impacts in the pulmonary arterial circulation. The consequences depend on the size of the embolus and the site at which it lodges.

A small embolus causes a localized pulmonary infarction and pleurisy if the periphery of the lung is involved. Small emboli may herald larger ones; repeated small emboli can cause pulmonary hypertension (Fig. 5a).

A large embolus blocks the main pulmonary arteries and thus causes a major block to the whole circulation. The effects are shown in Fig. 5(b). There is decreased output from the left ventricle and a rise in venous pressure.

Emboli imply the presence of deep venous thrombosis. In 50% of cases the site of the primary problem is not obvious.

Recognizing the pattern

A small embolus may cause pleuritic chest pain, haemoptysis and difficulty in breathing due to pain. However, it is often

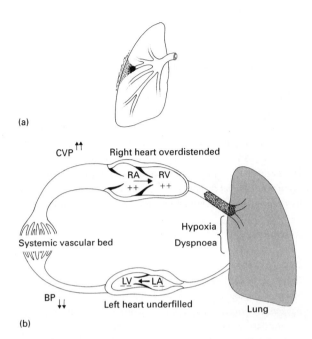

(a)

(b)

Fig. 5 (a) A minor embolus produces a pulmonary infarct. (b) A major pulmonary embolus affects the whole circulation.

silent. A large embolus may cause collapse, and is one of the common causes of sudden death postoperatively.

Usually there are no chest signs. The patient is almost always tachycardic. A life-threatening pulmonary embolism will give signs of a gallop rhythm, hypotension and right ventricular strain (e.g. raised JVP).

Proving the diagnosis
This is difficult and one must have a high index of suspicion.

It is worthwhile performing:

1 Arterial blood gases. There will be a lowered P_{O_2} due to the physiological shunt present. The P_{CO_2} will be low due to tachypnoea.

2 The ECG usually shows tachycardia, and may show an S wave in lead 1, a Q wave in lead 3 and an inverted T wave in lead 3 in the presence of right heart strain (S1, Q3, T3).

3 A chest X-ray is usually normal. Subtle signs may be present such as paucity of lung markings on the affected side, or a wedge-shaped opacity in the presence of pulmonary infarction.

4 Ventilation perfusion scans show areas of defects in perfusion which may be associated with defects of ventilation (matched defects), or they may not (V/Q mismatch). The scans report a probability that there has been an embolus. This ranges from low to moderate to high probability.

5 Emergency angiography. Pulmonary angiography is invasive and not without complications. However, it is the gold standard examination. A pulmonary angiogram can be performed by threading a catheter up any peripheral vein. This may show the presence of the clots in the major pulmonary arteries, confirming the diagnosis. The catheter can be used to infuse thrombolytic agents (see below). Whenever possible this investigation should be done if pulmonary embolectomy is to be carried out.

Management

Resuscitation

A large embolus can cause acute circulatory collapse and cardiac arrest. The patient may require intubating and ventilating with oxygen. An intravenous cannula should be inserted to provide a route for drugs. If the patient has a cardiac arrest, efficient heart massage may break up the clot and push it further into the pulmonary tree, thus allowing some circulation to be restored. Immediate embolectomy may be appropriate. This is discussed further below.

Analgesia

Non-steroidal analgesia is effective in pulmonary embolism. It may be dangerous to give any other analgesia because of the risk of exacerbating the hypotension.

Anticoagulation

The patient is heparinized and anticoagulated as on p. 112.

If the patient does not improve and cardiac failure persists, further measures to remove the clot are indicated. This may be attempted using thrombolytic agents or by open pulmonary artery embolectomy.

Thrombolytic agents

Many emboli can be dissolved by agents such as streptokinase, urokinase or tissue plasminogen activator. Thrombolytics may be given by direct infusion into the pulmonary artery or into the systemic circulation through a peripheral vein. They break up the embolus by activating plasminogen.

Thrombolytic therapy is dangerous in patients who are:

1 within 5 days of a major operation
2 within 10 days of a hip replacement
3 within 4 weeks of a diagnostic cannulation of a major artery
4 hypertensive
5 pregnant, within 10 days of delivery or lactating
6 in hepatic or renal failure
7 actively bleeding from the bowel or urinary tract.

These patients may be treated by pulmonary embolectomy, but the relative risks will have to be weighed up on an individual basis.

Pulmonary artery embolectomy

Massive pulmonary emboli can be removed surgically as an emergency. This is only indicated when the patient fails to respond to anticoagulation or thrombolytic therapy, when there is insufficient time to allow thrombolysis to work because of the patient's desperate condition, or when thrombolytic therapy is considered to be too dangerous.

The operation may be done in one of two ways.

OPERATION: INFLOW STASIS PULMONARY
EMBOLECTOMY

This operation is performed if there are no facilities for cardiopulmonary bypass. The superior and inferior vena cava are exposed through a midline sternotomy and controlled with tapes. The pulmonary artery is opened and the clot sucked out. The venous inflow can be restored and interrupted several times in order to remove all the emboli.

Codes

Blood .... 10 units as soon as possible
GA/LA .... GA
Opn time .... 1–2 h
Stay .... Variable
Drains out .... Chest drain 48 h, pericardial 4–5 days
Sutures out .... 7–10 days
Off work .... Variable, 2–3 months

OPERATION: CARDIOPULMONARY BYPASS

This is the safest way to remove major emboli surgically. The sternum is split and the right atrium and aorta cannulated. After cardiopulmonary bypass has been established the pulmonary artery is opened and all clot removed.

Codes

Blood .... 10 units
GA/LA .... GA
Opn time .... 2–4 h
Stay .... Variable
Drains out .... Chest drain 48 h, pericardial 4–5 days
Sutures out .... 7–10 days
Off work .... Variable, 2–3 months

1.8 Urinary Complications

Urinary tract infection

Urinary tract infection is a common complication in the post-operative period. Urinary catheterization is an important predisposing factor, although it can occur following any episode of hypovolaemia, with decreased renal perfusion, low urinary output and urinary stasis. The organism is commonly a Gram-negative bacillus such as *Escherichia coli*. Risk factors for the development of urinary tract infections in the non-hospitalized population include anatomical abnormalities leading to urinary stasis or urinary reflux into the upper tracts (ureter and kidney), bladder outflow obstruction with consequent postmicturition residual urine, stones, bladder diverticulum, bladder carcinoma, pregnancy and diabetes mellitus.

Recognizing the pattern

Women are more frequently affected than men. The patient complains of frequency and urgency of micturition, and burning dysuria. She is usually pyrexial and this may be the first sign if a catheter is in place. Other symptoms include suprapubic pain and pain in the renal angle due to ascending infection. Advanced infection can result in septicaemia and rigors. The urine looks cloudy and may smell offensive. There may be haematuria.

Proving the diagnosis

The white cell count is elevated with a neutrophil leucocytosis. Microscopic examination of a specimen of urine shows white cells and protein casts. The causative organism may be cultured.

Management

The patient is encouraged to drink as much as possible (e.g. 4–5 L/day). Antibiotics are commenced once the bacteriological specimen has been taken. The choice of drug is discussed on p. 111. Any indwelling catheter should be removed if this is feasible.

Further investigations, such as an intravenous urogram (IVU) and cystoscopy, are indicated if the infection does not settle or recurs.

Postoperative retention of urine

This is a common postoperative problem and the most frequent cause of oliguria following surgery. The patient finds it difficult to initiate micturition while under the influence of drugs, in strange surroundings, when movements are painful and when he is immobilized in bed. Benign prostatic hypertrophy is an important predisposing cause, although postoperative urinary retention also occurs in women. Patients at risk should be recognized during the initial clerking. Other causes of acute retention are mentioned on p. 469.

Recognizing the pattern

The patient in classical acute retention is anuric and in great discomfort with an intense desire to micturate. The bladder is palpable as a tender mass arising out of the pelvis.

This classic picture is not, however, always present and the condition can be difficult to diagnose. Elderly patients, in particular, may develop acute confusion, without other symptoms indicative of acute urinary retention. Furthermore, the patient may not be anuric. In acute retention with overflow the patient produces urine but the amounts are small (50–100 mL) and passed very frequently. This pattern, recorded on the fluid chart, should alert you to the possible diagnosis. An abdominal incision covered with dressings may make it impossible to palpate the enlarged bladder and thus obscure the cause of pain. Suprapubic dullness to percussion can be a useful sign in these circumstances. Finally patients with chronic retention may not be in any discomfort, but have a distended bladder and frequency.

Proving the diagnosis

The diagnosis is proved by passing a urethral catheter and releasing a large volume of urine (more than 500 mL in an adult). Very occasionally an ultrasound examination can be helpful to define the enlarged bladder.

Patients at risk should not be subjected to continual questions about whether they have passed urine or not. Privacy, reassurance and adequate analgesia are helpful. If retention is developing, a tranquillizer (such as diazepam 5–10 mg i.m.) can be useful and conservative measures, such as sitting in a hot bath, and allowing the patient to sit out on the toilet, should be tried.

There are two indications for catheterization:

1 The patient is in pain from the distended bladder and demands relief.

2 There is doubt about the diagnosis and renal failure must be excluded.

In other circumstances it is always worth waiting for the patient to pass urine naturally.

The method of passing a urethral or suprapubic catheter is described on p. 470. If there is very little urine in the bladder and adequate amounts are not produced after catheterization, the patient may be in renal failure and should be managed accordingly (see below).

Patients who have been in retention should have the catheter removed after 24–48 h. In elderly males, if two trials of catheter removal are unsuccessful, the patient should be considered for a prostatectomy (p. 476).

Postoperative renal failure

Failure to produce urine after an operation, once obstruction has been excluded, may be due to prerenal failure (Fig. 6).

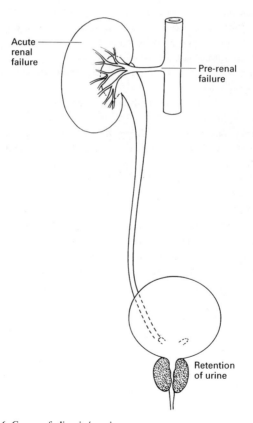

Fig. 6 Causes of oliguria/anuria.

Prerenal failure

The blood supply to the kidneys may become inadequate postoperatively due to dehydration, blood loss or systemic hypotension. These causes are reversible, but if they are not dealt with early the condition may progress to acute renal failure.

Making the diagnosis

An adequate urine output, in the postoperative period, is generally accepted to be at least 30 mL/h, for a 70-kg man. Elderly patients, children and patients with lower weights may pass less urine than this, but this figure is generally considered a useful yardstick. Having established that the urine output is inadequate, if necessary by insertion of a catheter, the diagnosis of prerenal failure is made by finding concentrated urine, signs of a cause, and excluding acute renal failure.

Examine the patient looking for hypotension, dehydration (dry tongue, skin turgor) or cardiac failure (JVP, CVP). Assess the peripheral perfusion (warm or cold hands?).

Inspect the charts, looking for a negative fluid balance, and check whether there has been any excess blood loss or a period of hypotension.

Check the renal function and measure the urine specific gravity. In prerenal failure, the plasma creatinine should be normal, but the serum urea may be high, indicating dehydration. The urine will be very concentrated (specific gravity over 1020).

Management

Administer crystalloid or colloid fluids, or blood, intravenously, in order to restore urine output. In the elderly or those with haemodynamic instability it is wise to monitor the CVP via a central line (p. 98), aiming to get it to the upper limit of normal. If the urine output remains poor, urine production can be stimulated by the use of an intravenous low dose dopamine infusion (2–5 μg/kg/min) or an intravenous bolus of frusemide (20–250 mg). These drugs do not prevent the development of acute renal failure, but may overcome anuria/oliguria, making the patient's fluid balance easier to manage.

Acute renal failure

In a surgical patient this usually follows a period of renal hypoperfusion (prerenal failure) as above. It can also be a complication of incompatible blood transfusion, extensive trauma or drug therapy. The condition is associated with acute necrosis of the renal tubules (acute tubular necrosis).

Making the diagnosis

The diagnosis is made after catheterization has excluded retention, and careful fluid status assessment and correction have excluded renal hypoperfusion. If the urine output remains less than 30 mL/h, acute tubular necrosis has occurred. This should be confirmed by finding a rising plasma urea and creatinine concentration. A urine specimen should be sent for biochemical analysis. Typical findings are low urine sodium, potassium and urea concentrations and a low osmolarity.

Management

1 Insert a central line to assist with the careful management of the patient's fluid status. Aim to keep the CVP at the upper limit of normal, avoiding fluid overload.

2 Administer an intravenous infusion of low-dose dopamine or an intravenous bolus of frusemide as this may restart urine production.

3 Treat hyperkalaemia. If the plasma potassium concentration is dangerously high ($[K^+] > 7.0$ mmol/L) administer calcium gluconate 10 mg intravenously while monitoring the ECG. Administer an intravenous bolus of 50 ml of 50% dextrose with 16 units of insulin and commence an intravenous dextrose/insulin infusion. Lower plasma potassium concentrations may be reduced by administration of an enteral potassium chelating agent (e.g. calcium resonium 15 mg q.d.s. orally or rectally).

4 The further management of established renal failure is complex and best described in medical textbooks. It includes:

(a) restricted fluid intake: 500 mL/day plus any fluid losses

(b) restricted protein intake (less than 20 g/day)

(c) adequate carbohydrate intake (3000 kcal/day)

(d) daily assessment of blood and urinary electrolytes and adjustment of electrolyte intake accordingly. Sodium losses are replaced but potassium is not given

(e) peritoneal dialysis or haemodialysis if necessary. Peritoneal dialysis can be used in a patient who has had laparotomy from about 4 or 5 days after the wound has been closed. Continuous haemofiltration is preferred in the intensively ill patient.

Urinary fistula

This either follows breakdown of a urinary tract anastomosis or accidental damage to the ureters during operation.

Recognizing the pattern

The condition presents with an increased discharge through the wound or drain site. This has a characteristic appearance and smell of urine. There is less constitutional upset than with an intestinal fistula.

Proving the diagnosis

The urea content of the fluid is high (like urine) and above the level of the patient's serum urea. If further proof is necessary it can be obtained by giving an intravenous injection of indigo carmine, which is excreted by the kidney and will appear through the fistula.

Management

Urinary fistula will close spontaneously (like bowel fistulae, p. 74) providing there is no distal obstruction. Such closure may take several weeks. The presence or absence of distal obstruction can be ascertained by performing a 'fistulogram'.

If the fistula fails to heal, operation is needed and the precise nature of this depends on the site of the fistula. Free distal urine drainage must always, however, be established.

Urinoma

This occurs for the same reasons as a urinary fistula, but does not drain spontaneously. An intra-abdominal collection of urine develops. This may become infected.

Recognizing the pattern

The condition presents with abdominal discomfort due to pressure and local inflammation. The patient may have a fever and a mass may be palpable.

Proving the diagnosis

The presence of a fluid collection is best demonstrated using ultrasound or a CT scan, which will have a characteristic appearance. The diagnosis is confirmed by demonstrating urine on aspiration (see below).

Management

A suspected urinoma should be drained percutaneously, under ultrasound or CT guidance. Distal obstruction should be excluded by performing an IVU.

1.9 Infections, Abscesses and Fistulae

Wound infection

Infection complicates between 1 and 40% of surgical incisions, depending on the type of procedure being performed (Fig. 7). A wide variety of organisms may be involved.

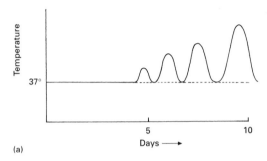

(a)

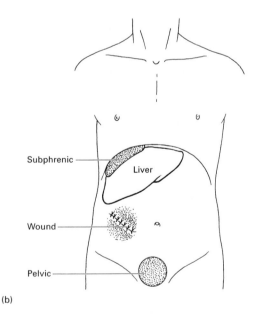

(b)

Fig. 7 (a) Postoperative sepsis. (b) Sites of postoperative abdominal sepsis.

Predisposing factors

1 Preoperative:
   (a) malnutrition
   (b) diabetes
   (c) carcinomatosis
   (d) infection near the site of incision
   (e) immunosuppressive therapy.
2 Operative:
   (a) the incidence of wound infection depends on the amount of operative contamination:
   - clean wounds: 1%
   - clean–contaminated: 1–5%
   - contaminated: 5–30%
   - dirty wounds: > 30%
   (b) infection from staff, instruments or air-borne agents
   (c) poor surgical technique, e.g. haematoma formation, devitalized tissue in wound or closure under tension.
3 Postoperative: infection on the ward (either from the patient himself, other patients or the staff).

Recognizing the pattern

There is a history of increasing pain and tenderness in the wound.

On examination the patient has a climbing, swinging pyrexia with localized tenderness in the wound, which is also swollen, hot and red. There may be fluctuation on palpation or pus may discharge.

Proving the diagnosis

1 White cell count. This will be elevated in active infection.
2 A specimen of pus must be sent to microbiology for culture.

Management

1 The collection should be drained. Remove some of the stitches and probe the wound to let out all the pus. Sometimes an anaesthetic is required to achieve adequate drainage.
2 The wound is dressed daily, or more frequently if dressings become saturated. The wound is not resutured but left to heal by secondary intention.
3 Analgesia.
4 If the patient has systemic illness or spreading cellulitis, then antibiotics should be given.

Wound dehiscence

Breakdown of the wound may be either partial or complete
(Fig. 8). In partial breakdown the skin closure holds, but break-
down of the muscle layers gives rise to an incisional hernia later.
In complete dehiscence the abdominal incision bursts open to

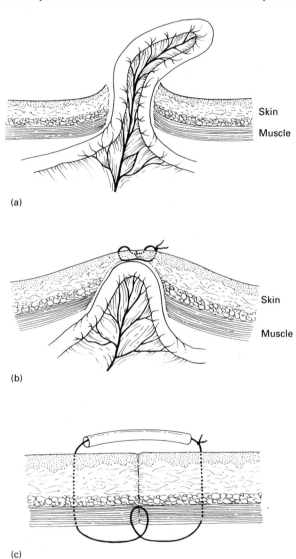

Fig. 8 (a) Complete wound dehiscence. (b) Incomplete (partial)
wound dehiscence. (c) Figure-of-eight suture.

reveal bowel. The aetiology is similar to that for wound infection. Exacerbating factors include obesity, raised intra-abdominal pressure (from coughing, difficulty in passing urine or constipation), ascites draining through the wound, wound infection and haematoma. However, most wound dehiscences are due to faulty technique. Factors include pulling the sutures too tight, inserting sutures too close to the edge of the muscle, and insecure knots. Wound dehiscence is much less common since deep-tension, one-layer, monofilament-suture techniques have been used.

Making the diagnosis

This occurs typically 4–10 days after operation. The patient may feel something 'give' in the wound. There is a sudden increase in pain and a pink fluid discharge from the wound. In complete dehiscence there is protrusion of loops of bowel. The patient becomes shocked and distressed.

Management

1 Lie the patient down and give reassurance
2 Strong opiate analgesia is required
3 Cover the wound with a sterile pack soaked in warm saline
4 The wound requires urgent resuture in theatre with deep-tension sutures.

OPERATION: RESUTURE OF ABDOMINAL WOUND
The dressings and sutures are removed and the whole wound is reopened. All the muscle layer sutures are taken out. A laparotomy is performed and any intraperitoneal pus is removed. Bacteriological specimens are collected for aerobic and anaerobic culture. The abdomen is then closed in one layer with deep-tension figure-of-eight sutures tied over either gauze or rubber to prevent them cutting into the skin (Fig. 8c). The subcutaneous layer is usually drained.

Codes

Blood	0
GA/LA	GA
Opn time	1 h
Stay	2 weeks or more
Drains out	3–5 days
Sutures out	14–21 days
Off work	6 weeks

Postoperative care

The sutures are left in place for at least 14 days. The wound tends to discharge and may require regular dressing. Antibiotics should be started at the operation and continued as long as necessary. They can be modified according to the results of the culture.

Infected intravenous drip site

A drip site may become infected and is one of the causes of postoperative pyrexia. The organism is often a staphylococci.

Recognizing the pattern

The patient complains of pain in the limb that is being infused. The intravenous infusion usually slows or stops completely.

The patient is pyrexial and the involved skin is red, swollen and tender. There may be spreading cellulitis over the vein proximally, and even pus around the entry of the cannula. Regional lymph nodes may become enlarged, tender and in-flamed.

Management

The cannula must be removed and the tip cultured. If the infusion is still required, resite the drip in the other arm. Flucloxacillin is given. Systemic analgesia is often needed and a poultice applied to the inflamed vein is comforting.

Subphrenic abscess

A subphrenic abscess commonly follows generalized peritonitis, particularly after acute appendicitis or a perforated peptic ulcer. It may also occur through infection of a haematoma after an operation such as splenectomy. Such abscesses are commonly just underneath the hemi-diaphragm but may also occur beneath the liver in the lesser sac or in the hepatorenal pouch.

Recognizing the pattern

The patient initially recovers from the operation and then 7–21 days later develops a swinging fever and general malaise, nausea and loss of weight. He may complain of pain in the upper abdomen which can radiate to the shoulder tip. He may also become breathless due to a pleural effusion above the abscess or collapse of the lower lobe of one lung.

On examination there is a swinging pyrexia for which no obvious cause is found. Occasionally, there may be tenderness or even oedema in the abdominal wall in the subcostal region. The liver may be displaced downwards and there may be physical signs of a pleural effusion or collapse of the lung.

Proving the diagnosis

The old aphorism 'pus somewhere, pus nowhere else, pus under the diaphragm' is a useful reminder of the possibility of a subphrenic abscess. The presenting symptoms and signs do not always suggest this possibility. Investigations which can be helpful are as follows.

1 A CT scan is effective in localizing the collection of pus
2 The white cell count is typically high.

Management

The best management is drainage but an early subphrenic abscess with no air or fluid level may be treated with broad-spectrum antibiotics (e.g. gentamicin, benzylpenicillin and metronidazole). Such treatment not infrequently leads to gradual resolution of the abscess. Gentamycin levels should be monitored especially in renal failure. If the patient remains toxic and ill for more than 5 days, conservative management should be abandoned and the abscess drained.

Drainage can often be performed percutaneously using radiological guidance, but an operation is occasionally required.

OPERATION: DRAINAGE OF SUBPHRENIC ABSCESS
The abscess may be approached by a posterior or anterior route.

Posterior approach
The patient is positioned lying on his side with the abscess uppermost. The 12th rib is removed and the subhepatic space or subphrenic space approached retroperitoneally. When the abscess is encountered it is opened and drained in the most dependent direction.

Anterior approach
The abdomen is opened through a subcostal incision and the abscess approached extraperitoneally and drained.

Once the abscess has been opened, covering antibiotics can be given, although they are not essential. Large abscess cavities are usually drained using a large silicone tube to encourage track formation.

Codes

Blood 0
GA/LA .... GA
Opn time .... 1 h
Stay .... 1–2 weeks
Drains out .... 10–14 days
Sutures out .... 7 days
Off work .... 4 weeks

Postoperative care
If the abscess is large, sinograms may be performed down the drain after 10 days and the progress of the cavity followed. The drain can then be gradually withdrawn as the abscess heals up behind it.

Hepatic abscess

This often occurs as metastatic infection from intraperitoneal sepsis, usually in a debilitated patient. The abscess may be single or multiple. The incidence is low since antibiotic treatment was introduced. The more common causes of hepatic abscesses include appendicitis, diverticular disease, ulcerative colitis and ascending cholangitis.

Recognizing the pattern
The patient is usually very ill with a high swinging fever and rigors. He may complain of right upper quadrant pain and develop mild jaundice. The liver may be enlarged and tender.

Proving the diagnosis
1 The white cell count is raised.
2 Liver function tests are abnormal. In particular the alanine transaminase (ALT) is raised.
3 The abscess cavity may be demonstrated on ultrasound or CT scan.
4 An erect chest X-ray shows a high right diaphragm and fluid in the pleura above it.
5 Blood cultures may occasionally be positive.

Management
The patient should be given broad-spectrum antibiotics and the abscess drained as soon as it is localized. Ideally this is done percutaneously under ultrasound or CT guidance. Open operation may be necessary.

OPERATION: DRAINAGE OF HEPATIC ABSCESS

The abscess is usually approached through an extrahepatic route over the right lobe of the liver. As the abscess is approached, oedema and fibrosis are encountered and this may be broken into, opening up the cavity in the liver. A red rubber drain is inserted.

Codes

Blood	2–4 units
GA/LA	GA
Opn time	1 h
Stay	14–21 days
Drains out	10–21 days
Sutures out	7 days
Off work	6–12 weeks

Postoperative care

The postoperative care is similar to that described above for a subphrenic abscess.

Pelvic abscess

This is an abscess in the rectovesical pouch commonly following peritonitis, e.g. after a pelvic appendicitis or colonic perforation. Infection of a pelvic haematoma following poor haemostasis is another common cause.

Making the diagnosis

A patient who has had generalized peritonitis becomes unwell with pyrexia and malaise 4–10 days postoperatively. There may be a history of mucus discharged per rectum. The abscess may rupture through the rectum or vagina.

On examination the patient has a swinging pyrexia, and rectal or vaginal examination may reveal a palpable mass which may be pointing and may indeed burst on examination.

Management

Daily rectal examinations should be performed to monitor the progress of the developing abscess. The abscess may point up into the wound or down into the rectum. When a fluctuant area is felt in the rectum it can be broken into with a finger under a short general anaesthetic. If the patient has systemic symptoms antibiotics may be given but these delay the ripening and discharge of the abscess. Premature attempts to drain the abscess through the rectum may damage adjacent loops of bowel, leading to fistula formation. An alternative route for drainage in women is through the posterior fornix of the vagina.

External intestinal fistula

This is a communication between the bowel lumen and the body surface. It develops postoperatively due to the following factors:

1 Disruption of a bowel anastomosis (due to tension, ischaemia, infection or distal obstruction)

2 Inclusion of the bowel when suturing the abdominal wall

3 Erosion of the bowel by an abdominal drain

4 Perforation of ischaemic bowel (e.g. due to damage to the mesentery at operation or after strangulation in a hernia).

Recognizing the pattern

Five to 10 days after operation there is an increased discharge through the wound or down a drain which becomes faecal and offensive. Persistent discharge causes general malaise, dehydration, hypoproteinaemia and weight loss. If the track is not completely walled off generalized peritonitis may occur.

Proving the diagnosis

The presence of a fistula can be demonstrated by radiological studies involving the use of water-soluble contrast.

Management

Fistulae tend to heal spontaneously providing there is no distal obstruction and providing the patient can be kept in positive nitrogen balance. Healing usually takes 3–6 weeks. A fistula will not heal under the conditions listed below.

1 The tract becomes epithelialized.

2 There is obstruction beyond the fistula site.

3 In the presence of persistent infection (e.g. tuberculosis, a foreign body, Crohn's disease, actinomycosis or an abscess in the fistula tract).

4 In the presence of malignant disease along the tract.

In the absence of these problems, conservative management should be followed:

1 Protect the skin from autodigestion (especially with a high intestinal or pancreatic fistula). This can be achieved by covering the surrounding skin with stomahesive and attaching an ileostomy bag to the fistulous opening.

2 Parenteral nutrition. This has transformed the management of intestinal fistulae. When a fistula is diagnosed a CVP line

should be set up in almost all instances. Oral feeding can then be restricted and the patient's nutritional state maintained until the fistula heals (see p. 96).

3 Adequate fluid and electrolyte replacement of the volume lost down the fistulous track must be given. Daily electrolyte estimations should be performed.

4 Octratide, a synthetic somatostatin analogue, may be used to convert a high output fistula (> 400 mL/day) to a low output fistula (< 400 mL/day). This reduces complications and may reduce the time to spontaneous closure.

5 Surgical closure may be required if the fistula fails to close off with the above conservative treatment. In that case it will be necessary to excise the fistulous track and deal with any obstruction, or other cause of failure to heal.

OPERATION: EXCISION OF FISTULA

The skin is incised around the external opening and the track dissected out and removed. Any obstructive lesion must be dealt with. The defect in the bowel is oversewn and the abdominal wall closed. A drain is put down to the fistula site. In the presence of persistent peritonitis it may be safer to bring out the bowel opening as an ileostomy (to be closed later). A repair of a large bowel fistula may need covering with a proximal colostomy.

Codes
Blood .... 2 units
GA/LA .... GA
Opn time .... 1–2 h
Stay .... 10–14 days
Drains out .... Wound drain and intra-abdominal drain 7–10 days
Sutures out .... 7–10 days
Off work .... 4–6 weeks

Bed sores

Bed sores occur over pressure areas in patients who are immobilized in bed for a long period. Five factors play a part: pressure, moisture, anaemia, malnutrition and injury.

Making the diagnosis

The area initially becomes erythematous and does not blanch on pressure. The skin then ulcerates and may become secondarily infected.

Management

Bed sores are avoided by good nursing care with regular attention to pressure areas and regular turning in bed. The patient should not be allowed to lie on damp sheets. Sheepskin pads under the heels and sacrum help. Patients who are going to be immobilized for a long period of time should be nursed on a water bed or ripple mattress.

For established bed sores, avoid pressure on the area. Regular gentle massage to the surrounding skin is necessary. Infrared therapy may help. Keep the area dry either with dressings or by leaving the wound open to the air. Antibiotics are required if there is spreading cellulitis or systemic illness and the patient must be mobilized as soon as possible.

Extensive chronic bed sores may require excision and rotational skin grafting.

Septicaemia

This is an overwhelming infection spreading from the primary source into the bloodstream due to Gram-negative organisms, staphylococci or streptococci. Gram-negative septicaemia is common after biliary or urological surgery.

Recognizing the pattern

The patient is collapsed with a pyrexia (39–40°C), a tachycardia and a normal or low blood pressure. The extremities are initially warm due to vasodilatation, but may later become cold due to hypoperfusion. The patient may have rigors.

Look for a cause. Inspect the urine; is it cloudy and thick? Examine the chest and abdomen; is there a CVP line that may be infected?

Proving the diagnosis

1 Blood cultures. Take two specimens of blood each of 10 mL minimum, from different sites. Inoculate the culture set provided (which may contain identifiable aerobic and anaerobic bottles). The blood should be taken using a strict aseptic technique. The forearm vein should first be identified and the skin then cleansed. The site of the venepuncture should not be contaminated again after this. The tops of the bottles should be cleaned unless they are already sterile. If the vein is not clearly visible, a heat-sensitive strip which changes colour over the vein may be useful. Otherwise use sterile gloves if further palpation is needed.

The blood collected is injected into the anaerobic bottle first. As the injection is made, avoid introducing any bubbles into the syringe. At this point you can also check that there is a good vacuum. The needles should not be changed unless a resheathing protector is available (because of the risk of needle-stick injury). The aerobic bottle is injected. Specimens should be sent to the laboratory as soon as possible for incubation.

2 Other microbiology samples should be sent depending on the suspected site of infection.

3 If there is a CVP line in use and it is suspected that this is the source of the infection, it should be removed and the tip cultured. Resite it if required.

4 Perform a white cell count.

Management

1 Intravenous antibiotics. These must be started immediately after the blood cultures have been taken. The choice depends on the sort of surgery which has been undertaken. For gut-related septicaemia penicillin, gentamicin and metronidazole or a cephalosporin and metronidazole provide broad cover. For urological surgery the metronidazole is unnecessary. If staphylococcal sepsis is likely, flucloxacillin should be substituted for penicillin (or vancomycin if methicillin-resistant *Staphylococcus aureus* (MRSA) is locally common). The initial antibiotics are modified when the sensitivities of the organism are known.

2 Intravenous support of the circulation. In severe cases a CVP line is used to monitor this.

3 Watch the urine output. The patient should be catheterized.

4 It is well worth while discussing the case with the microbiologists, particularly if the origin of the organism found is not known.

5 Treat the cause of the septicaemia as required.

1.10 Laparoscopic and Endoscopic Surgery

The development of endoscopic operations which do not require major incisions in the body wall is changing the practice of surgery. Endoscopic surgery has existed in gynaecology, urology and orthopaedics for several years, but the endoscopic techniques for operating in the abdomen (laparoscopy), chest (thoracoscopy) and other soft tissue spaces, have now begun to transform general surgery. The best established of these procedures is laparoscopic cholecystectomy and this and other endoscopic operations are now included in the relevant sections of this book. The modern housesurgeon requires a working knowledge of these techniques in order to explain them to patients, relatives and other health workers, and to assist in the care of patients undergoing the procedures.

General points about laparoscopic surgery

Because the operation is carried out through small incisions (usually less than 1 cm in diameter) there is much less trauma to the body wall. This is associated with less pain, less analgesic requirements and a more rapid recovery as far as the patient is concerned. There is also less scarring so the cosmetic result is superior. Patients usually enjoy a more rapid discharge from hospital. This may mean that complications then develop at home and may therefore be more difficult to spot, especially as such complications are rare. Before the operation the patient will need a clear explanation of what is intended. It can be very difficult for a patient to understand the gravity of their operation when they see very small scars on the skin afterwards.

Techniques

Endoscopic surgery relies on viewing the inside of the body using an image on a video screen. This image is used by the surgeon to perform the operation rather than looking at the body tissues directly, as in conventional surgery. Operating using an image has advantages. It can be obtained using a telescope through a very small incision, and is easy to magnify facilitating very detailed surgery. The image can also be enhanced in various ways and other information can be fed to the video screen including images from X-ray machines and other equipment.

A disadvantage is that modern video screens only produce a two-dimensional image so the surgeon's ability to distinguish depth is diminished (i.e. you also lose much of your normal tactile feedback, though it is still possible to 'feel' a certain amount through the shaft of the instruments).

Equipment

Instruments are placed into the body cavity through 'ports'. The body cavity has to be expanded in order to achieve a view. In the case of the peritoneum this may be done by insufflation with gas (carbon dioxide). It is also possible to produce a cavity by allowing air into a space produced by traction on the body wall. If, as is usually the case, the cavity is maintained by positive pressure then the ports need to contain valves so that the positive pressure does not escape.

Instruments have to be long and thin to extend through the ports and into the body to reach the target organ. The effector ends (graspers, scissors, etc.) are controlled by external handles on the outer end of the shaft. The surgeon will generally make use of one port for his left-hand instruments and one for his right-hand instruments. Other ports may be inserted to achieve a different direction of access or for positioning retractors or other special instruments. It is useful for you to know roughly how many ports are intended so that you can explain this to the patient before the operation.

In order to produce the colour image a high quality camera chip is required. Some cameras use a chip for each major colour (three-chip cameras) and this gives a higher resolution. The image is usually transmitted from the body cavity through a telescope (laparoscope) and the camera is attached to the outside end of this. Find out how it is attached so that you can disconnect and reconnect it for the surgeon if necessary. The quality of the image is critical for a good operation and both the camera lens and ends of the telescope must be kept clean. If you are holding the camera and telescope, avoid contact of the internal end with fatty tissue or blood. The chip in the camera transmits an electrical image to a 'camera box' which is usually situated on a trolley together with other equipment next to the operating table. This camera box develops the image into one that can be seen on a video screen. It is also possible to increase the brightness of the image by increasing the 'gain'. This uses a button either on the camera box or on the camera head itself and you should learn where it is. Using the gain brightens the image but decreases the resolution. It is often necessary to perform a 'white balance' for the camera so that its colour sensitivity is set to read white correctly and thus balance the other colours.

The operative site is illuminated with light transmitted down the telescope. The telescope is joined to the light source by a fibreoptic flexible light cable. This is also situated on the equipment trolley and you should learn which piece of equipment is which. The brightness of the light source can be varied by a control situated on the light source box. The optic fibres in the telescope and especially those in the light lead are fragile. The light cable must be treated with extreme care and replaced if sufficient fibres become broken.

As explained above, many endoscopic operations will require the maintenance of a tissue space using pressurized CO_2. For this purpose an insufflator is used and again you should familiarize yourself with its controls. CO_2 is usually provided by a cylinder attached to the back of the insufflator. There may be a reservoir in the insufflator with a read-out to say how much CO_2 it contains. Other instruments indicate the pressure of the CO_2 in the delivery line, and the rate of flow (in l/min). The pressure can be preset and there will be an instrument to indicate this. In normal laparoscopic operations the pressure is preset between 12 and 15 mmHg and should not exceed 15 mmHg. Every now and again during the operation you should check that the CO_2 pressure is being maintained and that the gas cylinder is not empty. This may be indicated by a low pressure and no gas flow. There should always be a full spare CO_2 cylinder in the theatre.

In order to obtain a clear view the surgeon usually makes use of suction and irrigation. These two modalities are normally delivered through a single probe and the flows are controlled with valves on the probe. The suction is connected to the theatre sucker. Irrigation is usually by saline (which may contain a little heparin) and this is pressurized in a separate irrigation apparatus.

Video

The image is viewed on a video screen, which, like any television apparatus, has various controls to adjust the brightness, colour and contrast of the image. By and large these are best left alone but they may need to be reset to a neutral position on occasions. In addition the surgeon may wish to record the operation on a video tape recorder which will be similar to those in domestic use. You should find out how to switch it to record, and how to start and rerun the tape. Make sure there is a fresh tape in the machine if a recording is to be made. Finally there may also be a machine to capture still video or digital images and produce them as prints. These may be filed in the patient's notes, kept by the surgeon or given to the patient.

Assisting at laparoscopic surgery

As a houseman you will often be required to hold and manipulate the camera. This is an important task as the surgeon can only carry out an accurate operation if he is given a good view. You should hold the camera steadily and avoid excessive movements. Only adjust the position when an adjustment is required. Learn where the focusing mechanism is and keep the image in focus. Learn how to move the camera and telescope into the abdomen (zoom) and how to move it out again. This may mean releasing the valve in the port so that the port does not move during this manoeuvre. You may also be required to hold instruments to retract organs.

Postoperative care of the patient

Generally speaking this is straightforward. Particular points are dealt with under the specific operations. The patients usually recover very quickly and have minimal pain. They may require analgesics which can usually be of the mild variety (paracetamol, codeine). Non-steroidal analgesics are useful for moderate pain but opiates are rarely needed. If the patient is discharged rapidly, tell them to get in touch with you if they develop increasing pain once they are home. This is unusual and should be taken seriously. It is often best to readmit them to check whether there is a serious problem.

1.11 The Intensive Care Unit

The houseman's role in the intensive care unit

Intensive care units are designed to look after the very ill. The department is often organized by the anaesthetic department, and run by senior specialized nursing staff.

The care of the patient is undertaken jointly by the surgeon and the intensive care staff, but the ultimate responsibility for a surgical patient normally resides with the consultant surgeon. In the intensive care unit the housesurgeon's role is to act as a coordinator and to monitor all aspects of patient care, making sure that nothing is left out. Although most of the management decisions are made by others, it is important to keep everybody in touch with events and to keep up to date with the patient's progress yourself.

The intensive care unit often seems very impersonal, with a large part of the management based on observation charts, results and machinery. In the midst of all this do not forget to examine the patient. Also remember that even if patients cannot speak (because they are intubated) they may well be able to see and hear all that is going on. Make sure you keep them fully informed about how they are progressing and avoid discussion or teaching within earshot.

The intensive care unit chart

The information and observations about each patient are usually recorded on a large chart and you should rapidly make yourself familiar with the layout of the one used in your hospital (Fig. 9). It is usually divided up into sections covering circulation and respiration, neurological observations and fluid balance.

Daily management of patients on the intensive care unit

The chart

Inspect the chart, thinking in terms of systems.

1 Circulation. Are the pulse, blood pressure and CVP stable and, if not, why not? Has there been any response to therapy given in the last 24 h?

2 Respiration. If the patient is on a ventilator, the tidal volume,

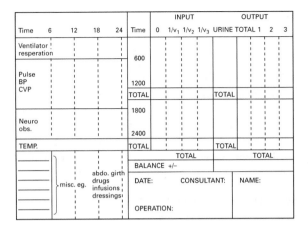

Time	6	12	18	24	Time	INPUT					OUTPUT				
						0	$1/v_1$	$1/v_2$	$1/v_3$	URINE	TOTAL	1	2	3	
Ventilator resperation					600										
Pulse BP CVP					1200										
					TOTAL					TOTAL					
					1800										
Neuro obs.					2400										
TEMP.					TOTAL					TOTAL					
						TOTAL				TOTAL					
			abdo. girth drugs infusions dressings	misc. eg.	BALANCE +/-										
					DATE:	CONSULTANT:				NAME:					
					OPERATION:										

Fig. 9 The type of chart used in the intensive care unit.

minute volume, respiratory rate and ventilator pressure are recorded. Check the blood gases. These will give an indication of whether or not the ventilation is satisfactory. The anaesthetist usually makes decisions about this but you should keep yourself in the picture. The blood gases are usually recorded separately on the result sheet.

3 Fluid balance. Check the total input versus the total output in the last 24 h. If there has been excessive loss, is this being replaced? Is the urine output adequate? A patient in intensive care should produce at least 0.5 mL/kg body weight/h (35 mL/h for a 70-kg patient) and preferably two to three times this volume.

4 Intravenous regimen. Has it been written up for the next 24 h and does it need adjusting according to the fluid balance?

5 Investigations. Check the day's results, particularly the urea and electrolytes, the haemoglobin and the most recent chest X-ray. The intravenous chart may well need further adjustment after looking at the electrolytes. Check the serum albumin; low values cause a fall in oncotic pressure and predispose to pulmonary oedema. Check whether the patient's blood clotting studies and platelet numbers are satisfactory.

6 Drug treatment. Review the analgesia given and ascertain whether it has been satisfactory either by communicating with the patient or the nurses, or by checking the effect of analgesia on the pulse rate and blood pressure. Is the patient on antibiotics? Review any bacteriological results. Should they be started, stopped, continued or changed?

7 Temperature. What is the source of any pyrexia?

The patient

Having looked at the chart to assess the patient's progress over the previous 24 h, examine the patient. Take particular note of the character of the pulse, the JVP, the lung bases and any evidence of peripheral oedema. Note his state of hydration. Check for bowel sounds and that the wound is satisfactory, and feel if there is any localized tenderness in the calf muscles. Watch closely for any evidence of neurological deterioration or signs of mental strain. At the end of this examination you should have formed a clear idea as to whether the patient's state reflects what is expected from the readings on the chart.

Surgical management

Keep a close eye on the following:

1 Wound dressings.
2 Abdominal or wound drains.
3 Stitches; when should they be removed (these tend to be forgotten in intensive care)?
4 State of postoperative ileus.

As the patient recovers he should generally be moved off the intensive care unit as soon as it is practicable. Patients get little rest while being intensively cared for and the mental strain is considerable. Make sure a bed is being kept somewhere for the patient to return to in the general ward.

If there is one overriding rule, it is to keep in constant liaison with the intensive care registrar and, through him, to keep the rest of your team informed.

2 Prescriptions and Other Tasks

2.1 Management of Intravenous Fluids

The indications for setting up an intravenous infusion in a surgical patient are as follows:

1 To give the normal fluid and electrolyte requirement to a postoperative patient who is unable to drink.

2 To replace abnormal losses, e.g. haemorrhage or vomiting.

3 As a route for intravenous drugs.

4 To give parenteral feeding.

A useful approximation for checking the fluid and electrolyte intake against body weight is:

1 40 mL fluid/kg adult body weight (babies need more, old people less).

2 2 mmol sodium/kg.

3 1 mmol potassium/kg.

The diagrams in this section will illustrate the contents of a litre unit.

Normal daily requirements (Fig. 10)

The replacement of fluid volume, and of electrolytes should be considered separately. The normal volume requirement for an adult has to replace:

1 The 'insensible' loss of water in faeces and from the lungs — about 500 mL.

2 Urinary output — about 1000 mL.

3 Insensible loss from the skin plus perspiration — 500–3000 mL depending on the patient's temperature and environmental conditions.

Abnormal losses

Abnormal losses have to be added to these. They can be external

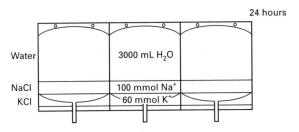

Fig. 10 Daily requirements for water, sodium and potassium ions.

or sequestrated within the body. External losses are usually more or less isotonic (vomiting, diarrhoea, fistulae) but may contain proteins (e.g. from nephrotic kidneys) or even blood cells. Fluid can also be sequestered internally in the so-called third space. Such losses are not immediately obvious and are often underestimated. They occur in diseases which induce a severe inflammatory reaction like pancreatitis, peritonitis and burns, but also after operative trauma. Isotonic fluid then leaks into the interstitial tissue (in wounds or generalized oedema) and gut (e.g. in paralytic ileus). These losses are temporary and with patient recovery the volume will be reabsorbed and excreted as urine producing a negative daily fluid balance.

Intravenous feeding

Intravenous feeding is needed in:

1 Patients who have no oral intake for more than 4–5 days (after major surgery).

2 Patients whose digestive system is not functioning due to ileus, malabsorption or fistulae.

3 Patients who require extreme amounts of calories because of multiple injuries or severe burns.

4 Patients who are candidates for parenteral nutrition.

Commonly used intravenous fluids

Crystalloid preparations

These are solutions of electrolytes in water. They disperse throughout the extracellular fluid space and are not confined to the circulation. They are dispensed in 500 or 1000 mL units.

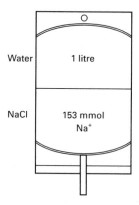

Fig. 11 One litre of normal saline.

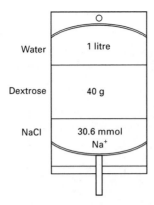

Fig. 12 One litre of 4% dextrose, 0.18% saline.

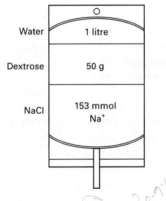

Fig. 13 One litre of 5% dextrose, 9% saline.

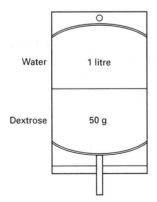

Fig. 14 One litre of 5% dextrose.

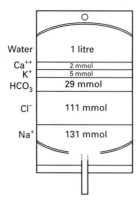

Fig. 15 One litre of Hartmann's solution.

Hartmann's solution is more 'physiological' than the others and contains potassium, calcium and lactate as well as sodium chloride. It mimics the electrolyte content of extracellular fluid, the lactate being metabolized to bicarbonate.

Normal saline (0.9%) is traditionally the most commonly used. It has, however, the disadvantage of inducing hyperchloraemic metabolic acidosis if given in large volumes.

Dextrose is readily taken up by cells. Pure dextrose solution is therefore effectively water, i.e. volume replacement only.

Dextrose saline (4% dextrose + 0.18% saline) is a solution designed to simplify the continuous replacement of volume and electrolytes, and balance normal losses. There are formulations of 'dextrose saline' which are in fact 0.9% saline with 5% dextrose (see Fig. 13). They are hyperosmolar. Be aware of this and prescribe the percentage clearly on the fluid chart.

Any of these fluids may have additional potassium added, usually in 10-mmol batches of KCl.

Other types of intravenous fluid

Whereas crystalloid solutions distribute in the entire extracellular volume, colloid solutions stay in the blood circulation. They are therefore useful to replace losses of blood volume, though apart from blood, they have no oxygen-carrying capacity. They are electrolyte solutions which also contain albumin or other macromolecules in place of albumin (Table 4). Because of the increase in colloid osmotic pressure they draw fluid from the tissues into the circulation in addition to the actually added volume.

Plasma protein fraction should be given through a filter but carries no hepatitis risk. Its main use is in volume resuscitation

Table 4 Contents of colloid solutions.

	Na⁺	K⁺	Ca⁺	Cl⁻	Protein or polyglycan
Plasma protein fraction	145	0.25	–	145	50 g (95% albumin)
Haemaccel	145	5.1	6.25	145	35 g (polygeline)
HAES 6%	153	–	–	153	60 g (pentastarch)
Dextran (in normal saline)	153	–	–	153	100 g (dextran)

in young children and patients with burns. Because of the rapid turnover of albumin the effect lasts for 24–36 h only. It is therefore of little use in treating a low serum albumin.

Gelatine solutions (Haemaccel (Fig. 16) and Gelofusine) are solutions of partially degraded gelatin. They have a half-life in the circulation of 3–4 h. There is a possibility of anaphylactic reactions because of their protein nature, but this is not as common as was previously thought.

HAES (hydroxyethyl starch) is made from amylopectin and because of its similarity to glycogen anaphylactic reactions are rare. HAES expands to a volume of 145–200% of the infused volume and has an effect on volume and microcirculation for 3–4 h. It is degraded by serum amylase and can lead to elevation of amylase estimation in blood.

Dextrans are polymers of glucose with an average molecular weight of either 40 or 70 kDa dissolved in either isotonic saline or 5% glucose. They are being superseded by the above two groups. Dextran interferes with cross-matching of blood once in the circulation and therefore any serum for cross-matching should be taken before the infusion is started.

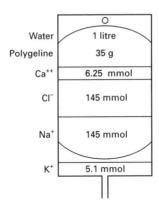

Water	1 litre
Polygeline	35 g
Ca⁺⁺	6.25 mmol
Cl⁻	145 mmol
Na⁺	145 mmol
K⁺	5.1 mmol

Fig. 16 One litre Haemaccel.

Blood

Blood is used to replace loss of red blood cells. Whole blood may be used or the volume may be reduced by infusing packed red cells. The latter are useful for treating chronically anaemic patients and have the advantage that the valuable plasma protein fraction can be used for other patients.

Blood contains sodium and potassium as well as citrate, phosphate, dextrose and sometimes adenine. After several weeks storage it also holds significant amounts of cellular debris, free haemoglobin, phosphate and ammonia. It has then lost most of its clotting factors and platelets. If large amounts of blood are transfused very quickly it is important to observe the serum potassium. The serum calcium can also become depressed due to the infusion of excess citrate in the stored blood. More common problems are hypothermia from rapidly transfused cold blood, and alkalosis because citrate is metabolized to bi-carbonate. Blood should always be given through a filter. Finally, the clotting factors are diluted by large transfusions of stored blood and should be assessed after such therapy. Additional fresh frozen plasma (FFP) with active clotting factors needs to be given during massive transfusions. Even small transfusions carry the risk of infection, transfusion reactions and immuno-suppression.

Prescribing the daily requirement

Replacement of normal losses

A suitable basic intravenous regime including electrolytes, for a fit 70-kg adult is:

1 Water 3 L
2 Sodium 100 mmol
3 Potassium 60 mmol.

This is usually given in one of two regimes, A or B.

Regime A (Fig. 17)

This gives the patient some energy in the form of dextrose: 2 L of 5% dextrose solution = 100 g of dextrose, which yields 410 kcal. Although this is insufficient for energy requirements postoperatively, it is all right in the short term as the body utilizes endogenous stores. However, should the patient be off oral fluids for more than 4–5 days, intravenous nutrition must be considered.

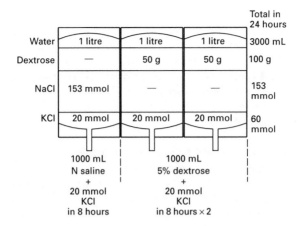

Fig. 17 Regime A: 2 L of 5% dextrose and 1 L of normal saline in 24 h.

Regime B (Fig. 18)

An alternative regime gives the patient 3 L a day, 90 mmol of sodium, 60 mmol of potassium and 120 g of dextrose. As can be seen, this contains slightly less sodium and supplies glucose in a more continuous fashion.

Replacement of abnormal losses

In certain circumstances the above basic regimes have to be modified to take account of abnormal losses. These are replaced

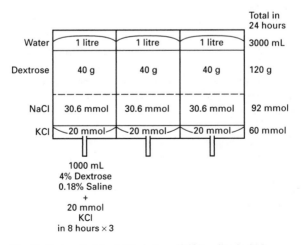

Fig. 18 Regime B: 3 L of 4% dextrose/0.18% saline in 24 h.

according to their composition. This usually means using an isotonic balanced electrolyte solution (Hartmann's). In vomiting from pyloric stenosis chloride and hydrogen ions are the main losses and are replaced with isotonic saline. Pyrexia (250 mL/degree of fever) and artificial ventilation increase insensible losses which contain minimal electrolytes. In extensive burns the capillaries also leak proteins, and resuscitation has to include albumin.

Extra volume and electrolytes (crystalloids)

Extra electrolytes are required when the patient is suffering from losses of fluid rich in salt. This occurs in vomiting, diarrhoea and intestinal fistulae. More insidiously extracellular fluid containing electrolytes is sequestered into the peritoneum and gut after abdominal operations and into the interstitium in severe inflammatory conditions such as pancreatitis. Losses of intestinal contents and from sequestration should usually be replaced with Hartmann's solution.

Extra volume (water)

When the patient is pyrexial or the weather is hot, insensible salt-free losses increase. Extra water without electrolytes is required. An intake of 3000 mL/day does cover some increased losses as commonly required by postoperative patients. If more is required the rate of infusion is simply increased and additional 5% dextrose prescribed.

Less fluid

In the first 24 h postoperatively the metabolic response to the trauma of surgery causes increased aldosterone and increased antidiuretic hormone release. This causes both salt and water retention and because of this some surgeons or anaesthetists prefer to give less fluid and no salt in the first 24 h, e.g. 5% dextrose 1 L 12-hourly (Fig. 19). This is then followed by regime A or B (see above) on day 2.

Extra potassium

Most of the body potassium is in the cells and the serum potassium is not a good guide to overall depletion. The serum potassium may only fall when a large deficit has occurred. Those patients who may require extra potassium include the following:
1 Patients receiving certain diuretics (frusemide, bendrofluazide).
2 Patients with large volumes of gastric aspirate or prolonged vomiting.

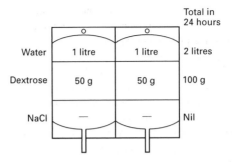

Fig. 19 Five per cent dextrose 1 L 12-hourly.

3 Patients with a fistula from the biliary tract or small bowel.
4 Patients with diarrhoea (e.g. ulcerative colitis or villous adenoma).

The amount of potassium required depends on the volume lost. For every 500 mL of gastrointestinal loss, consider an extra 5–10 mmol of potassium.

Special cases

Acute rehydration

More intensive intravenous fluid therapy is required in the dehydrated patient, especially if an operation is imminent. Any regime for such a patient is 'tailor-made' to suit his calculated deficit as judged by the history, clinical state and biochemical results. It may be necessary to infuse, for instance, Hartmann's solution at a rate of 1 L/h for a limited period. Clearly the state of the patient's kidneys and heart will dictate how safely such rapid replacement can be given. In these cases the decision about what should be given will have to be made by the registrar or consultant.

Children

The management of babies and very small children is undertaken jointly between the surgeons and the paediatricians and is not discussed further here.

Elderly patients

The elderly patient on intravenous fluids requires close monitoring because of the risk of precipitating left ventricular failure. It is essential that you assess any elderly patient carefully before prescribing intravenous fluids. The hydration status is best assessed by clinical signs. Ideally these patients are given a regime with less volume and no more sodium than is necessary. The following prescription may be suitable:

1 0.9% saline: 1 L + 40 mmol KCl in 12 h

2 5% dextrose: 1 L + 20 mmol KCl in 12 h.

This gives 2 L of fluid/day with 153 mmol of sodium and 60 mmol of potassium. Patients may need more fluid if they become dehydrated. Many elderly patients are on diuretics or digitalis and therefore a close eye must be kept on the electrolytes. Do not forget to change these drugs to intravenous injections if the patient does not drink.

Haemorrhage

Blood loss should ideally be replaced by blood and after a certain point this is vital to maintain the oxygen-carrying capacity. With rapid losses, however, while blood is being cross-matched, the circulating volume may be maintained with a colloid, e.g. Haemaccel, Hespan, plasma protein fraction or even type-specific uncross-matched blood.

Acute renal failure

Here intravenous fluids must be severely restricted but must still replace the necessary constituents. The volume usually prescribed covers the daily insensible fluid loss plus the previous day's urinary output. Fluids may be written by the hour in this situation to allow closer control, e.g. 30 mL/h plus the previous hour's output. The electrolytes must be watched carefully and usually the urinary electrolyte loss is measured twice a day. Sodium is replaced in proportion to the previous day's urinary loss. Potassium must not be given as it is usually retained.

Intravenous feeding

Most of these patients requiring intravenous feeding are catabolic and the aim is to reverse this catabolism by giving the patient protein and energy. Sufficient energy derived from non-protein sources, e.g. carbohydrate or fat ensures that the protein given is used for protein anabolism and is not itself broken down to provide a substrate for glycolysis.

A typical surgical patient needs 12–16 g nitrogen/day (80–90 g protein) and 3000 kcal. The energy may either be given as concentrated dextrose (4.1 kcal/g) or as fat, e.g. Intralipid (9.3 kcal/g). These fluids are hypertonic and acid and need to be given through a central vein. They are given slowly as they may be toxic to the heart.

In addition to the provision of energy, total parenteral nutrition takes into account the replacement of water, electrolytes, some trace elements and vitamins. The daily requirements are often calculated by a nutrition nurse and may be provided in a ready mixed form by the hospital pharmacy.

Intravenous feeding needs to be monitored by daily measurement of the urea, electrolytes and blood sugar. The liver function tests and haemoglobin are measured every third day.

In patients with an intact intestinal tract, a better alternative to parenteral feeding is assisted enteral feeding, using a fine-bore nasogastric tube or surgical gastrostomy and continuous infusion into the gut. This is easier, carries less risk of infection, has a positive effect on the immune system and reduces the risk of duodenal stress ulcers. However, it may be complicated by incomplete absorption and diarrhoea.

Monitoring the effect of infusion therapy

Whatever regime is chosen the effects must be constantly monitored. Low and high extracellular volume should be diagnosed clinically. Biochemistry tests are helpful to detect concentration and composition changes of the serum (and extracellular space). Therefore assess the following parameters:

1 Cardiovascular signs: pulse, blood pressure, jugular vein pulse (JVP).

2 Central nervous signs: drowsiness, coma.

3 Tissue signs: skin turgor, dry tongue and mucous membranes, oedema.

4 Urine output: the minimum acceptable urine output is 0.5 mL/kg/h. It should preferably be 1 mL/kg/h. This means 35–70 mL/h or 800–1600 mL/day in a 70-kg patient.

5 Fluid balance (i.e. input compared with output). Check the totals on the observation charts. It is the houseman's duty to ensure that the nursing staff keep these records accurately and up to date.

6 Measurement of the urea and electrolytes: these are usually performed every 2 days.

7 CVP measurement: this gives a good indication of the degree of filling of the venous side of the circulation. It also provides information about cardiac function. A central venous pressure (CVP) line is generally required in any patient requiring intensive fluid therapy who is at higher risk because of reduced heart or kidney function.

CVP

OPERATION: SETTING UP A CVP LINE

The objective is to place a long intravenous cannula or catheter with its tip in the superior vena cava. A strict aseptic technique is used and the patient is placed slightly head down. The skin of the selected entry site is cleaned and isolated using sterile towels. A bleb of local anaesthetic is inserted at the puncture site. Various entry points can be used as follows:

1 The basilic vein lying medially in the antecubital fossa.

2 The subclavian vein beneath the clavicle. The introducing cannula is inserted at a point 2 cm below the middle of the clavicle aiming at the centre of the suprasternal notch. The needle is kept horizontal and advanced while maintaining suction on the syringe. Blood appears in the syringe as the vein is entered. A catheter is then inserted through the lumen of the introducing cannula and threaded down the correct distance. This may be judged by marking the cannula previously.

3 Internal jugular vein. The vessel is cannulated just behind the sternocleidomastoid muscle in the neck. The vein can be fixed by grasping the muscle and elevating it slightly. The needle is inserted half-way between the mastoid process and the head of the clavicle. It is advanced deep to the medial border of the clavicle in the direction of the nipple in a male. This approach is easier in the anaesthetized patient.

Once in place the catheter should be fixed with a suture or adhesive tape and the entry site dressed with antiseptic spray and dry gauze. The catheter is attached to a three-way tap. One limb of the tap is attached to a manometer and the other to a saline infusion. When the manometer line is switched to the patient the meniscus should fluctuate with respiration. Switch to the saline and lower the bag below the patient to check that blood will run back up the line ('flashback'). The saline is run slowly at a rate sufficient to keep the vein open (e.g. 1 L over 16–24 h).

A chest X-ray is always taken to confirm that the catheter tip lies in the superior vena cava, and to check that there is no pneumothorax.

Complications

1 Infection of the catheter tip and septicaemia. If symptoms of septicaemia occur with no other known primary infection, the catheter should be removed and the tip cultured.

2 Pneumothorax. This may follow the cannulation of internal jugular or subclavian veins by any approach. Patients should be

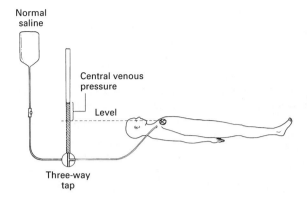

Fig. 20 Measuring the CVP.

observed for dyspnoea and chest pain following the cannulation.
3 Hydrothorax. This occurs if the catheter lies in the pleural cavity.
4 Phlebothrombosis.
5 Air embolus. Accidental disconnection of a CVP line in an upright patient will lead to air aspiration. Lie the patient flat whenever making connections.

Measurement of the CVP (Fig. 20)
The scale of the manometer is set to a fixed reference point on the patient, with the aid of a spirit level. The usual reference point is the mid-axillary line. Mark the point clearly on the skin and use it for all subsequent readings. The patient should be in the same position each time.

Having set the zero of the manometer scale to that level, continue as follows:
1 Fill the manometer with fluid.
2 Connect the manometer tube to the patient, closing off the saline infusion.
3 The meniscus should move up and down with respiration. Initially it will drop steadily until the meniscus is moving above and below a mean pressure. The lowest reading to which the meniscus falls is recorded.
4 Reconnect the saline infusion isolating the manometer.

The normal value for the CVP at the mid-axillary line in the supine patient is +1 to +9 cmH$_2$O. The reading is elevated if there is any right-sided cardiac failure or if the patient is being ventilated. It will be low in the hypovolaemic patient. A series of readings is more valuable than a single measurement. Due to the variation in venous tone in the normal patient, a trend will give a more accurate estimate of the venous filling of the heart and its response to therapy.

Removing the line
Tilt the bed in the Trendelenburg position. Cut the holding suture, apply pressure over the entry point into the vein, and withdraw the line. Using a no-touch technique, cut off the tip and send it for culture.

2.2 Prescribing Drugs for Surgical Patients

How to write a prescription

Prescribing drugs for patients is the houseman's responsibility. It is most important that the prescription should be written clearly and correctly. You will have to prescribe both those drugs the patient was taking before coming into hospital, and also any others that are to be given during admission.

Prescriptions will generally be written on the drug chart. Outpatient prescriptions are made on a specially designed form (EC10) but may be written on any headed notepaper. A specimen suitable for outpatient prescribing is shown in Fig. 21.

There are certain requirements which must be observed when prescribing drugs.

1 Identify the patient. The prescription must be clearly labelled with the patient's name, address, hospital number and date of birth. If there are two or more patients with the same name, then extra care is needed to avoid confusion.

2 Date.

3 Drug. Use the approved name of the drug and not its trade name.

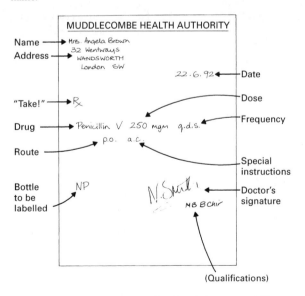

Fig. 21 A specimen prescription (for abbreviations see p. 102).

Table 5 Abbreviations used in prescribing.

Abbreviation	Latin/meaning	Translation
Rx	recipe	take
Site	–	–
p.o.	*per os*	by mouth
p.r.	per rectum	by rectal administration
i.m.	intramuscular	by intramuscular injection
i.v.	intravenous	by intravenous injection
s.c.	subcutaneous	by subcutaneous injection
s.l.	sublinguum	sublingual
frequency	–	–
stat.	*statim*	immediately
o.d.	*omni die*	every day (once a day)
b.d./b.i.d.	*bis die/bis in die*	twice a day
t.d.s	*ter die sumendus*	to be taken three times a day
q.d.s.	*quater die sumendus*	to be taken four times a day
o.m.	*omne mane*	morning
o.n.	*omne nocte*	evening
s.o.s	*si opus sit*	if there is need, if necessary (usually a single dose)
p.r.n.	*pro re nata*	occasionally, when required. Add the maximum frequency as well, e.g. p.r.n. 4-hourly (usually used for multiple doses)
Other terms		
a.c.	*ante cibum*	before food
p.c.	*post cibum*	after food
iu		international unit
tab.	*tabletta/tabella*	a tablet
mist.	*mistura*	a mixture
gtt.	*guttae*	drops
supp.	*suppositorium*	a suppository
tr./tinct.	*tinctura*	a tincture
ung.	*unguentum*	ointment
n.p.	*nomen proprium*	the proper name. (Usually means the dispenser should label the prescription with the proper name)
BNF		British National Formulary
BP		British Pharmacopoeia
BPC		British Pharmaceutical Codex

4 Dose.

5 Route.

6 Rate or frequency of administration.

7 Duration of treatment with that drug or maximum number of doses.

8 Signature of a qualified doctor. This is a legal requirement. In addition it is usual to put your registered qualifications when you are prescribing on headed notepaper rather than the usual prescription form. Outpatient prescriptions require the doctor's address.

Abbreviations commonly used in prescriptions are shown in Table 5.

Controlled drugs

Drugs such as narcotic analgesics, because they are open to abuse, are controlled by the Misuse of Drugs Regulations (1973). These are known as 'controlled drugs'. The regulations state that the prescription must carry the following (Fig. 22):

1 Patient's name

2 Date

3 Prescriber's full signature in his own handwriting

4 Name of the drug in full

5 Form of the drug (e.g. tablets, elixir)

6 Strength of the prescription

7 Total quantity of the preparation in both words and figures.

Pharmacists are not allowed to dispense controlled drugs on an incomplete prescription, or on an 'and repeat' basis.

Review

Make it a rule to review the drug chart every day during the ward round. Any drugs that are no longer required should be

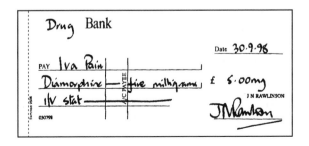

Fig. 22 In many respects a controlled drug prescription is like a cheque.

crossed off (e.g. antibiotics). Other drugs may need changing, e.g. from intravenous to oral or from a stronger to a weaker analgesic.

Discharge

When the patient is discharged from hospital he must be given sufficient drugs to last him until he can obtain more from his own doctor. Usually hospital pharmacies will supply drugs to last the patient a maximum of 2 weeks. It is important to tell the GP as soon as possible what drugs the patient has been given to take home. Point out any new drugs given for the present illness and how long they should be prescribed. Also note any change made to the patient's previous therapy. This is best done by a note sent to the GP (with the patient if this is possible) on the day of discharge.

Drug management

The following are short notes on the use of analgesics, antibiotics and sedatives in surgical practice.

Analgesics

Adequate pain relief after operation is important as it helps the patient to move and cough and thus lowers the risk of thromboembolism and pulmonary collapse. A patient will not always complain when he is in pain and you should enquire about this rather than wait for him to ask for drugs. Also ask him if the pain killers he has been given are adequate. Occasionally patients do not like to take pain killers at all and feel they should be able to do without them. They need firm reassurance that no harm will come from the drugs and indeed they will benefit from using them. If analgesia is written up 'p.r.n.' (as required) the patient should be informed of this so that he can ask for it when required. Analgesia must be sufficient to allow the patient to cough with the minimum of discomfort.

Pain reduction can be achieved by:
1 Local anaesthetics
2 Systemic drugs.

Local anaesthetics

In modern surgical practice, with the advent of long-acting anaesthetics such as bupivacaine (Marcain), local analgesia has become the method of choice for pain reduction after many surgical procedures. Excellent analgesia can be achieved for 8–10 h. It may be given:

1 By local infiltration of the wound at the time of surgery. This can be useful in the smaller operations such as removal of skin lumps, hernia repairs and so forth.

2 By regional nerve block. Examples include intercostal nerve blocks for abdominal and thoracic operations, and ring blocks of toes and fingers.

3 Epidural analgesia may be used, but requires high-dependency nursing, especially if combined with epidural opiates.

If regional local anaesthesia is used for day-case surgery, warn patients that they can damage the area anaesthetized without realizing it, and should be careful to avoid such damage.

Systemic analgesic drugs

Systemic analgesics are chosen in a step-wise fashion depending on the severity of the pain.

Relief of acute pain

Severe pain

Opiates are the drugs of choice. These are all strong analgesics and narcotics. Morphine and Pethidine are the standard drugs in this group. Omnopon is a mixture of opiates, about 50% of which is morphine. Pethidine is a weaker analgesic than morphine. All three are very effective in the short term.

1 Morphine (10–20 mg i.m./i.v. 3–4-hourly). Occasionally it is useful to give a small dose (e.g. 5 mg i.v. 2–3-hourly) so as to provide analgesia but avoid the side-effects seen soon after the administration of a larger 4-hourly dose. A normal dose of morphine for a 70-kg man with an abdominal incision would be 10–20 mg i.m. 4-hourly.

2 Pethidine (75–100 mg i.m./i.v. 4-hourly). The normal dose for a 70-kg man would be 100 mg i.m. 4-hourly.

3 Papaveretum (Omnopon) (10–20 mg i.m., orally, or i.v. 3–4-hourly). A normal dose for a 70-kg man with an abdominal incision would be 15–20 mg 4-hourly.

Patient-controlled analgesia systems (PCAS)
Intravenous infusions of opiates may give improved pain control. They are given as a basic continuous infusion with intermittent boluses on demand. For boluses the patient presses a button on the PCAS. The lock-out time between boluses, the basic rate and the bolus dose can be adjusted.

Side-effects

Opiates have side-effects. Dependence and tolerance do develop, although this is never a problem in the patient immediately after surgery. The following, however, are of importance in the surgical patient:

1 Nausea and vomiting. Prochlorperazine (Stemetil) 12.5 mg i.m. 8-hourly is the main antiemetic prophylactically prescribed, but it can, especially in children and the elderly, cause extrapyramidal dyskinesias.

2 Respiratory and cough suppression. Nurses are advised to check patient alertness and respiration rate before administration of every opiate dose.

3 Constipation and prolonged ileus (less with Pethidine). This should be treated prophylactically in patients with oral intake. A combination of a stimulant with a softening agent (e.g. codanthramer, 2 capsules at night) is the most effective.

4 Biliary tract spasm, particularly closure of the sphincter of Oddi. This occurs with all three drugs, though less so with Pethidine.

Remember that these opioids cause miosis, so avoid using them for patients with a head injury. If narcotic analgesia is required in these cases, codeine phosphate should be given.

Contraindications

1 Respiratory disease — narcotics may precipitate respiratory failure.

2 Hepatic failure — small doses may precipitate hepatic encephalopathy.

3 Hypothyroidism, hypopituitarism, Addison's disease — use of narcotics may lead to coma.

4 Raised intracranial pressure — narcotics may lead to coma.

5 Patients on monoamine oxidase inhibitors — these drugs potentiate narcotics.

Moderate pain

An example is somatic pain from the wound after the first 2–3 days.

1 Dihydrocodeine (DF118) (25–50 mg i.m. 4–6-hourly; 30–60 mg orally 4–6-hourly). Dihydrocodeine is midway between morphine and codeine in potency and its main side-effect is constipation. With prolonged use the patient may require laxatives.

2 Codeine (30–60 mg orally 4-hourly). This is an analgesic which is partly converted to morphine in the body. It has only

one-quarter to one-sixth of the analgesic power of morphine and the side-effects are even less. Dependence does not usually occur, but it is very constipating.

3 Diclofenac (25–50 mg orally t.d.s. or 75 mg i.m. b.d.) is a strong non-steroidal anti-inflammatory drug with good postoperative analgesic effects. It has however, the typical side-effects causing gastric erosions and ulcers and must not be given to asthmatics or to patients with renal impairment.

Mild pain

Fashions vary widely in the drugs which are popular at any one time for relief of mild pain. Some suggestions follow:

1 Co-proxamol (1–2 tablets 4–6-hourly). Each tablet of co-proxamol contains 32.5 mg dextropropoxyphene (related to methadone) and 325 mg paracetamol. There is a known incidence of side-effects and toxicity (respiratory and cardiac depression) due to the dextropropoxyphene and its metabolite norpropoxyphene. It is an opioid analgesic and dependence is believed to occur. Although few trials have been done there is little evidence that it is superior to paracetamol in its analgesic effect. It is contraindicated in patients with poor renal function due to the accumulation of norpropoxyphene.

2 Paracetamol (0.5–1 g (1–2 tablets) 4–6-hourly). This is a good analgesic with very little in the way of side-effects.

3 Aspirin (300–600 mg (1–2 tablets) orally 4–6-hourly). The use of this drug is contraindicated in patients with a past history of stomach disorders.

Most mild analgesics must be given orally. Rectal preparations are available for paracetamol and Diclofenac. Diclofenac may also be given intramuscularly.

Control of chronic pain

The control of chronic pain is a speciality in itself. A few points can be noted here:

1 In a patient with incurable disease the aim is to prevent the pain, not to treat it once it occurs. Prevention is not only better for the patient but requires less analgesia. It is kind to leave the patient with some tablets by his bedside at night in case he wakes up with pain.

2 Opiates are usually required. In a terminally ill patient the danger of dependence is unimportant. However, tolerance develops, so the dose will need to be increased as time passes. The priority is to keep the patient free of pain.

3 Attempt, if possible, to control pain with oral or rectal drugs to save the repeated discomfort of injections. Some examples of drugs used are the following:

(a) oral morphine/diamorphine, e.g. 10 mg 4-hourly and increase as required. An antiemetic should be prescribed and a laxative may also be required

(b) 'Brompton's cocktail' is an elixir made of morphine, chlorpromazine and cocaine. It has mixed analgesic and tranquillizing effects and can be very useful. Many hospital pharmacies have their own version of this cocktail and so ask them for advice as to the dose prescribed

(c) Levorphanol (1.5–4.5 mg one to two times daily). This is a synthetic morphine-like drug which is well absorbed orally and causes less sedation than morphine

(d) Oxycodone (Proladone) suppositories. These contain 30 mg of oxycodone pectinate. This is an opiate. One is useful at night as the drug is longer acting than morphine. The effect is equal to 20 mg of morphine orally and it lasts about 8 h

(e) buprenorphine (Temgesic, dose 400 µg 6–8-hourly). This is a long-acting analgesic and has both agonist and antagonist properties with opiates. It therefore must not be used with other opiates. It may be given sublingually.

Hypnotics and sedatives

Surgery, however minor, is always associated with anxiety. While drugs can be no substitute for gentle reassurance and explanation by both the housesurgeon and nursing staff, hypnotics and sedatives do have a use. The more rested and relaxed a patient is, the better he will tolerate the operation. It is a good idea to prescribe night sedation for every patient, to be taken if required. The patient must be told that this is available. He may require reassurance that he will come to no harm by taking sleeping tablets for a few nights.

The following are short notes on some of the drugs commonly used:

1 Diazepam (Valium) (2, 5 or 10 mg orally or i.m.). This drug is a benzodiazepine and is a tranquillizer and muscle relaxant. It can be used to relieve general anxiety during the day, often in small doses (e.g. 2 mg 8-hourly). It can also be used as an adjunct to pain killers for relief of pain from an abdominal wound when this pain is due to muscle spasm. It may be taken orally or intramuscularly. It is a very safe drug, although drowsiness and confusion can occur, especially in the elderly patient.

2 Nitrazepam (Mogadon) (5–10 mg orally *nocte*). This is also a benzodiazepine and is marketed as a hypnotic. It is safe and effective although it does cause a slight 'hangover' the next day and may well cause confusion in elderly patients.

3 Temazepam and flurazepam (dose temazepam 10–30 mg *nocte*, flurazepam 15–30 mg *nocte*). These are two other benzodiazepines which are used as hypnotics. Both have shorter half-lives. Temazepam, in particular, causes less 'hangover' and is suitable for the elderly.

All benzodiazepines can cause respiratory depression and are contraindicated in patients with chronic respiratory disease.

4 Dichloralphenazone (Welldorm, 1.3–1.95 g (2–3 tablets) *nocte*). This is a useful hypnotic, related to chloral hydrate, and is less likely than nitrazepam to cause confusion in the elderly patient. It is a safe drug, although it does interact with oral anticoagulants, displacing them from their binding proteins. This increases their effect and their rate of elimination.

5 Chlormethiazole (Heminevrin). This is a useful second-line drug for the relief of insomnia and is particularly good for agitation in the elderly patient: for insomnia, 2 capsules *nocte*; for sedation, 1 capsule 8-hourly (each capsule contains 192 mg of chlormethiazole in *Arachis* oil).

Antibiotics

Antibiotics are used either for prophylaxis or treatment.

Antibiotic prophylaxis

Prophylactic antibiotics are timed to be present in wound fluids when the patient is most at risk from infection. Generally this means the peroperative period and the antibiotics are given just before the operation. The choice of drug is usually made by the consultant as part of his routine management. Some suggestions are shown in Table 6 although it is realized that these will rapidly become out of date. The reader may then wish to fill in the drugs that are at present used in his unit for his own future reference.

Patients on gentamicin are at risk from damage to kidneys and the acoustic nerve if levels rise too high. Levels should be measured before and after the third dose and then twice weekly. Acceptable levels are less than 2 mg/L before, and 6–10 mg/L 1 h after, injection.

Antibiotics for acute infections

The antibiotic used will depend on the suspected site of infec-

Table 6 Prophylactic antibiotics.

Procedure	Organism	Prophylaxis	Alternatives
Large bowel surgery[*]	Anaerobes, coliforms, *Streptococcus milleri*	Gentamicin 120 mg i.v. plus metronidazole 500 mg i.v. plus benzylpenicillin 1.2 g i.v. at induction	Cefotaxime 1 g, i.v. plus metronidazole 500 mg i.v. or ciprofloxacin 200 mg, i.v. plus metronidazole 500 mg i.v.
Appendicitis	Anaerobes	Metronidazole 1 g p.r. 2–3 h preoperatively	
Biliary surgery	Coliforms	Cefotaxime 1 g i.v. at induction	Ciprofloxacin 200 mg i.v.
Arterial surgery	*Streptococcus* or *Staphylococcus*	Gentamicin 120 mg and flucloxacillin 500 mg i.v. at induction, continue for 3 doses with 80 mg gentamicin	
Amputations	*Clostridium* (gas gangrene in stump)	Benzylpenicillin 1.2 g i.v. at induction	
Insertion of orthopaedic metal implants	*Staphylococcus aureus*, *Staphylococcus epidermidis*	Flucloxacillin 1 g i.v. at induction	Cefotaxime 1 g i.v.
Urinary tract surgery	*Escherichia coli*, *Proteus*, faecal *Streptococcus*, *Pseudomonas*, *Klebsiella*, enterobacter	Benzylpenicillin 1.2 g i.v. plus gentamicin 120 mg i.v. at induction (choice also depends on urine culture)	

[*]If faecal contamination has occurred then continue a 2–5 day course of medication. The dose of gentamicin is then 80 mg t.d.s.

tion and thus on the predicted organism. Confirmation of the causative organism and its antibiotic sensitivity will be obtained when a bacteriological culture has been performed. It is useful to send appropriate specimens (urine, swabs, sputum, blood culture) before starting treatment.

Table 7 Antibiotics for acute infections.

Condition	Likely organism	Initial antibiotic therapy
Wound infection		
Indurated, localized, white pus	? *Staphylococcus*	Flucloxacillin 250 mg q.d.s. p.o.
Indurated, spreading cellulitis	? *Streptococcus*	Phenoxymethylpenicillin 500 mg q.d.s. p.o.
Foul-smelling pus	? Anaerobes	Metronidazole, e.g. 400 mg t.d.s. p.o. or 1 g supp. t.d.s. p.r.
Infected drip site	*Staphylococcus*	Flucloxacillin 250 mg q.d.s. p.o.
Chest infection		
Pneumonia at admission (community acquired)	*Pneumococcus*	Benzylpenicillin 600 mg q.d.s. i.v.
Pneumonia post-operatively (hospital acquired)	*Haemophilus influenzae*	Cefuroxime 750 mg t.d.s. i.v.
Pneumonia after aspiration	Gram-negative rods and anaerobes	Cefotaxime, 1 g b.d. i.v. and metronidazole 500 mg t.d.s. i.v.
Urinary tract infection		
Uncomplicated		Norfloxacin 400 mg b.d. p.o., or augmentin 375 mg t.d.s.
Severe, i.e. fever over 38.5°C, rigors, acute pyelonephritis		Benzylpenicillin 1.2 g i.v., and gentamicin 80 mg 8-hourly i.m. or i.v. initially (24 h), then norfloxacin 400 mg p.o b.d.
With indwelling catheter (no symptoms, positive culture only)		No treatment (see p. 472)

In Table 7 some common sites of perioperative infections are shown, together with the possible initial antibiotics to use. Specific surgical infections (e.g. acute cholecystitis) are discussed in the appropriate section.

Anticoagulants

The usual drugs used for anticoagulation are heparin, low molecular weight heparins and warfarin.

Heparin

Prophylaxis of deep vein thromboses

Heparin (5000 units, s.c. b.d.) and its low molecular variants (e.g. Enoxaparin, 20 mg s.c. daily) reduce the risk of deep vein thrombosis, especially in patients who are obese, on bed rest, are elderly, have lower limb surgery or a debilitating disease such as sepsis or cancer. Do not forget to institute physical means of prophylaxis such as compression stockings, leg exercises and raising the foot of the bed.

Treatment of deep vein thrombosis

Anticoagulation for established deep vein thrombosis has a less proven benefit on survival or later complications than prophylaxis, but is generally used. Initial treatment is with heparin given intravenously in a dose of 100–150 iu/kg body weight immediately, followed by an intravenous infusion of 30 000–40 000 units/day. The level of anticoagulation should be monitored with daily partial thromboplastin times (PTT) and these should be kept at 1.5–2.5 times the normal level by adjusting the rate of the infusion. For uncomplicated deep vein thromboses subcutaneous tinzaparin (175 units/kg body weight s.c. daily) can be used, which avoids having to check the prothrombin time.

Warfarin

Long-term anticoagulation may be maintained with warfarin. It is commenced after 3–7 days of heparinization. This drug takes 48–72 h to take effect and therefore a loading dose is given while the patient is still on heparin. A suitable regime is as follows:

1 Prescribe a loading dose of warfarin. This is usually 10 mg/day orally given at 6 p.m. for 2 consecutive days. A lower dose may be required for patients with a low body weight, the elderly or those with hepatic disease.

2 On the morning of day 3, test the coagulation times. The prothrombin time is used to assess the effect of warfarin and expressed as the international normalized ratio (INR). The INR times should be 2.5–4.5. Less than 2.5 denotes under-anticoagulation and more than 4.5 over-anticoagulation. If the INR is in the expected range stop the heparin.

3 Prescribe further warfarin on the basis of this test and recheck the clotting values 1–2 days later. The dose to be given is adjusted according to the value of the INR. The blood tests are taken in the morning and the warfarin is prescribed in the evening. Continue to check the INR until it is in a therapeutic range with constant warfarin doses.

The main side-effect of over-anticoagulation is haemorrhage, particularly into the urinary and alimentary tract. If haemorrhage occurs, the drug should be stopped and the INR checked. If bleeding is significant, FFP 2–4 units should be given. Phytomenadione (vitamin K_1) (10–21 mg i.v.) also reverses warfarin but takes some hours to work and prevents re-anticoagulation for 7–10 days. Should the patient have a heart valve replacement get urgent advice from a haematologist before any intervention.

Many drugs and conditions affect the activity of warfarin and the INR must be reviewed regularly after changes in the concurrent drug therapy.

1 Some drugs displace warfarin from plasma proteins, increasing the anticoagulation effect, e.g. aspirin, phenylbutazone and clofibrate.

2 Liver disease potentiates warfarin activity.

3 Low vitamin K (in association with jaundice or antibiotic treatment) also increases warfarin activity.

4 Liver enzyme induction, e.g. by chronic alcoholism or phenobarbitone therapy increases the rate of metabolism of warfarin and a higher dose is required. The dose must be reduced when the inducing agent is withdrawn.

Anticoagulation is contraindicated if there is a recent history of haematemesis, peptic ulceration, ulcerative colitis, haematuria, cerebral haemorrhage or hypertension and in women in the first trimester or last 4 weeks of pregnancy. These contraindications are not absolute and the risks must be balanced against the benefits.

Thrombolytic therapy

Thrombi, once formed, may be dissolved using thrombolytic agents such as streptokinase or tissue plasminogen activator (TPA). These are dealt with on p. 56.

Bowel preparation

The aim of preparing the bowel before abdominal surgery is to clear the colon of exogenous material and lower the number of infective organisms. Such bowel preparation is essential before a colonic resection.

Emptying the bowel

Left-sided lesions

The patient is started on a low-residue diet 2 days before the operation. The day before operation he may have clear fluids. The usual drug given to empty the bowel is Picolax (one sachet at 8 a.m. and at 2 p.m. each, orally). This causes severe diarrhoea, so advise the patient to drink 2–3 L for rehydration that day.

Right-sided lesions

Transit time is faster on the right and preparation can be gentler. The patient is given clear fluids only for 24 h before operation. The contents of the bowel are evacuated using Picolax (1 sachet at 2 p.m. orally).

Haemorrhoidectomy and minor anal procedures

The rectum is emptied with phosphate enemas given 4–6 h before theatre. Do not give enemas to patients immediately before an operation, for example in day surgery. Liquid faeces may contaminate the operating field.

If there is a colostomy or ileostomy planned or if there is only a remote chance of this being required, the patient has to be seen by a stoma nurse. She will explain the handling of the stoma to the patient and mark the most convenient site.

Non-absorbable antibiotics used to be given to disinfect the bowel. They are rarely used now.

2.3 Sutures and Drains

Sutures

It is useful to be familiar with the various types of suture, their uses and their effect on the management of wounds. Generally, a suture may be either absorbable or non-absorbable, and has either a braided, twisted or monofilament structure. It can be made from natural or synthetic material.

Types of suture

Absorbable sutures are broken down in the body tissues over a varying number of days either by enzymes or by hydrolysis by the tissue fluid. It is important to differentiate between the times of loss of tensile strength and of disappearance of the material as these are not necessarily the same. An increasing range of suture materials with planned absorption times is becoming available.

Non-absorbable sutures remain in place for some years unless they are removed.

Braided sutures (where the strands are plaited together) and twisted sutures (where the separate strands are twisted round each other) are very flexible and therefore easy to handle and knot. The knots usually hold and are secure. The disadvantage of these types of suture is that fluid can seep between the strands (capillarity) and microorganisms can get into the interstices of the yarn, giving rise to long-term infections. Most braided sutures are proofed or coated in an attempt to prevent this.

Conversely, monofilament sutures consist of only one strand of material. They tend to be less flexible and more 'slippery'. They are therefore less easy to handle and knot, and the knots need more throws to be secure. The only nidus provided for infection is within the interstices of a knot.

Absorbable sutures

Absorbable sutures are used if no permanent support is required, especially if the knot as a foreign body could lead to complications.

1 Tying off small arteries and veins near the skin (knot could erode skin).

2 Stitches in the ureter, urinary tract, or biliary tract (where permanent sutures form a focus for stone formation).

Table 8 Absorbable sutures sorted by time until loss of 50% strength.

Trade name	Material	50% loss of strength (days)	Other features
Plain catgut	Sheep or cow intestine	3	Absorbed by tissue proteases
Chromic catgut	Sheep intestine soaked in chromic salts	5–7	Tanning delays breakdown and results in less tissue reaction
Monocryl (Ethicon)	Poliglecaprone 25	7	New development, monofilament
Vicryl (Ethicon)	Polyglaclin 910	14	Braided, good knotting properties, minimal tissue reaction, most commonly used
Dexon (Davis & Geck)	Polyglycolic acid	20	Braided, similar to Vicryl
PDS (Ethicon)	Polydioxanone	28	Monofilament, very little tissue reaction, absorbed by hydrolysis, beginning to replace nylon for closure of abdominal wounds
Maxon (Davis & Geck)	Polyglyconate	~ 35	Similar to PDS, monofilament

3 Closing off tissue spaces, e.g. subcutaneous space.

4 For closing the skin when it is an advantage not to have to remove the stitches (children, day surgery, scrotum).

5 In small bowel anastomosis or stomach mucosal anastomosis (non-absorbable sutures in the stomach can cause long-term ulceration).

The most common types of absorbable suture are listed in Table 8.

Table 9 Non-absorbable sutures.

Trade name	Material	Features
Ethilon (Ethicon)	Nylon	Monofilament, very slowly degraded (~15%/year), minimal scarring.
Dermalon (Davis & Geck)		
Surgilon (Davis & Geck)	Nylon	Braided, minimal tissue reaction
Neurilon (Ethicon)		
Silk	Silk	Braided or twisted, loses 80% strength in 80 days
Prolene (Ethicon)	Polypropylene	Monofilament, strong, most permanent suture, least tissue reaction
Mersilene (Ethicon)	Polyester fibre	Braided, particularly strong, well tolerated by tissues
Ethibond (Ethicon)	Polyester with polybutylate coating	As above, braided, slides better through tissues because of coating
Goretex (Gore & Assoc.)	Expanded PTFE	Strong, specially designed for knot security and used for vascular anastomoses
Steel	Stainless steel	Extremely strong, does fragment over period of years, used in orthopaedics and in cardiothoracic surgery for closure of sternum

Non-absorbable sutures

If the loss of strength of a suture might have severe consequences (as in vascular anastomoses, heart valve replacements, ligation of major vessels or closure of the abdominal wall), non-absorbable sutures are generally used. Non-absorbable material is also often used in tissues which heal slowly like tendons and ligaments. The materials commonly used are reviewed in Table 9.

Table 10 Sizes of synthetic sutures.

Size	Metric scale (mm × 10)	Diameter (mm)
4	6.0	0.6
3	5.5	0.55
2	5.0	0.5
1	4.0	0.4
0	3.5	0.35
2/0 (00)	3.0	0.3
3/0 (000)	2.0	0.2
4/0 (etc.)	1.5	0.15
5/0	1.0	0.1
6/0	0.75	0.075
7/0	0.5	0.05
8/0	0.4	0.04
9/0	0.3	0.03
10/0	0.2	0.02

Sizes of sutures

The size of the suture refers (non-linear) to the diameter and therefore to its strength. Examples of suture sizes for synthetic materials are given in Table 10. Natural collagen tends to be slightly larger. During the operation the choice of size depends on the necessary strength. To give a few examples:

1 Size 0 silk is used for tying off larger arteries.

2 Vicryl size 2/0 and 3/0 provides the standard ties for other vessels.

3 Skin is usually closed with 3/0 or 4/0 material down to 6/0 in plastic surgery.

4 Size 5/0 and 6/0 are fine sutures used in arterial surgery.

5 Size 10/0 is only just visible to the naked eye and is used in microvascular surgery and nerve repairs.

Suture removal

The time of suture removal depends on the site of the incision and the general state of the patient.

1 Head and neck. Wounds in the head and neck heal rapidly. A cosmetic result is also needed and therefore early suture removal is an advantage. Sutures in this area are generally removed within 3–5 days, e.g. thyroid scar 3 days, face scar 4 days.

2 Abdomen and thorax. Transverse or oblique incisions 5–7 days. Vertical incisions 7–10 days.

3 In patients who are cachectic, i.e. those with carcinomatosis, on steroid therapy, with severe infection, or with hepatic or renal failure, the tissue healing can be delayed and therefore the sutures must be left longer (10–14 days or longer).

Table 11 Needles.

Curved	Small—used with needle holders
Straight	Large—hand needles
Eyed	Suture material must be threaded through the eye
Atraumatic	The suture material is built into the end of the needle and the needle puncture therefore causes only a minimally larger hole than the suture itself
Round-bodied	The needle has a round shape and is only sharp at its tip. Used for suturing peritoneum, fat, bowel, liver, etc.
Taper-cut	The needle also has a round shape but is sharpened on several sides towards the tip, giving it cutting properties. This type of needle is useful for passage through tough tissues where it important to keep the needle track size to a minimum
With cutting edge	These are flattened and 'sword-like' and cut through the tissues as they are passed. They can be used on tough fibrous tissue (e.g. breast) or the skin, may cause haemorrhage by cutting neighbouring blood vessels
With blunt taperpoint	This type of needle was developed to reduce the risk of needle-stick injuries. It is used to suture the abdominal wall, but does not penetrate skin

Needles

Needles are either curved or straight; eyed or atraumatic; round-bodied, taper-cut or with a cutting edge (Table 11).

Drains

Drains are put in by the surgeon to allow any fluid or air collecting at the operation site or in the wound to drain to the surface while allowing the main wound to heal. Fluids to be drained include blood, pus, urine, faeces, bile or lymph. Drains are also used in interventional radiology to tap collections of these fluids.

Drains may be superficial (i.e. in the wound), or deep.

1 Intraperitoneal, e.g. next to an intestinal anastomosis
2 In a hollow organ or duct, e.g. a T-tube in the bile duct
3 In an abnormal channel, e.g. a fistula
4 To drain a deep cavity, e.g. an abscess or haematoma.

In addition drains are either open, i.e. draining into a dressing or bag open to the air, or closed, i.e. draining into a sterilized air-tight tube and container. The drainage system can be:

1 On free drainage, e.g. drainage of ascites by gravity
2 On suction, e.g. Redivac drains
3 Controlled by a one-way valve, e.g. an underwater seal or chest drains (see p. 253).

Types of drains and their uses

Open drains

Corrugated rubber drain (Fig. 23a). Rubber causes a tissue re-action and the drain track caused by this material persists longer than when inert materials are used. The drain is fixed by a suture at the end of the wound and a safety pin must be placed through the end to prevent the drain slipping inwards. Corrugated rubber drains can be used either for the wound or for deep drainage.

Yates' drain (Fig. 23b). This is a corrugated drain made of a series of capillary tubes joined side to side. It is generally made of polyethylene which is less reactive than rubber. The drain site therefore tends to close more quickly once the drain has been removed. Its uses are similar to corrugated rubber drains and it is secured as described above.

Closed drains

Redivac drain (Fig. 23c). This is a fine tube, with many holes at the end, which is attached to an evacuated glass bottle pro-viding continuous suction. It is used to drain blood beneath the skin, e.g. after mastectomy or thyroidectomy, or from deep spaces, e.g. around a vascular anastomosis.

'Shirley' wound drainage or sump drain. This is a suction drain with an intake tube supplying air to the bottom of the main tube. This allows continuous suction and the flow of air prevents the tube getting blocked.

Silastic tube drain. Silastic is a polymeric silicone and incites little tissue inflammation. Therefore, once this type of drain is

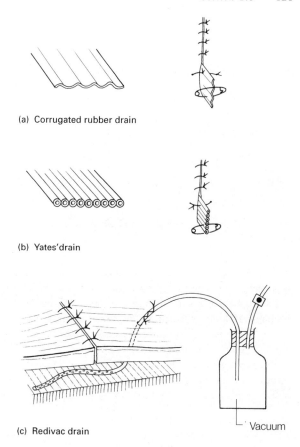

(a) Corrugated rubber drain

(b) Yates'drain

(c) Redivac drain

Vacuum

Fig. 23 Various types of wound drain.

removed the track closes rapidly. A Silastic tube drain can be used to provide closed drainage to deep anastomoses, e.g. of the bowel (Fig. 24).

Red rubber tube drain. This causes an intense tissue reaction and fibrosis. The track will therefore persist for some time after the drain is removed. This feature can be useful for drainage of chronic abscess cavities such as an empyema or hepatic abscess.

T-tube drains. After bile duct surgery a T-tube is inserted in the bile duct, which allows bile to drain while the sphincter of Oddi is in spasm (Fig. 25). Once this relaxes the bile can drain normally down the common bile duct into the duodenum. T-tubes are made of a variety of materials and surgeons vary in the design they prefer.

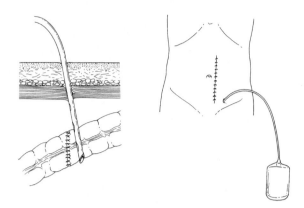

Fig. 24 Deep closed drainage of a colonic anastomosis.

Removal of drains

A drain is removed as soon as it is no longer required. Hence it is necessary to know the purpose for which it was inserted and you should ascertain this from the surgeon at the time of operation. If fluid is still draining the drain is serving a purpose. Check the drainage chart and consider carefully before removing it. The following are general guidelines:

1 Drains put in to cover perioperative bleeding and haematoma formation, can come out after 24–48 h.

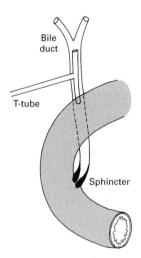

Fig. 25 A T-tube allows bile to drain if the sphincter of Oddi is in spasm.

2 Drains put in to cover serous collections can come out after 3–5 days.

3 Where a drain has been put in because the wound may later become infected, it should be left for 1–5 days.

4 Drains put in to cover intestinal anastomoses should not be removed until after 5–7 days.

5 A T-tube can be removed after 6–10 days. Before this is done, a T-tube cholangiogram must be performed to make sure that there is distal patency in the common bile duct (see p. 335). Some surgeons clamp the T-tube for 24 h before it is removed

6 Chest drains — see management of thoracotomy (p. 257).

2.4 Relatives, Discharges, Deaths and Documents

Dealing with relatives

It is an important part of the houseman's job to answer enquiries from relatives as to the nature of the disease, the type of operation that is intended and the prognosis. The relatives will view any operation as a very major undertaking and will often be dreading the outcome. Keeping them informed is not just a humanitarian exercise. If the relatives are happy about a patient's management, they will pass on this confidence to the patient and this can be a great help to you as his doctor. Also, most compensation claims have their basis in a lack of communication and mutual understanding. It is worthwhile setting aside two periods a week when you will be available on the ward for any relatives to come and see you. Tell the nursing staff when these will be.

The personal touch

It is better if only one person deals with the relatives. Otherwise misunderstandings may arise. This is occasionally difficult to achieve where a system of cross-cover is operated and the on-call houseman looks after patients on other wards as well.

Continuity is important because only you know what you have already told the relatives. If you know that they are visiting one evening, stay on the ward until you have seen them. This often takes less time than repairing the damage caused by an interview with someone who does not know the case.

If you are asked to see the relatives of a patient on another ward about whom you know nothing, start by asking them what they have been told so far and apologise that the doctor they normally see is not available. Before the interview look at the notes, not only to find out about the case, but also to see if any record has been made of previous conversations.

Documentation

After you have spoken to a patient about a diagnosis that may cause concern, or spoken to a patient's relatives, write down what you have told them in the notes and comment on any difficulty or reaction from those listening. For example, 'Mother told that her son has a malignant growth on the leg. Very upset. Has requested that the son should not be told. She is coming

124

tomorrow with husband and would like to be seen again. Would also like an appointment with the consultant in the next clinic.' Tell the senior members of your surgical unit about the interview.

Patient discharge

When discharging a patient you must give them instructions on the following:

1 Stitches. When and how stitches are to be removed if this has not been done already.

2 Activity. How active he can be in the postoperative period and when he may go back to work. This depends on the nature of his job. Guidance on this topic is given in the 'codes' for individual operations later in this book.

3 Drugs. The patient should usually be given the drugs which he was on when he came into hospital together with any others which may be necessary as part of his present treatment. He should be told clearly how long he needs to take these. His GP must be informed of the therapy as soon as the patient is discharged from hospital. This is best done by giving him a note to take home.

4 Follow-up. When is the patient to be seen again?

Discharge summary

A summary of the patient's admission should be completed as soon as possible after the time of discharge and sent to the patient's GP. This can be produced from data entered into a computer and sent by fax. A copy is filed in the notes. The letter should carry a printed legible name and contact telephone number and should include concise relevant information under the following headings:

1 Patient details (name, registry number, GP, address, date of birth).

2 Admission details (ward, date, emergency/elective, consultant, etc.).

3 Diagnoses.

4 Reason for admission.

5 Investigations (summary of inpatient results).

6 Operation details (very brief).

7 Non-operative treatment.

8 Postoperative details (problems, complications).

9 Information given to patient/relatives — very important, especially if the prognosis is grave.

10 Method of discharge (home, transferred, died, etc.).

11 Drugs and other discharge treatment.

12 Follow-up arrangements — does the patient know when they will be seen, or how they can find out?

13 Other comments.

Dealing with death

The houseman often has the task of telling relatives that a patient is going to die or has died. He is also responsible for the care of these terminally ill patients. This is a delicate job and each individual doctor will develop his own methods. Below are written some ideas, aimed to help you formulate your own approach.

Informing the relatives that a patient is going to die

The relatives will need to be told if the patient is likely to die. This is best done by taking them into a quiet room and explaining that nothing further can be done usefully to prolong life. Arrange not to be disturbed.

It is often best to start by asking the relatives what they feel is going to happen. Using this as a guide, the patient's situation must be explained honestly, clearly and slowly. Generally it is important to be absolutely truthful. There are very few situations, if any, where hiding the truth from the relatives is the more appropriate course of action. Try to be positive, rather than negative, emphasizing what you can still do to help the patient. Often the one comfort that you can give is to say that their relative will be given sufficient analgesia to stay free of pain. Point out what the relatives can do themselves to help the patient through this inevitable period of life, i.e. to remain cheerful and positive rather than to show sadness.

A situation has become increasingly common where there are the means to keep a patient 'alive' although this would clearly be inappropriate (i.e. in cases of brain death). This may be difficult to explain to relatives. You may have to explain the hopelessness of the situation and the loss of dignity that keeping a patient 'alive' with brain death entails. Usually the relatives will understand and agree that the right thing to do is what is suggested. When the relatives remain worried and further guidance is needed, arrange for them to see your consultant. In this situation he is likely to wish to see them anyway.

Care of the terminally ill patient

A terminally ill patient also needs to know what is going on.

Choose a time to talk privately. Again it is better to be totally honest in what you say, although in this case there are a few situations where hiding the truth is more appropriate. Patients are not always ready to face the prospect of death and may have to be brought gently round to this over several interviews. A few patients make it clear that they never wish to discuss the possibility of death and you must be sensitive to this and respect their wishes.

Once the patient has accepted that death is imminent, they will often ask, 'How long do I have, doctor?' It is best to be truthful and tell them that you do not know. If they persist, talk in terms of 'a matter of days, weeks or months' as seems appropriate. You will usually be wrong.

The everyday care of a dying patient is a nursing speciality, requiring great sensitivity and skill. The houseman must make certain that the pain relief is adequate. Added sedation at night is often necessary. Otherwise the purpose of treatment is the control of symptoms with the minimum of discomfort. The patient should still be seen regularly, especially when he or she is dying. Most patients know the situation and take a lack of visits by the houseman as evidence that they have been forgotten and are already regarded as deceased.

Confirming death

A doctor is required to verify death. The four signs to confirm are as follows.
1 No pulse
2 No heart sounds
3 No breath sounds
4 Pupils fixed and dilated.

Sufficient time must be spent listening for heart and breath sounds to confidently exclude a very slow cardiac rate or intermittent breathing. Be particularly careful if the patient has taken an overdose or has been on sedative drugs.

If you are uncertain (e.g. in an obese patient in a deep coma, in whom you might not be able to feel the pulse or hear the heart sounds anyway), do the following:
1 Look in the optic fundi — the blood in the retinal veins becomes separated when circulation stops.
2 Perform an electrocardiogram (ECG) or an electroencephalogram (EEG).

As you leave the patient and are approached by the relatives, you must be absolutely certain whether or not death has occurred.

Informing the relatives of a patient who has died

The death may be expected or unexpected. Telling relatives about an expected death is usually straightforward. Giving information about an unexpected death often results in great distress and is a difficult situation to handle.

Again privacy is important when talking to the relatives. Leave your bleep outside and ask not to be disturbed. Speak clearly, slowly and truthfully and usually the best line to take is to tell them of the death early and then talk a little about the reasons of why and how it happened. Offer comfort where possible, saying, for example, that the patient died peacefully and was not in pain. Relatives will usually demand to know why the death has occurred and ask, 'What has gone wrong?'. Try not to be defensive about the care the patient has received and make the seriousness of the patient's illness clear. Emphasize that prolonged suffering has been avoided if this is the case. After that it is useful to sit briefly in silence allowing the relatives to take it all in. Where appropriate, physical contact like grasping a hand does more good than 10 minutes of talking.

It is a help to ask a senior nurse to come in and arrange for refreshments to be brought. However, much the surgical team may have done for the patient, at that moment the relative sees you as the conveyor of bad news, and there may come a point when it is best to leave the relative in the company of a nurse who can sit, talk quietly and comfort them.

The postmortem

Postmortems are performed for two reasons. Firstly, all cases referred to the coroner undergo a postmortem unless he is fully satisfied about the cause of death. This is done as a routine and is a legal requirement.

Secondly, postmortems are performed to obtain information about a death, information which may be of value in treating other patients later. An autopsy should ideally be performed on all patients dying in hospital. Such a postmortem is requested by the consultant responsible for the case and requires the permission of the relatives. You may have to obtain this. It is best to tell the relatives that postmortems are usually done on patients who die in hospital and ask for their permission, pointing out that the information obtained will benefit other patients. Most relatives understand the need but they do not wish to discuss details at a time of great distress. They also wish to be reassured that the funeral arrangements will not be delayed.

The housesurgeon must then send the case notes, any relevant investigations, the form of consent and usually another form with a brief synopsis of the patient's history and progress while in hospital, down to the postmortem room. It is worthwhile finding out when the postmortem is to be held so that you can attend. Often you are the only member of the surgical team who is able to do so.

Death certificates, the coroner and cremation forms

Death certificates

When one of your patients dies, you are legally required to fill in a death certificate and send this to the Registrar of Births and Deaths. The information is used to prepare national statistics about causes of death.

You can only fill in the death certificate if you attended the deceased before death. If you see the body for the first time after death you are not qualified to sign the certificate. It cannot be signed by someone else on your behalf either. Any medical practitioner who signs a death certificate must be registered. Provisional registration entitles a housesurgeon to sign death certificates only in cases arising out of his duties in an approved hospital while working for a fully registered practitioner.

Ideally a certificate should be issued for all deaths, even those that are also being referred to the coroner. In this case Box A on the back of the certificate must be initialled informing the registrar that he must wait for the coroner's decision before allowing the body to be buried or cremated.

In addition, a separate form must be signed and given to the informant saying that the death certificate has been issued. The informant, usually a relative of the deceased (other persons entitled to perform this role are listed on the back of the death certificate), is legally required to take the death certificate sealed in an envelope to the registrar within 5 days (8 days in Scotland). The informant will also be required to state certain particulars relating to the deceased's life. A counterfoil is filled in to be kept by the hospital.

The death certificate starts by stating the patient's particulars. There then follows a section where the housesurgeon is required to state whether he saw the body after death. This is not a legal requirement, although it is a sensible thing to do in order to avoid cases of mistaken identity.

Statement of cause of death

This is in two parts.

Part 1

Part 1 records the sequence of conditions and diseases that led to the patient's death. This is written in sequential order, starting with the condition that actually caused death, and going on to the underlying disease. This sequence must be causally linked. Each condition entered at the top of the list should occur as a consequence of the condition written immediately below it, eventually ending up with the underlying cause.

For example, a patient with chronic peptic ulceration who dies of peritonitis a few days after an operation for perforation of a duodenal ulcer would be entered as follows:

1 Peritonitis, due to
2 Perforation of duodenal ulcer [operation and date], due to
3 Peptic ulcer of the duodenum.

The terms used must be precise. Words like 'pulmonary oedema' or 'coma' are not accurate enough. Words like 'cirrhosis' imply alcohol toxicity and, whether or not this is true, the registrar will refer the case to the coroner. If the condition was infectious, the site, causal organism and duration of infection must be stated. If a tumour occurs in the list, state the histology and whether it was malignant or benign, the anatomical site, and whether it was primary or secondary. If it was a secondary tumour, indicate the site of the primary and whether this had been removed or not.

Part 2

Part 2 records other conditions that may have contributed to the death, but are not related to the causal sequence of disease described in part 1. For example, the above patient's form might be completed with 'Part 2: Chronic bronchitis'.

Other examples are available for guidance in the book of death certificates. There is also a list of unacceptable terms.

On the back of the death certificate there are two boxes. Box A has already been described. Box B is a box that must be initialled by the practitioner if he is still awaiting results of laboratory tests which may aid the diagnosis that he has put on the certificate.

It is most important that this death certificate is filled in legibly and correctly. Otherwise it will be rejected by the registrar and delay the arrangements for burial or cremation. There is no significant variation in the form of death certificate in Scotland, Wales or Northern Ireland.

If you feel that the patient's death is unexplained, you cannot sign the death certificate and the case must be referred to the coroner.

Referral to the coroner

The role of the coroner is to investigate death. He does this in order to ensure that the cause of death was natural and to identify deaths where further enquiry is necessary. Such deaths include those where a crime may have been committed, where there is an accusation of negligence on behalf of the police authorities or medical profession, or where claims for compensation might follow. All the facts necessary to answer any such enquiry must be available before the disposal of the body.

Cases that need reporting

Below is a list of circumstances where a death should be reported to the coroner. The Registrar of Births and Deaths is under a statutory obligation to report such cases. Medical practitioners, however, are not, although in practice it saves time and establishes a close working relationship between the medical profession and the coroner's office if they do so. It is also the duty in common law of anyone to report such cases, although this is not enforceable. Circumstances in which a death should be reported to the coroner are:

1 Where the cause of death is unknown.

2 Where no doctor has treated the deceased in their terminal illness, or where the deceased's medical practitioner did not attend the patient within 14 days of death.

3 Where death is associated with medical treatment, e.g. deaths occurring during an operation or during recovery from a general anaesthetic. Generally, any death occurring in the 24 h after an anaesthetic is reportable, although there is some variation with different coroners. Also, cases where any form of medical treatment, including drug therapy, has contributed to a patient's death should be reported.

4 Sudden, unexplained or suspicious death. This includes death occurring within 24 h of emergency admission to hospital.

5 Death from industrial accident or disease, road traffic accidents, domestic accidents (e.g. death following a fall causing fractured neck of femur), deaths from violence or neglect, death following abortion, death from poisoning (including alcohol), and cases of suicide.

6 Any case where, following death, there is a definite or suspected claim for negligence either against the doctors or nursing

staff. In such a case medical practitioners must not only inform the coroner but also inform their defence union immediately and give no verbal or written statement to the injured party until this is done.

7 Death while a patient was in legal custody. For instance, you might be involved in treating a case which has been brought in from police custody, having been found unconscious.

In cases where you are uncertain whether or not you ought to report the case to the coroner, always telephone him or his officer and discuss it. After hearing your story he may well give permission for you to write a death certificate.

The coroner has three courses of action in dealing with the case. Firstly, he may, after considering the facts, be satisfied that the cause of death was natural and no postmortem is required. He will then allow a death certificate to be issued.

Secondly, he may require that a postmortem be carried out, usually by a coroner's pathologist. If the result shows that the death was from natural causes then there is no need for an inquest and the death certificate can be issued.

Thirdly, he may feel, following a postmortem, that an inquest should be held. This includes all criminal cases, suicides, death from accidents or industrial mishap, deaths in custody and deaths where claims of negligence have been put forward. In cases where negligence is claimed against a medical practitioner, he must be legally represented by his defence society.

The system in Scotland and Northern Ireland is broadly similar, although in Scotland the role of the coroner is performed by the procurator-fiscal.

Cremation forms

Once the registrar has received the death certificate and approved it and providing that no further evidence is required from the body, he authorizes its disposal and issues a certificate for this. This may be by either burial or cremation. Cremation is under very strict control. This ensures that medicolegal evidence is not destroyed and that cremation is not performed against the wishes of the relatives or of the deceased.

The cremation form is in two parts, each signed by a separate doctor. These doctors must not be related and should not be partners of the same practice. In hospital the two doctors should not belong to the same 'firm'.

The first part (form B) is usually signed by the doctor who issued the death certificate. In this case the doctor is legally required to examine the body after death and give details of the mode of dying, in addition to the clinical diagnosis and cause of death. It also asks if the patient has a cardiac pacemaker or radioactive implants. If these are present they must be removed before cremation.

The second part (form C) is signed by a doctor who must have been fully registered for at least 5 years. He must not be related to the deceased. He must also see the body after death and question the doctor signing form B.

The purpose of this procedure is that both doctors must certify the cause of death, confirm that it is natural, and agree that further examination or enquiry is unnecessary.

Other medical certificates and legal statements

A doctor may be required to provide statements on a patient's health for insurance companies, for employment or to be used as evidence by the police. In the latter case, housesurgeons must discuss the case with their consultant, who is ultimately responsible for that patient. In casualty, statements are commonly required on victims of assault and the house officers are often the only people who have seen and treated the patient concerned. In this case they must write the report themselves. Any such statement should be factual and truthful. Keep to the medical facts and avoid laying the blame on anyone. Try to include measurements and figures where possible when describing injuries. In cases of difficulty the doctor's defence union will be able to advise.

Surgical audit

Carrying out a regular audit of medical activity is now a requirement for all units in the UK. You will be partly responsible for collecting data for this.

The data required for audit are virtually identical to the information provided in the discharge letter and will include details of the following:

1 Patient: address, GP, date of birth, sex, etc.

2 Admission: emergency/elective, consultant, ward, source, etc.

3 Diagnosis: find out who is supposed to choose diagnoses and what system of verification (if any) is in use.

4 Operation: enough details are required to allow this to be coded for later analysis.

5 Complications: record anything which has been a problem during admission.

These data will subsequently be used for presentation at

regular audit meetings when the total workload and any problems arising from it will be reviewed and discussed. You can make this process considerably easier by making sure accurate and relevant data are recorded during the patient's admission. Trying to ascertain facts after the patient has left the hospital is much more time-consuming.

Find out what system is in use on your unit. Keep up with the work by clearing notes each day. A huge pile of notes awaiting processing after patient discharge can become a depressing burden.

Coding

In order to allow accurate analysis the diagnosis, operation and often the complications will need to be coded. This is the doctor's responsibility. It is more and more done using computers and is based on agreed lists of diagnoses such as the International Classification of Diseases (Revision 10) (ICD-10) or the READ code. Be accurate in coding as this information will be used for analyses and research by some of your colleagues for many years ahead. When in doubt about what diagnosis to choose ask your registrar or consultant.

3 Head and Neck Surgery

3.1 Lumps in the Head and Neck

An important early step in the diagnosis of lumps in the head and neck is to decide whether the lump is in the skin or deep to the skin.

Lumps in the skin include those peculiar to this area, such as cervical auricle (see below), and others common anywhere in the skin such as sebaceous cysts, dermoids, lipomas, fibromas, basal cell carcinomas and squamous cell carcinomas. The latter are dealt with in section 13.

If the lump is deep to the skin you will have to decide in which anatomical region it belongs and particularly whether it is behind, beneath or in front of the sternomastoid muscle. The important anatomical regions are the parotid, the submandibular, the pretracheal area, and the anterior and posterior triangles of the neck (see Fig. 26). Lumps in these regions are dealt with on the following pages:

1 Cervical auricle
2 Lumps in the parotid region (pp. 138–142)
3 Lumps in the submandibular region (pp. 142–145)

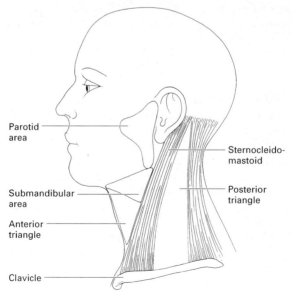

Parotid area

Sternocleido-mastoid

Submandibular area

Posterior triangle

Anterior triangle

Clavicle

Fig. 26 Some important anatomical areas in the head and neck.

4 Lumps in the anterior triangle
  (a) branchial sinus (p. 145)
  (b) branchial cyst (p. 146)
  (c) carotid body tumour (p. 148)
  (d) pharyngeal pouch (p. 149)
5 Lumps in the posterior triangle
  (a) cervical rib (p. 151)
6 Pretracheal area
  (a) thyroid (section 4.1, p. 181)
  (b) parathyroid (section 4.2, p. 198)
7 All areas
  (a) cervical lymphadenopathy (p. 153)
  (b) malignant lymphoma (p. 155)
  (c) cystic hygroma (p. 157).

Cervical auricle

This is an accessory ear lobe and is situated low in the neck anterior to the sternomastoid. It consists of a cartilaginous skeleton covered with skin, and is easy to diagnose providing the clinician is familiar with it.

Treatment is by cosmetic removal.

Lumps in the parotid region

You must be familiar with the normal extent of the parotid gland (see Fig. 26). If the swelling is in this area and deep to the skin, then it is in the parotid gland until proved otherwise. Swellings of the parotid are of two kinds.
1 Generalized, involving the whole gland
2 Localized, i.e. lumps within the gland.

Generalized enlargement of the parotid

The parotid is enlarged secondary to either inflammatory disease or obstruction of the main parotid duct.

Viral parotitis — mumps

This disease is common in children and causes bilateral parotid swelling. Occasionally it may affect only one side. The parotid duct opening looks inflamed, but there is no pus. There is usually a history of contact with the disease about 3 weeks previously. Check whether the patient has had mumps in the past as second attacks are very rare. The virus may also cause orchitis and pancreatitis. In doubtful cases, two mumps virus antibody titres taken 1 week apart may be helpful. No specific treatment is required and the swelling usually resolves over 7–10 days.

Bacterial parotitis

Acute bacterial parotitis used to be common in surgical wards. The condition is usually secondary to obstruction of the duct by viscid secretions. Embolization during septicaemia has also been implicated. The condition is now much rarer but may be seen occasionally. The usual organisms are *Staphylococcus*, *Streptococcus* or *Pneumococcus*.

Recognizing the pattern

It occurs in dehydrated patients postoperatively, particularly in the elderly. The history is of a dull throbbing pain and swelling on the side of the face. The pain is worse on speaking or eating. Examination of the inside of the mouth may show pus extruding from the opening of the parotid duct. The whole gland becomes acutely inflamed and very tender and the patient looks toxic and ill.

Management

A pus swab is taken for culture and antibiotic sensitivity. The treatment is with antibiotics (ampicillin and flucloxacillin). The patient must be adequately rehydrated, and the mouth kept clean. Occasionally an abscess forms and may require drainage.

Autoimmune parotitis

Autoimmune disease usually affects both the other salivary glands and the lachrymal glands, causing symmetrical, painless progressive enlargement. Mikulicz's disease is enlargement of the salivary glands and lachrymal glands associated with a dry mouth. Sjögren's disease is similar but the syndrome also includes dry eyes and arthritis. The diagnosis and management of these conditions are beyond the scope of this book.

Obstruction of the parotid duct

Obstruction of the parotid duct due to stones is unusual as the parotid secretion is watery and the duct is wide. It is more often due to stenosis of the opening of the parotid duct. This may occur due to trauma of the inside of the cheek secondary to ill-fitting dentures. Often the duct has an irregular pattern similar to bronchiectasis, described as sialectasis. This results in sludging of secretions and obstruction, with secondary infection.

Recognizing the pattern

The patient is usually adult and complains of painful swelling of the parotid gland during meals. Inspection of the opening of the duct opposite the second upper molar tooth may reveal the stenosis.

Proving the diagnosis
A sialogram may be helpful in excluding the presence of stones and may also show 'sialectasis'. This is dilatation of the ducts within the gland due to chronic obstruction and previous inflammatory episodes.

Management

This is usually conservative and the patient is taught to 'milk' the duct contents forward by massaging the cheek and thus preventing stasis in the duct. If the stenosis is severe, it may be dilated using lachrymal duct dilators under a local anaesthetic. Antibiotics are given if infection is present.

Localized lumps in the parotid

Sixty per cent of parotid lumps eventually prove to be benign mixed tumours (pleomorphic adenomas, see below).

An adenolymphoma (also called Warthin's tumour) is benign but may be bilateral or multiple. This tumour accounts for 10% of parotid neoplasms. The tumour is soft and may feel cystic.

Other tumours are less common and include the mucoepidermoid tumour and acinic cell tumour. Both of these are usually benign but may recur locally and occasionally undergo malignant change.

The adenoid cystic carcinoma (cylindroma) is a malignant lesion and has a tendency to spread along nerve sheaths.

Carcinoma of the parotid is a highly malignant lesion which may arise from a mixed cell tumour. By the time it presents there may already be extensive local infiltration with or without nerve paralysis.

The most common non-neoplastic solitary nodule is a cyst.

Mixed tumours of the parotid

Mixed tumours are so called because they contain adenoma cells surrounded by pools of mucin, which look like cartilage on histological sections. These tumours are benign but have an incomplete capsule and consequently have a high rate of local recurrence if incompletely removed. There is also a risk of malignant change in the long term. Because of these factors it is very important to excise the tumour by performing a formal parotidectomy.

Recognizing the pattern

The history is of a slowly growing painless swelling on the side of the face. The patient may be of any age beyond the teens. There is a firm, smooth lump in the parotid area, usually in the lower anterior part of the gland just above the angle of the jaw. This may appear to be quite superficial, but careful examination will show that the skin moves over it. Establish that the lump is indeed in the parotid gland and not attached deeply to bone or muscle. Look for extensions inside the mouth or pharynx, and check whether the facial nerve is involved by observing facial movements. Look for involved lymph nodes on both sides of the neck. If any of these are found the lesion may be malignant.

Proving the diagnosis

The diagnosis is proved by fine-needle aspiration cytology.

Deep lobe involvement and spread to the parapharyngeal space can be assessed by computed tomography (CT) or magnetic resonance imaging (MRI) scanning.

Management

A suspected mixed tumour of the parotid should be removed by superficial parotidectomy.

Preoperative management

The patient should be warned of the slight possibility of a facial weakness postoperatively, although this is usually transient. Loss of sensation in the distribution of the greater auricular nerve (ear-lobe region) should be discussed. A nerve stimulator may be required during the operation and theatre should be informed of this.

OPERATION: SUPERFICIAL PAROTIDECTOMY

An incision is made anterior to the ear, extending as an S-shaped curve into the upper neck. The facial nerve trunk is firstly identified and its branches are then traced forwards in the parotid gland and all tissue superficial to them excised together with the tumour. If the tumour is deep to the facial nerve it can be excised by displacing the nerve branches. The wound is usually drained using a suction drain.

Codes

Blood 0

GA/LA ....GA

Opn time ....2–3 h

Stay ....3–5 days

Drains out ....24–48 h

Sutures out ....3–5 days

Off work ....2–3 weeks

Postoperative care

Check and record the movements of the facial muscles supplied by each individual branch of the facial nerve, i.e. temporal, orbital, buccal, mandibular and cervical. If there is any weakness, note whether it is partial (in which case full recovery is likely). If it is complete, recovery is also likely unless a nerve is known to have been divided at operation. Recovery takes 6–8 weeks.

The clips or sutures are removed, leaving those in any unhealed area until the last. If the tumour is malignant, radiotherapy will probably be given. Occasionally radiotherapy is also given to mixed tumours of the parotid, particularly if the surgery is being done for recurrent disease. With mixed tumours of the parotid, regular follow-up is advisable.

Management of other parotid lumps

Because of the possibility of neoplasia, these lumps will usually be excised to establish an exact diagnosis. However, fine-needle aspiration cytology should be performed prior to any form of open biopsy. If the lump is obviously malignant then biopsy and radiotherapy may be the only possible treatment. For lesions of unknown aetiology, however, biopsy alone is not advisable as it may result in local implantation of a neoplasm. Most lesions of the parotid are therefore removed by superficial parotidectomy.

Lumps in the submandibular region

The submandibular salivary gland measures about 4–3 cm and is situated beneath the angle of the jaw. Its superficial portion is in the neck outside the mylohyoid muscle and its deep portion lies in the floor of the mouth deep to the mylohyoid. Its duct drains from the deep part of the gland forwards to the floor of the mouth beneath the tip of the tongue (Fig. 27).

As in the parotid, enlargements are either generalized or localized.

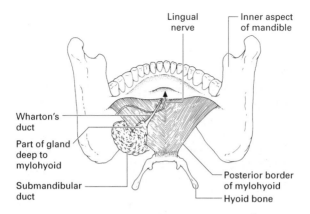

Fig. 27 The anatomy of the submandibular gland. The floor of the mouth viewed posteriorly (tongue removed).

Generalized enlargement of the gland is commonly secondary to stone formation. It also occurs in autoimmune syndromes (as in the parotid gland).

Localized enlargements are of the same aetiology as those already described for the parotid gland (p. 140), although a greater proportion are malignant.

Submandibular stones

The secretion of this gland is more viscous than that of the parotid and the duct is narrower, so stone formation and obstruction are relatively common. Secondary infection (usually with *Staphylococcus*, *Streptococcus* or *Pneumococcus*) is dangerous because of the risk of swelling and oedema in the floor of the mouth and consequent respiratory obstruction (Ludwig's angina).

Recognizing the pattern

The condition can occur at any age and is common in young adults. The history is of intermittent painful swelling beneath the jaw occurring with meals. The patient may also have noticed 'gravel' in the mouth. The gland is palpable and tender during these episodes. A stone may be palpable in the duct in the floor of the mouth beneath the tongue.

Proving the diagnosis

Most stones are radio-opaque and may be seen on a plain X-ray of the floor of the mouth. A submandibular duct sialogram will also confirm the presence of the stone, and detect any sialectasis within the gland (p. 139). The stone may be palpable.

Management

In a few patients the stone will pass spontaneously. If it has been giving symptoms for 3 or 4 weeks, it can be removed from the duct using a local anaesthetic. Where the condition has become chronic, where stones are recurrent, or where the stone is situated in the gland itself, removal of the submandibular gland is preferable.

OPERATION: REMOVAL OF STONE FROM SUBMANDIBULAR DUCT

Local anaesthetic is infiltrated in the floor of the mouth and a silk suture is passed around the duct proximal to the stone. This prevents the stone slipping back into the main gland. The buccal mucosa and the duct are incised over the stone and the stone removed. The wound in the floor of the mouth is not sutured.

Codes

Blood	0
GA/LA	LA (GA if the stone is small and will be difficult to find)
Opn time	30 min
Stay	Day case
Drains out	0
Sutures out	0
Off work	1 day

Postoperative care

Mouthwashes should be given.

OPERATION: REMOVAL OF SUBMANDIBULAR GLAND

Preoperative management

No special preparation is necessary. Warn the patient of possible transient weakness of the corner of the mouth (see below). A nerve stimulator can be useful at operation but it is not essential.

Operation.   An incision is made 2.5 cm below the angle of the jaw over the gland. The mandibular branch of the facial nerve curves up over the jaw at this point, lying on the facial artery. It can be damaged if the incision is too high. It can also be damaged by retraction. This damage results in weakness of the corner of the mouth and care should be taken to avoid this.

When the deep portion of the gland is removed, care is taken not to damage the lingual or hypoglossal nerves which lie deep to it. The wound is usually drained.

Codes

Blood	0
GA/LA	GA or LA
Opn time	1–2 h
Stay	48 h
Drains out	About 48 h
Sutures out	3–4 days
Off work	About 1 week

Lumps in the anterior triangle of the neck

These include the following:

1 Branchial sinus
2 Branchial cyst
3 Carotid body tumour
4 Pharyngeal pouch.

Branchial sinus

During fetal life the second arch skin grows over the branchial clefts closing them off: if this closure is incomplete a fistula, sinus or cyst may result along the tract. A branchial sinus usually opens as a tiny hole in the lower part of the neck. Although the external opening may seem very small there is frequently a track running up the neck, which may go as high as the posterior pillar of the fauces in the pharynx (forming a fistula).

Recognizing the pattern

The patient is almost always a child, often in the first year of life. The sinus has usually been present from birth and the mother notices the discharge. On examination the opening is situated in front of the anterior border of the sternomastoid, one-third of the way up from the origin of the muscle. It discharges glairy fluid intermittently.

Proving the diagnosis

The above history and signs are quite characteristic and no further investigation is necessary.

Management

The treatment is surgical removal of the whole sinus or fistula. The operation is best performed early in life before the child's neck grows. In a baby it is often possible to excise even a long tract through one incision. The optimum time for operation is between the ages of 6 months and a year.

PREOPERATIVE MANAGEMENT

With an older child the mother should be warned that more than one incision may be necessary to remove the whole tract. She will be surprised to hear this as the external lesion looks so insignificant.

OPERATION: REMOVAL OF BRANCHIAL
FISTULA/SINUS

The external opening is mobilized with an ellipse of skin. The tract is followed up in the neck using a lachrymal probe in its lumen as a guide. Some surgeons use methylene blue to outline the tract. The tract is dissected out as high as possible and then, if necessary, a second transverse incision is made, usually at about the level of the hyoid bone. The tract is then followed up between the internal and external carotid arteries, until it reaches the pharyngeal epithelium. Frequently it peters out before this. The wound is usually drained.

Codes

Blood	Group and save serum
GA/LA	GA
Opn time	30–90 min depending on extent
Stay	24–48 h
Drains out	24 h
Sutures out	3–5 days

Branchial cyst

A branchial cyst (Fig. 28) is thought to be formed by squamous cell inclusions within cervical lymph nodes, or less frequently from an isolated remnant of a branchial cleft in the neck. Its

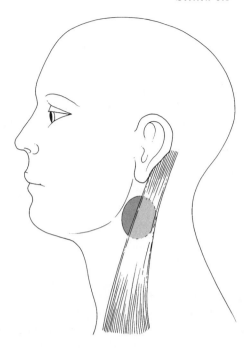

Fig. 28 A branchial cyst.

wall contains lymphoid tissue and it may become inflamed in any generalized lymphadenopathy in the neck. Not infrequently the cyst contents become purulent and it may present as a cervical abscess.

Recognizing the pattern
The cyst usually makes its appearance in childhood or early adult life. It frequently appears as a swelling during an upper respiratory tract infection. It may be painful. The swelling persists once the infection has subsided. Abscess formation causes severe pain, which is worse on moving the head. On examination it is usually about 5–10 cm in diameter and lies deep to the sternomastoid muscle, appearing beneath its anterior border. It is frequently related to the upper third of this muscle behind the angle of the jaw (see Fig. 28). It fluctuates, but does not transilluminate as its contents are opaque.

Proving the diagnosis
The diagnosis is made on the history and the site of the swelling and no other tests are necessary. Fine-needle cytology can be helpful.

Management

OPERATION: REMOVAL OF BRANCHIAL CYST

A transverse incision is made over the lump and deepened until the cyst is encountered. It is then excised. Care is taken to avoid damage to the carotid vessels, internal jugular vein and hypoglossal nerve which usually lie deep to the swelling.

Codes

Blood 0
GA/LA .... GA
Opn time .... 30–60 min
Stay .... 24 h
Drains out .... 24 h
Sutures out .... 3–5 days
Off work .... 3–7 days

Carotid body tumour

This tumour is a chemodectoma arising from the cells in the carotid body. It grows very slowly over many years. Histologically it is a non-chromaffin paraganglionoma.

Recognizing the pattern

The patient is usually aged over 50, although the condition can present earlier. He may notice the lump himself or it may be found at a routine medical examination. The lump is hard and transmits pulsation rather than being pulsatile itself. It is situated at the carotid bifurcation and appears as a tumour beneath the anterior border of the sternomastoid. It is mobile from side to side but not up and down.

Proving the diagnosis

MRI and a carotid angiogram may be helpful both in defining the extent of the tumour and in establishing that there is an adequate collateral through the opposite carotid artery.

Management

The tumour is usually removed. It can, however, be safely watched for many years and this course may be preferable in the elderly, frail patient.

PREOPERATIVE MANAGEMENT

Some surgeons may require the use of a carotid shunt (see p. 547).

OPERATION: REMOVAL OF CAROTID BODY
TUMOUR

A vertical incision anterior to the sternomastoid is usually
employed. The lesion is carefully dissected from the carotid
artery. (this can be a very haemorrhagic procedure). Alternatively, it can be excised and a graft placed between the
common and internal carotid arteries. A suction drain is
used. The wound is closed with clips or sutures.

Codes

Blood .... 4 units
GA/LA .... GA
Opn time .... 3–4 h
Stay .... 5–7 days
Drains out .... 24–48 h
Sutures out .... 5 days
Off work .... 3–4 weeks

Postoperative care

See carotid artery surgery (p. 547). The blood pressure should
be monitored regularly and may tend to fall lower than
preoperatively. This should be maintained by transfusing
blood as necessary.

Pharyngeal pouch

A pharyngeal pouch is a pulsion diverticulum of the pharyngeal
mucosa, probably arising as a result of a relative obstruction at
the level of the cricopharyngeus muscle. There is frequently a
previous history of heartburn and reflux due to hiatus hernia
and it is possible that the obstruction is due to hypertrophy in
an attempt to prevent overspill of refluxing gastro–oesophageal
contents into the larynx. The mucosa protrudes through Killian's
dehiscence (Fig. 29).

Recognizing the pattern

The condition occurs in elderly patients and it is more common
in males. The story is one of dysphagia. Characteristically the
first mouthful is easily swallowed but thereafter the pouch fills
up with food and obstructs the upper oesophagus. The patient
is then unable to swallow further food and will regurgitate the
contents of the pouch. Inhalation of regurgitated contents, especially at night, causes fits of coughing and episodes of
pulmonary infection.

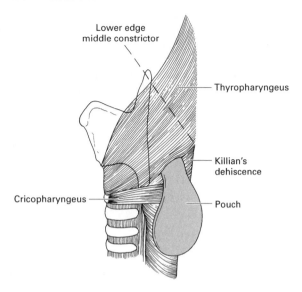

Fig. 29 The anatomy of a pharyngeal pouch.

Proving the diagnosis

The pouch is easily demonstrated on a barium swallow. Ask the radiologist to look specifically in the upper neck.

Management

The management is to excise the pouch externally and release the cricopharyngeal spasm, or use endoscopic surgical, laser or stapling techniques to bypass the pouch.

Preoperative management

The patient should be put on fluids only for 24 h pre-operatively. The patient is warned about potential pharyngeal perforation and damage to the recurrent laryngeal nerves.

OPERATION: EXCISION OF PHARYNGEAL POUCH
An incision is made at the level of the hyoid bone usually on the left side. The mucosal pouch is found and excised and the mucosal defect closed. The cricopharyngeus muscle is divided longitudinally (myotomy). The wound is drained and a nasogastric tube is passed down into the stomach. Endoscopic techniques usually result in a shorter hospital stay and recovery period.

Codes

Blood	0
GA/LA	GA
Opn time	1–2 h
Stay	5–7 days
Drains out	2–3 days
Sutures out	5 days
Off work	3 weeks

Postoperative care

The patient is fed through a nasogastric tube and a barium swallow is performed on the fifth day. If this shows no leakage, normal feeding can be instituted. If leakage is demonstrated feeding continues with a nasogastric tube until a repeat barium swallow shows the pharyngeal wound has healed.

Lumps in the posterior triangle

Cervical rib

In approximately 1 in 200 people the costal element of the seventh cervical vertebra overdevelops to a varying degree. The result is a cervical rib which, when fully formed, is bony and attached to the first normal rib. It may, however, be nothing more than a fibrous strand. In half the cases the condition is unilateral, usually on the right side. The subclavian artery and first thoracic nerve pass over the cervical rib to gain access to the upper limb. The artery may be narrowed over the rib and dilated distally. In the latter case mural thrombus may form and give rise to distal emboli. The first thoracic nerve can also be damaged by direct pressure. Very often a thin fibrous strand causes more symptoms than a fully formed cervical rib.

Recognizing the pattern

The condition may occur in either sex and symptoms usually begin in the late teens when the neck extends and the shoulders droop. The patient may notice a swelling or tenderness in the neck on the affected side. There may be pain due to vascular insufficiency. This is worse on exercise, especially if the arm is elevated. There may be distal ischaemia with a cold pale hand and occasional numbness or even trophic changes in the fingers. More rarely the patient may complain of neurological symptoms, which include numbness and paraesthesiae in the forearm and weakness of the hands. Palpation of the neck may reveal the abnormal rib. There may be signs of ischaemia or emboli in the hand. The radial pulse may disappear if the arm is fully elevated. Look for wasting in the hypothenar or thenar muscles and motor and sensory changes in the first thoracic nerve distribution. There may be a bruit over the subclavian artery.

Proving the diagnosis

An X-ray of the cervical spine will demonstrate the presence of a bony cervical rib or an enlarged anterior tubercle of the seventh cervical vertebra (associated with a fibrous band).

Arteriography may demonstrate a constriction and post-stenotic dilatation in the region of the cervical rib, especially if the angiogram is taken with the arm elevated.

Management

A cervical rib causing neurological symptoms may be managed conservatively with physiotherapy to improve the muscles that elevate and support the upper limb girdle. A cervical rib causing vascular problems or well-marked neurological problems should be treated surgically.

OPERATION: REMOVAL OF A CERVICAL RIB

The cervical rib is approached through a skin crease incision and removed, including its periosteal covering. If this covering is not removed there is a danger of recurrence. A fibrous band may also be excised. In some cases it is only necessary to split the scalenous anterior to relieve the pressure.

Codes

Blood .... 2 units
GA/LA .... GA
Opn time .... 1–2 h
Stay .... 3–5 days
Drains out .... Suction 24 h
Sutures out .... 4 days
Off work .... 2–3 weeks depending on occupation

Postoperative care

The postoperative course is usually uncomplicated. The patient should have a chest X-ray in the first few hours to exclude a pneumothorax.

3.2 Cervical Lymphadenopathy

Enlarged lymph nodes and lymphatic conditions

Enlarged cervical lymph nodes are the most common palpable lumps in the head and neck. The nodes may be enlarged due to either inflammatory or neoplastic processes and the precise node involved depends on the site of the primary pathology. It is therefore important to know which areas of the head and neck drain to the various lymph nodes (Fig. 30 and Table 12).

Inflammatory causes of enlarged lymph nodes may be acute or chronic. Acute inflammations are common in children and may be due to viruses or bacteria. The latter may progress to pus formation and present as a cervical abscess.

A typical chronic inflammatory cause of cervical lymphadenopathy is tuberculosis. These lymph nodes become very indurated and tend to give rise to sinuses.

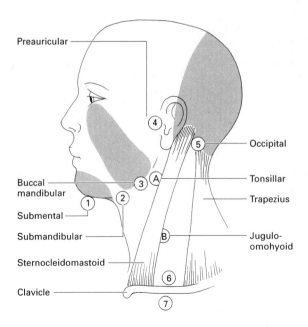

Fig. 30 The cervical lymph nodes and their areas of drainage. See Table 12 for key.

Table 12 The cervical lymph nodes and their areas of drainage.

Name	Area of drainage
1 Submental group	Tip of tongue, anterior end of lower lip, floor of mouth and lower gum, bilateral drainage
2 Submandibular group	Submental group, centre of forehead, nose, paranasal sinuses, front of neck, lips, anterior two-thirds of tongue
3 Buccal and mandibular group	Cheek, lower eyelid
4 Preauricular group	Temple, vertex, eyelids, orbit, external acoustic meatus
5 Occipital group	Back of scalp, posterior edge of pinna
6 Supraclavicular group	Occipital nodes, axillary nodes, breast, body wall
7 Infraclavicular group	Lower neck, preaxial border of upper limb, body wall, breast
A tonsillar node (anterosuperior deep cervical node)	Subcutaneous nodes, tonsil
B jugulo-omohyoid node (posteroinferior deep cervical node)	Submental group, submandibular group, posterior third of the tongue. These nodes therefore receive all the lymph drainage from the tongue

Neoplasms producing enlarged cervical lymph nodes include primary disease of the lymphatic system and secondary metastases from head and neck squamous carcinomas or thoracic or abdominal carcinomas. Hodgkin's disease is a primary lymphoma commonly presenting in the neck.

Sarcoidosis may also present as cervical lymphadenopathy.

Making the diagnosis

It is important to look for the possible primary sites of disease. Look inside the mouth, including the fauces, tonsils, tongue and teeth. A full ear, nose and throat (ENT) examination should be carried out. Nodes low down in the neck may arise from intra-thoracic or intra-abdominal pathology (Virchow's node). Look for enlarged nodes elsewhere and hepatosplenomegaly.

Screening tests indicated in any lymphadenopathy include a full blood count, erythrocyte sedimentation rate (ESR), virology screen including infectious mononucleosis and chest X-ray.

Management
Open biopsy is only done after repeated fine-needle aspiration and a formal panendoscopy has excluded a primary squamous carcinoma of the upper aerodigestive tract.

OPERATION: BIOPSY OF CERVICAL LYMPH NODE
An incision is made over the enlarged node and it is removed. If the node is very large or infected a drain may be used. Remember to send part of the node for bacteriological culture, including tuberculosis, as well as for histological examination.

Codes
Blood 0
GA/LA .... LA or GA
Opn time .... 15–45 min: depends on size and adherence of node
Stay .... Depends on cause
Drains out .... 24 h
Sutures out .... 5 days
Off work .... Variable

Postoperative care
The cause of the lymphadenopathy will have to be treated.

Acute inflammatory lymphadenopathy
The correct treatment in the first 24 h is antibiotics, but once pus formation occurs (after 48 h) drainage becomes necessary. Treating a cervical abscess with antibiotics leads to a chronic swelling (antibioma).

Tuberculous lymphadenitis
Modern treatment is with antituberculous therapy and excision of lymph nodes if they fail to settle.

Malignant lymphoma
Lymphomas are malignant neoplasms of lymphoid tissue. They are divided on a histological basis into Hodgkin's disease and non-Hodgkin's lymphoma. Further subdivisions of lymphomas are made on histological and immunological criteria. These

subgroups have different prognoses and may require different approaches to treatment.

A lymphoma typically presents with asymptomatic lymphadenopathy which may or may not be localized. Some patients have systemic symptoms which may include fever, weight loss and night sweats (type B symptoms). Other symptoms include malaise, pruritis and alcohol-induced pain. The diagnosis is confirmed by biopsy of an enlarged node. It is essential to send fresh unfixed material to the laboratory.

Staging the disease

Once the diagnosis has been made, further investigation is performed to stage the disease. This is done to determine what type of treatment is required and to predict the prognosis. The staging is as follows:

Stage I: a single group of nodes involved

Stage IE: a single extralymphatic organ or site, e.g. skin (rare)

Stage II: two or more lymph node sites are involved on the same side of the diaphragm

Stage III: lymph node sites are involved on both sides of the diaphragm. This includes involvement of the spleen

Stage IV: extralymphatic organ involvement (e.g. liver, bone marrow or lung).

Each stage is subdivided into A or B depending on the absence (type A) or presence (type B) of symptoms.

Investigations

The patients are usually worked up on a medical or haematological unit. The investigations may include the following:

1 Full blood count, erythrocyte sedimentation rate (ESR), liver function tests and plasma proteins.

2 Chest X-rays.

3 CT of the chest and abdomen.

4 Bone marrow biopsy.

5 Lymphangiogram — this is now rarely used.

6 Bone scan and/or liver and spleen scan.

7 Liver biopsy. This is done if there is significant hepatomegaly (more than 3.5 cm). A positive result means stage IV disease and makes laparotomy unnecessary.

8 Staging laparotomy. This used to be carried out to look for abdominal spread if the above investigations failed to show definite stage IV disease. It has since been outdated by improved imaging techniques.

9 MRI scanning may be useful for imaging glands in the high cervical region and assessing node involvement.

Management

Lymphomas may be treated by radiotherapy, combination chemotherapy or both, the choice depending on the stage of the disease and histological subtype, and whether the patient has significant symptoms.

Radiotherapy may be given either to the group of involved nodes (involved field) or to wider areas (extended field, e.g. 'mantle' or 'inverted Y').

Chemotherapy is given systemically either with a single drug or more usually with a combination of drugs. The choice depends on the stage of the disease, the patient's age, the ESR, the bulk of the disease and the histological grading. The present principles of treatment are outlined below.

Stages IA and IIA of Hodgkin's disease are treated with radiotherapy (involved field or extended field). Adjuvant chemotherapy is increasingly used, even in limited stage disease.

All other stages are treated with combination chemotherapy.

Non-Hodgkin's lymphomas are treated on similar lines, although chemotherapy is introduced at an earlier stage, with combination chemotherapy for the higher histological grades and single agents for lower grade lymphomas. Radiation may be used to control local sites of disease.

Cystic hygroma

This is a congenital lesion made up of lymph-filled spaces which arise from an embryonic remnant of the jugular lymph sac. Its correct name is a cavernous lymphangioma. It occurs in the base of the neck, both in the posterior triangle and anteriorly. It may extend up to the jaw, over the anterior chest wall, and down into the axilla. Very occasionally it may occur in the axilla alone.

Recognizing the pattern

The lesion occurs in young children and is often noticed at birth. On examination there is a soft, cystic and compressible lump just beneath the skin, superficial to the neck muscles. It transilluminates brilliantly, tends to vary in size and may have a lobular surface.

Management

The lesion is best treated by surgical excision. Sclerosants have been used.

Continued on p. 158

Continued.

Preoperative management
The patient or parent should be warned of the slight possibility of damage to branches of the brachial plexus and that some of the lesion may have to be left behind in order to avoid this. If this is the case, there will be a possibility of recurrence.

OPERATION: EXCISION OF CYSTIC HYGROMA
Removal of a large lesion can be tedious as it may ramify amongst the branches of the brachial plexus. It should be removed completely if possible, or it will recur. Occasionally a cystic hygroma extends into the axilla and in that case a separate incision is needed to remove it.

Codes
Blood .... 1 unit in babies, otherwise group and save
GA/LA .... GA
Opn time .... Depends on extent: 1–2 h
Stay .... 2–5 days
Drains out .... 2–5 days
Sutures out .... 3–5 days

Postoperative care
This is usually uncomplicated. The main problem is that fluid and blood tend to collect at the site of the cystic hygroma and the suction drains therefore need to be left for a long time. If fluid continues to collect after they are removed, it will have to be aspirated until the cavity heals completely. The length of hospital stay depends on the extent of the lesion.

Solitary lymph cyst
This is a variant of the cystic hygroma in which only one cyst is present. It is treated by simple excision.

3.3 Conditions of the Mouth

Those conditions of the mouth to be considered include the following:
1 Cleft lip and palate (p. 159)
2 Cysts in the mouth (p. 160)
3 Malignant tumours of the mouth (p. 164)
4 Conditions of the tongue are dealt with on pp. 170–177.

Cleft lip and palate

The most common developmental abnormalities are cleft lip and palate. These occur when there is failure of fusion of the processes contributing to facial development (Fig. 31). Twelve per cent of cases are familial. The left side is more commonly affected than the right. Of those babies with abnormalities, one-quarter have a cleft lip alone and a further quarter a cleft palate alone. The other 50% have both lesions. Fifteen per cent of cleft lips are bilateral.

Making the diagnosis

All but the most minor abnormalities are seen at birth. The main problem is with sucking and therefore feeding. Speech and dentition are also affected when there is a cleft palate, while a cleft lip on its own leads to an abnormality of facial development. Fifty per cent of patients with cleft palates have some hearing loss due to oedema around the Eustachian tube.

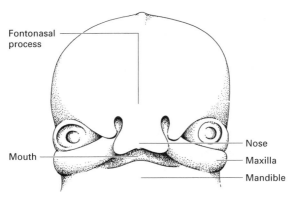

Fig. 31 Cleft lip and palate. The facial processes during development (7 weeks of gestation).

On examination note:

1 Whether the condition is unilateral or bilateral
2 Whether the palate is involved
3 How extensive the palatal lesion is.

Ten per cent of cases have other abnormalities so a thorough general examination should be undertaken.

Management

Treatment is surgical repair and is undertaken by a specialist plastic surgeon. In a cleft lip alone feeding is unimpaired and the lesion may be repaired at about the age of 6 months so that normal facial development may occur.

A cleft palate is associated with feeding problems and the baby will need to be either spoon-fed or fed with liquid dripped into the mouth. The lesion is usually repaired between 1 and 2 years of age to avoid significant speech impairment and dentition problems.

When both abnormalities exist together, the cleft lip is often repaired at the age of 8 weeks and the cleft palate at the age of 1 year.

Cysts in the mouth

Mucous retention cysts

When the duct of a mucous gland becomes blocked, mucus collects under the epithelium of the lip. Although these cysts may occur anywhere where there are mucous glands, they are usually on the lower lip or inside the buccal mucosa (Fig. 32).

Recognizing the pattern

The patient may be of any age and complains of a slowly growing lump which is painless. It may be accidentally bitten. On examination the cyst is a pale pink or blue colour with a glairy

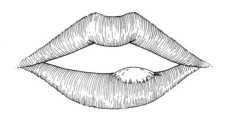

Fig. 32 A mucous retention cyst.

appearance. It usually measures between 0.5 and 2.0 cm in diameter and is not fixed to the underlying muscle.

Management: removal

OPERATION: REMOVAL OF MUCOUS RETENTION CYST

Although the operation may be carried out under a general anaesthetic (in a particularly nervous patient or in a child), it is usually done with local anaesthetic infiltration (e.g. 1% xylocaine with 1/200 000 adrenaline). The lip is incised and the cyst enucleated or deroofed.

Codes

Blood	0
GA/LA	LA
Opn time	15–30 min
Stay	Outpatient
Drains out	0
Sutures out	5 days or absorbable
Off work	2–3 h

Ranula

Ranula is Latin for a small frog. The term is used to describe a unilateral cystic swelling in the floor of the mouth formed either from a blocked mucous gland or from an accessory salivary gland.

Recognizing the pattern

The patient is usually a child or young adult of either sex who presents with a history of a swelling in the floor of the mouth. This develops over a few weeks and may fluctuate in size. There may be a past history of similar swellings. The lump is painless. On examination the swelling lies on one side of the floor of the mouth between the tongue and mandible. It is semitransparent, grey and up to 5 cm in diameter. It is smooth, spherical and cystic. It transilluminates. Rarely a ranula may possess a deep extension into the neck (possibly developing from the cervical sinus). The ranula is not attached to the overlying mucosa, mylohyoid or muscle of the tongue. The submandibular duct either overlies the lesion or is displaced to one side.

Management

Management is excision or marsupialization.

> OPERATION: EXCISION/MARSUPIALIZATION OF
> RANULA
>
> Ideally the cyst is completely excised. This is occasionally
> difficult and in that case it may be marsupialized, the re-
> mains of the cyst now becoming the floor of the mouth. If
> there is deep extension of the ranula below the mylohyoid,
> the cyst must be completely removed and it is approached
> from the neck as opposed to the floor of the mouth.

Codes

Blood 0
GA/LA .... GA
Opn time .... Proportional to extent and depth
Stay .... 2–5 days
Drains out 0
Sutures out .... Usually absorbable
Off work .... Variable

Dermoid cyst

This is a midline swelling on the floor of the mouth, originating
during development by entrapment of ectoderm beneath the
skin during fusion of the mandibular processes. It may be above
or below the mylohyoid.

Recognizing the pattern

A patient of either sex usually presents between the ages of 10
and 25 years complaining of a painless swelling under the floor
of the mouth. This may cause a double chin appearance. It may
occasionally become infected. On examination the swelling is in
the midline in the floor of the mouth or beneath the chin. It
is 2–5 cm in diameter and is spherical, smooth and cystic or
'putty'-like. The contents are opaque and it will not transilluminate.

> OPERATION: EXCISION OF DERMOID CYST IN
> THE MOUTH
>
> The cyst may be approached from an external incision beneath
> the mandible or a small one can be removed from within the
> mouth.

Codes

Blood 0
GA/LA .... GA
Opn time .... 30 min, depending on site

Stay .... Day case
Drains out .... 0–24 h
Sutures out .... Usually absorbable
Off work .... 1–2 weeks

Developmental cyst

This is a cyst, which forms in the same way as a dermoid cyst but occurs within bone. The commonest is the globular maxillary cyst, which occurs in the upper jaw between the premaxilla and the maxilla, i.e. between the incisor and canine. The treatment is excision.

Dental cyst

This is a cyst around the root of an erupted but decayed or infected tooth, which develops from epithelial cells of the enamel organ.

Making the diagnosis

The patient may be of any age or sex and presents with a diagnosis of painless swelling, usually of the upper jaw. There is a history of dental caries. The cyst may become infected and therefore painful.

The diagnosis is confirmed by X-ray.

Management

Treatment of dental cysts requires complete excision of the epithelial lining and is undertaken by an orodental surgeon. Obviously existing dental caries must also be treated.

Dentigerous cyst

This is a cyst containing an unerupted tooth and usually develops around the upper or lower third molar.

The patient is usually a young adult who presents with a painful swelling.

On examination there is swelling of the jaw, usually near the upper or lower third molar and this may have damaged the outer table of the bone. There will be one tooth missing.

Proving the diagnosis

The diagnosis is confirmed by X-ray.

Management

The cyst is excised by a dental surgeon (as under dental cyst above).

Alveolar abscess

This is an abscess formed around the root of a decaying tooth, often in a previous dental cyst. Under pressure the pus tracks out usually through the thinner lateral plate of the jaw, to form an abscess beneath the cheek or mandible.

Making the diagnosis

The patient is usually a child or young adult and presents with a dull, throbbing ache and swelling of the jaw. He may be generally unwell with a past history of dental caries. On examination the patient is pyrexial with a hot, tender, red swelling of the jaw, spreading either to the labial or buccal margin. When the patient still has his first dentition, either the upper or lower jaw may be affected. There is evidence of dental caries and there may be cervical lymphadenopathy.

Proving the diagnosis

The diagnosis is proved by X-ray.

> ### Management
> This consists of drainage and antibiotics. Advanced cases may be complicated by severe swelling of the floor of the mouth and the danger of incipient respiratory obstruction.

Benign tumours of the mouth

Epulis

Localized swelling of the gum.

Fibrous epulis

This is a fibroma developing from the periodontal membrane and presenting as a localized lesion between the gum and the tooth. Malignant change may occur, forming a friable, bleeding mass.

The management is removal. Histology should be requested.

Bony epulis

This is an osteoclastoma causing the overlying gum to become locally hyperaemic and oedematous. It is also referred to as a giant cell tumour. Depending on its size, it may be curetted out or may require excision of a large amount of mandible and bone grafting.

Granulomatous epulis

This is a mass of granulomatous tissue forming around a chronically infected or carious tooth or ill-fitting denture. The treatment is tooth extraction and curettage of the granulomatous tissue, which should be sent for histology.

Mixed salivary tumour (accessory pleomorphic adenoma)

There are accessory salivary glands in the oral cavity, particularly lining the hard palate, where salivary tumours can arise. As in the parotid gland, a mixed salivary tumour is benign but has an incomplete capsule. This may result in recurrence after simple enucleation. Malignant change is more common in accessory salivary glands than in the parotid.

Recognizing the pattern

The patient may be of either sex and is usually elderly. The lesion presents as a slowly growing but progressively enlarging painless lump in the palate. Eventually it may interfere with eating and speaking. On examination there is a smooth, hard lump beneath the mucous membrane. The mucosa is usually mobile over it. Initially the lump is also mobile over the mandible but it may later become attached. Alteration or a rapid increase in size suggests malignant change.

Proving the diagnosis

The diagnosis is proved by excision biopsy.

> **Management**
> Management is by excision with a margin of normal mucosa. It is unusual to have to remove palatal bone.

Malignant tumours of the mouth

Adamantinoma

This is a locally invasive tumour of epithelial cells derived from the enamel organ and it resembles a basal cell carcinoma in both histological appearance and behaviour. It usually forms multiloculated cysts.

Recognizing the pattern

The patient is usually a schoolchild or young adult, more commonly of African or Asian origin, who presents with a painless swelling of the jaw. There may be a past history of excision and recurrence. On examination there is swelling, usually of the molar region or the mandible, which may cause egg-shell cracking of the overlying bone.

Proving the diagnosis

The X-ray appearances are characteristic. There are large loculi in the bone, which has a honeycomb appearance. This differentiates it from the cysts described above.

Management

Local curettage is inadequate as the condition will recur. The tumour must be excised with a margin of normal bone either side and bone graft may be required postoperatively.

Carcinoma of the lip

This carcinoma is often called 'countryman's lip'. Histologically it is a keratinizing squamous cell carcinoma. Aetiological factors include pipe-smoking and long exposure to sunlight or severe weather.

Ninety-three per cent of the lesions occur in the lower lip. Five per cent occur in the upper lip and 2% at the angle of the mouth. The lymphatic drainage is to the submental nodes if the lesion is in the lower lip and to the submandibular nodes if the lesion is in the upper lip. Blood-borne spread to the liver and lungs is late and rare. Lesions in the angle of the mouth have a worse prognosis due to the involvement of two lymph fields.

Recognizing the pattern

Ninety per cent occur in men aged over 65 years. Most have led an active outdoor life or have been pipe-smokers. The history is of a chronic ulcer of the lip which enlarges and fails to heal. It may present as a warty growth or a fissure. More advanced lesions may be painful, become infected and disturb eating. On examination the ulcer usually has a characteristic raised rolled edge with blood-stained slough in the base.

Proving the diagnosis

This is done by biopsy.

Management

An early lesion may be treated by either surgery or radiotherapy. Some of these lesions are small and can be treated as an outpatient procedure under a local anaesthetic.

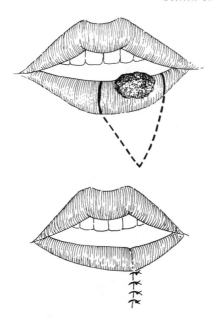

Fig. 33 Wedge excision of carcinoma of lip.

OPERATION: WEDGE EXCISION OF CARCINOMA
OF THE LIP
A simple wedge resection is performed (Fig. 33). There is
marked bleeding from the marginal artery of the lip and this
can be controlled by pressure on the lip while a suture is
inserted. It is important to remove an adequate margin of
normal tissue on either side. The cosmetic result is very
satisfactory.

An alternative to surgery is radiotherapy. There is a 75%
5-year survival with either form of treatment.

A larger lesion will require resection and plastic reconstruction of the lip.

Codes

Blood	0
GA/LA	GA or LA
Opn time	30–60 min
Stay	2–7 days
Drains out	0
Sutures out	7–10 days
Off work	3 days to 2 weeks depending on the size of the lesion

Squamous cell carcinoma

Squamous cell carcinoma or anaplastic variants of it can occur at any site in the mouth where there is stratified squamous epithelium. Carcinoma of the tongue is an example (p. 173). The presentation and management of lesions elsewhere depends on the precise site and extent of the lesion. The mainstay of treatment is either radiotherapy or excision with or without reconstructive surgery.

Malignant melanoma

Malignant melanoma can rarely occur in any part of the lining of the mouth. Its treatment is considered in the section on skin conditions (p. 580).

Tumours of the jaw

These may be either primary or secondary and both are rare.

Carcinoma of the maxillary antrum

The maxillary antrum is lined by respiratory epithelium. The usual type of carcinoma occurring in this site is a squamous cell carcinoma, although adenocarcinomas are also seen. Carcinoma in the nasal sinuses occurs in woodworkers after a long latent period.

Making the diagnosis

The patient is usually male and elderly. The primary is usually undetected whilst it remains within the sinus and only becomes evident when it has invaded the surrounding structures including either the orbit, the nasal cavity or the hard palate and upper jaw. In these situations it presents as a mass or an ulcerated lesion. On examination the tumour is then fixed to bone.

Proving the diagnosis

The diagnosis is confirmed by CT scanning and MRI.

> **Management**
> This consists of either radiotherapy, or excision and reconstruction. Combined therapy with radiotherapy and surgery is often used.

Malignant disease of the tonsil

Malignant disease of the tonsil is usually due to squamous cell carcinoma (85%) or a lymphosarcoma. The lymphoid tissue may also be involved in a more generalized lymphoma. A carcinoma of the tonsil spreads to adjacent structures such as the palate and base of the tongue and thence on to the deep cervical nodes.

Recognizing the pattern

The patient with squamous cell carcinoma is usually over the age of 60 years and presents with pain in the throat which radiates to the ear. There is progressive enlargement of the tonsil causing dysphagia and 'thickening' of the speech. Eventually the growth ulcerates causing bleeding and marked fetor oris.

In contrast, lymphosarcoma occurs in slightly younger patients between the ages of 50 and 65 years and the enlargement is usually painless. Ulceration and bleeding occur very late.

The ipsilateral deep cervical nodes may be enlarged due to secondary growth or due to infection secondary to a malignant ulcer.

Proving the diagnosis

The diagnosis is proved by biopsying the enlarged tonsil.

Management

Both types of tumour are treated by radiotherapy to the affected tonsil and the ipsilateral side of the neck. Large squamous cell tumours are occasionally treated by surgical resection combined with radiotherapy. Metastases in the cervical nodes may be treated by dissection of the neck (see p. 176).

3.4 Conditions of the Tongue

Chronic superficial glossitis

Chronic inflammation of the tongue is characterized by leuco-plakia (white matt patches seen on the normal stratified squamous epithelium). The condition is premalignant. Macroscopically there is epithelial hyperplasia (hyperkeratosis), widening of the prickle cell layer (acanthosis) and a chronic inflammatory cell infiltrate. The presence of atypical cells, loss of polarity, local mucosal invasion, and nucleated cells appearing close to the surface indicate malignant change.

Classically the aetiological factors are the six Ss: smoking, spirits, spices, syphilis, sharp tooth, sepsis.

Syphilis was once an important factor although it is now very rare in the UK. Pipe-smoking and chronic trauma due to bad teeth or ill-fitting dentures are now the most significant causes. Chronic superficial glossitis can also be 'idiopathic'.

Recognizing the pattern

The patient is frequently an elderly male. The presenting com-plaint is usually that the patient or his relatives have noticed a change in colour of the tongue or a new irregularity. Otherwise it causes very few symptoms (unlike acute glossitis which is painful). There may be a past medical history of venereal disease or dental problems. On examination typically it presents as patchy changes on the tongue and may be sited close to the cause (e.g. a sharp tooth).

There are four clinical stages.

1 A thin, grey, transparent film appears on the surface of the tongue.

2 Opaque white patches may develop (leucoplakia). With time these become yellow and may show cracks or fissures.

3 Further hyperplasia produces white nodules on the surfaces while desquamation in between leaves red, raw areas.

4 The development of a nodular or papillary growth may in-dicate _____ _ _____ _ _ _ _ _ _ _ _ *n situ*.

_____ and deep cervical lymph nodes should also

Management

If there is any suggestion of malignant change, a biopsy of the lesion should be performed. If there is only a small patch of leucoplakia, it may be removed completely; at the same time any known cause must be remedied. A Wassermann reaction is done to exclude syphilis. If the lesion is too large to remove completely and there are no suspicious areas, it can safely be left and should improve once the cause has been removed. The patient must be reviewed regularly to detect any evidence of malignant change.

Ulceration of the tongue

Tongue ulcers may be:

1 Traumatic
2 Aphthous
3 Tuberculous
4 Syphilitic
5 Chronic non-specific
6 Carcinomatous.

Traumatic ulceration

This is an ulcer on the side of the tongue caused by a sharp tooth or ill-fitting denture.

Recognizing the pattern

The patient is of any age and complains of a painful ulcer on the side of the tongue. On examination there is a chronic infected ulcer close to a cause such as a cracked tooth or an ill-fitting denture.

Management

When the cause is removed or remedied, the ulcer heals over a few days.

Aphthous ulceration

There are many causes of these small ulcers. In children both viral and fungal (*Candida*) infections are implicated. In adults this common type of ulcer is non-contagious and frequently shows a familial disposition.

Recognizing the pattern

The patient is usually an adolescent or young adult and the condition is more common in women than men. The ulcers are very painful. On examination there is a small, round, white ulcer on the tongue, gums or inner aspect of the lips. The ulcers may be multiple.

Management

The patient should be reassured that the condition is not serious. The ulcer will heal on its own over a period of about 10 days. Healing can be hastened by topical hydrocortisone tablets. Oral salicylate gel gives symptomatic relief. If the ulcer fails to heal, then the diagnosis should be reviewed and if necessary a biopsy performed.

Tuberculous ulcer

This is now a rare cause of tongue ulceration. It occurs in undiagnosed advanced pulmonary tuberculosis.

Recognizing the pattern

Multiple, very painful ulcers with undermined edges occur along the edges of the tongue.

Proving the diagnosis

The diagnosis of tuberculosis is proved on chest X-rays, sputum culture and microscopy.

Management

Treatment is antituberculous therapy.

Syphilitic ulcer

The typical lesions of the tongue are the chancre of primary syphilis, snail-track ulcers, Hutchinson's wart of secondary syphilis and the gumma of tertiary syphilis.

Treatment is with antibiotics (penicillin).

Chronic non-specific ulcer

This is a chronic ulcer which is usually situated on the anterior two-thirds of the tongue. No predisposing factor can be found. The lesion is usually painful. Syphilis and tuberculosis are excluded by investigation. The diagnosis is confirmed and the lesion cured by excision biopsy.

Neoplasms of the tongue

These may be either benign or malignant. Benign neoplasms of the tongue are rare. The following may occur:

1 Papilloma
2 Angioma
3 Lingual thyroid
4 Neurofibroma
5 Lipoma.

These are treated by excision. In the case of a lingual thyroid, it is important to be sure that there is other thyroid tissue lower down in the neck. A thyroid isotope scan will give this information.

Carcinoma of the tongue

This is usually a keratinizing squamous cell carcinoma. The aetiology is the same as that for chronic superficial glossitis and leucoplakia. The prognosis becomes worse the further back the lesion is on the tongue. Overall the 5-year survival is 25%.

Recognizing the pattern

The patient usually presents between the ages of 60 and 70 years. Carcinoma of the tongue used to be very much more common in men, but now, due to the declining incidence of syphilis and the disappearance of the clay pipe, the incidence in men and women is equal. There may be a past history of dental caries, pipe-smoking or venereal disease. More advanced carcinomas cause pain in the tongue, which may be referred to the ear. There may also be excessive salivation and defective tongue movement or difficulty with speech due to spread into the floor of the mouth. If the lesion becomes infected, fetor oris results. On examination the lesion may be one of the following:

1 A wart with a broad firm base and surrounding induration
2 An ulcer with typical everted rolled edge and infected bleeding slough in the base
3 A hard indistinct nodule.

The patient may have had a pad of cotton wool in his ear for the pain and there may be evidence of secondary lymph node involvement.

The extent of secondary spread must be assessed. The tip of the tongue and the posterior third have bilateral lymphatic drainage (Fig. 34) so examine both sides of the neck. Blood spread occurs late and almost always from carcinoma on the posterior third of the tongue.

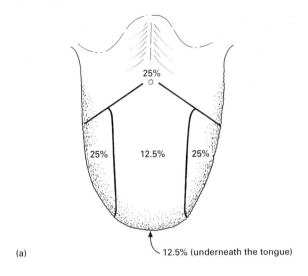

(a)

25%

25%   12.5%   25%

12.5% (underneath the tongue)

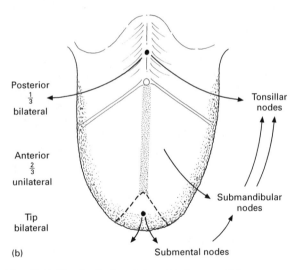

Posterior
⅓
bilateral

Anterior
⅔
unilateral

Tip
bilateral

(b)

Tonsillar
nodes

Submandibular
nodes

Submental nodes

Fig. 34 (a) The distribution of sites of malignancy of the tongue.
(b) The lymphatic drainage of the tongue.

Proving the diagnosis

The diagnosis is confirmed by biopsy. The differential diagnosis
includes that of other ulcers of the tongue (see p. 171) and other
solid lesions of the tongue (see p. 173).

Management

Treatment is by excision and/or radiotherapy. The latter can be administered either as external irradiation or by radioactive implants. The choice of type of therapy and operation depends on the extent of the lesion.

A small lesion less than 1 cm in diameter may be excised locally. Larger lesions are initially treated by radiotherapy but, if the lesion does not respond or recurs, then operation is required. This may be extensive and consist of either a partial glossectomy, a hemi-glossectomy or subtotal glossectomy (see below). If lymph nodes are involved, a dissection of the neck lymph nodes will be required.

Preoperative management
Investigations should include the following:
1 Full blood count and ESR
2 Wassermann reaction
3 Chest X-ray
4 CT or MRI scan and X-rays of the mandible if tumour extent and bone invasion are to be assessed.

Mouthwashes may help to clean up an infected lesion.

OPERATION: PARTIAL GLOSSECTOMY FOR CARCINOMA OF THE TONGUE
The amount of tissue removed depends on the size of the lesion and an adequate margin is necessary (at least 1 cm). Bleeding may be profuse and the assistant can help to control this by compressing one side of the tongue posteriorly to compress the lingual artery.

Codes
Blood .... Group and save serum
GA/LA .... GA
Opn time .... 1 h
Stay .... 3–5 days
Drains out 0
Sutures out .... Absorbable
Off work .... 1 month

Postoperative care
Regular daily mouthwashes are given.

OPERATION: HEMI-GLOSSECTOMY

In this operation half the tongue is removed. It is performed for lesions of the lateral border of the tongue that are clear of the mandible. A submandibular dissection may also be required and sometimes this is combined with a dissection of the neck on that side.

Codes

Blood .... 2 units
GA/LA .... GA
Opn time .... 1–3 h
Stay .... 10–14 days
Drains out .... 3–5 days
Off work .... 4–6 weeks

OPERATION: NECK DISSECTION

This operation is undertaken as part of an attempted radical cure of any lesion which has spread to the cervical lymph nodes. A variety of neck dissections can be performed, the most common being a radical neck dissection of the lymph nodes in continuity with the internal jugular vein and the sternomastoid muscle.

Codes

Blood .... 2 units
GA/LA .... GA
Opn time .... 3–5 h
Stay .... 7–10 days
Drains out .... 3–5 days
Sutures out .... 7 days
Off work .... 4–6 weeks

OPERATION: COMPOSITE RESECTION
(COMMANDO OPERATION)

In this procedure an extensive dissection of the neck, mouth and pharynx is carried out, including a segment of the body or ramus of the mandible. The intraoral defect is repaired, using a vascularized skin flap. The symphysis menti, geniohyoid and genioglossus muscles are disrupted, and the airway is in danger as the tongue is liable to fall back. Elective tracheostomy is required. A fine-bore nasogastric tube is used for feeding purposes.

Codes

Blood .... 4 units

GA/LA .... GA

Opn time .... 6 h

Stay .... 3–4 weeks

Drains out .... 3–5 days

Sutures out .... 7–10 days

Off work .... 3 months

4 Endocrine Surgery

4.1 Lumps in the Thyroid Gland and Goitres

General assessment of thyroid lumps

Faced with a lump in the pretracheal region of the neck, you have to decide on the following:

1 Is it in the thyroid?
2 Is it solitary or generalized?
3 Is the patient toxic, euthyroid or myxoedematous?

Is the lump in the thyroid gland?

The thyroid gland is situated behind the pretracheal fascia and, as this fascia is attached to the larynx, the gland moves up and down on swallowing. This feature, together with their midline situation, makes the diagnosis of thyroid swellings easy. The patient is given a glass of water and asked to raise his chin. The clinician first observes the lump from in front and then feels it standing behind the patient. The patient is asked to swallow and the movement of the lump is noted.

Is it solitary or generalized?

Is the enlargement of:

1 The whole gland (a goitre)? This is dealt with on p. 183.
2 A nodule within the gland (solitary nodule)? This is dealt with on pp. 189–192.

Thyroid status

The patient may be:

1 Thyrotoxic
2 Euthyroid, i.e. normal
3 Myxoedematous.

Thyrotoxicosis

Patients with an overactive thyroid gland have symptoms of tiredness, weight loss, anxiety, tremor, palpitations and amenorrhoea, and tend to prefer cold to hot weather.

On examination there is nervousness and agitation, a tachycardia of over 100, fine tremor of the fingers and lid lag. There may also be exophthalmos. A bruit is occasionally audible over a toxic goitre.

Myxoedema

Myxoedematous patients are slow in thought, speech and movement, are overweight, have thickened skin and tend to lose their hair. They have a slow pulse rate. They prefer warm weather.

Investigations for thyroid lumps

The following tests are used to investigate thyroid lumps:

1 Serum tri-iodothyronine and tetra-iodothyronine (T3 and T4). These are raised in thyrotoxicosis.

2 Thyroid-stimulating hormone (TSH). This gives an indication of the activity of the pituitary in stimulating the thyroid. There is a feedback mechanism whereby TSH is raised when the thyroid hormone level is below normal. An elevated TSH therefore confirms hypothyroidism. In hyperthyroidism it is depressed. The new sensitive immunoradiometric assay (IRMA) for TSH is very accurate, detecting hypo- and hyperthyroidism.

3 Thyrotrophin-releasing hormone test (TRH test). In this test thyrotrophin (TSH) levels are measured after a dose of TRH (200 μg in 2 mL i.v.). Normally this produces a rise in TSH by 20 min and levels fall again by 60 min after the injection. No such rise occurs in thyrotoxicosis because the pituitary is suppressed by the high T4 level. The rise is exaggerated in primary hypothyroidism.

4 Thyroid antibody estimation (see Hashimoto's disease, p. 183).

5 Computed tomography (CT) scan of neck and upper mediastinum. The important points to look for are whether the trachea is deviated by the nodule and whether it is narrow in either its anteroposterior or lateral diameter.

6 Fine-needle aspiration cytology. This has largely superseded radioactive and ultrasound scans in the investigation of thyroid disease.

7 Thyroid scan. The patient is given radioactive technetium to drink and the tissue uptake over the thyroid gland is plotted. A toxic gland shows a markedly increased uptake of radioactive tracer over the normal. This increased uptake may be generalized as in Graves' disease, or focal (a 'hot nodule') as in a toxic autonomous nodule. A cold (inactive) nodule suggests possible malignancy.

8 Ultrasound scan. This shows if the lump is solid or cystic and may show if it is solitary or part of a multinodular goitre.

Goitres

There are four main types:
1 Physiological
2 Nodular
3 Inflammatory
4 Toxic.

Physiological goitre

A physiological goitre occurs at puberty, during pregnancy and in conditions of iodine deficiency. Apart from the latter state, no treatment is necessary.

Nodular goitre

A nodular goitre can be a benign or malignant enlargement of the thyroid gland with areas of hyperplasia and involution. No treatment is necessary, unless:
1 The patient becomes thyrotoxic.
2 There is compression of other neck structures, resulting in dyspnoea or dysphagia.
3 The patient is particularly worried by the cosmetic appearance of the goitre.
4 A focal increase in size or the development of hoarseness (due to recurrent laryngeal nerve palsy) suggests malignant change.

In any of these cases subtotal thyroidectomy may be indicated (see below).

Inflammatory goitre

The usual causes of diffuse inflammation of the thyroid gland are Hashimoto's disease and De Quervain's thyroiditis. Riedel's thyroiditis is very rare.

Hashimoto's disease

In this condition antibodies are produced against thyroglobulin and microsomes.

Recognizing the pattern

The patient is usually a middle-aged female who presents with a goitre and is usually at first thyrotoxic and later myxoedematous. The gland is diffusely enlarged initially, but later becomes replaced by a small fibrotic remnant with a characteristic bosselated surface.

Proving the diagnosis

The diagnosis is proved by finding thyroid antibodies in the serum.

Management

In Hashimoto's disease operation should be avoided as this will hasten the onset of thyroid deficiency. Patients should be warned that they may eventually require thyroid hormone replacement. If they are already myxoedematous, this should be instituted (T4 50–200 µg/day). Thyroidectomy is occasionally required to relieve pressure symptoms, for cosmetic reasons or to establish a diagnosis.

De Quervain's thyroiditis

This is a non-suppurative inflammation of the gland due to a viral infection. The usual organism is the Coxsackie virus.

Recognizing the pattern

A patient of either sex (more commonly female) presents with an acutely swollen, tender gland, often preceded by a sore throat and mild constitutional upset. The patient becomes pyrexial and transiently thyrotoxic.

Proving the diagnosis

There may be a lymphocytosis and a raised erythrocyte sedimentation rate (ESR). Typically the T4 may be elevated in the acute state but the uptake of radioactive iodine by the inflamed gland is diminished. There are no thyroid antibodies in the serum.

Management

Mild analgesia is usually sufficient. More severe cases may be treated with three courses of prednisolone (10–20 mg/day). The condition settles spontaneously but may recur.
Hypothyroidism is very unlikely.

Riedel's thyroiditis

Riedel's thyroiditis is a rare condition of the thyroid in which the gland becomes hard and enlarged with infiltration of scar tissue, which then involves the surrounding tissues. It results in hypothyroidism, recurrent laryngeal nerve palsy and stridor. Because of these features, it mimics carcinoma of the thyroid. It often has to be biopsied in order to establish the diagnosis. The management, once the diagnosis is established, is to leave well alone and treat with T4 if the patient becomes myxoedematous.

Toxic goitre (thyrotoxicosis or Graves' disease)

Thyroid hormones regulate the basal metabolic rate. Their own level is controlled by TSH released by the pituitary.

Graves' thyrotoxicosis is now thought to be an autoimmune disease. Autoantibodies against the TSH receptor on thyroid membrane have been isolated, and these stimulate the gland. Long-acting thyroid stimulator-protector (LATS-P) is a human-specific immunoglobulin found in almost all patients. LATS itself is not human specific and is found in fewer patients. The TSH levels are abnormally low.

The condition has a familial incidence, and there is an association between it and other autoimmune diseases (e.g. myasthenia gravis, pernicious anaemia, Addison's disease). There is diffuse enlargement of the gland with hyperplasia and hypertrophy. There may be a lymphocyte and plasma cell infiltration. In approximately 25% of patients the disease is self-limiting.

Recognizing the pattern

Females are more often affected than males and the disease usually occurs between the ages of 15 and 45 years. Thyrotoxicosis may, however, occur in both younger and older patients.

The symptoms of toxicity are described on p. 181.

On examination

In a toxic goitre the gland is smoothly enlarged and the patient shows signs of thyrotoxicosis. The skin over the gland may be warm and there is often a systolic bruit. Thyrotoxicosis may also be associated with exophthalmos or pretibial myxoedema.

Management

There are three possible forms of management available for the thyrotoxic patient. These are as follows.

1 Medical treatment. This is the first-line treatment of Graves' disease in patients younger than 25, providing the goitre is not too large:

   (a) the production of thyroid hormones can be blocked using drugs such as carbimazole (5–10 mg 8-hourly) or propylthiouracil (100 mg 8-hourly). The drugs are stopped after 18–24 months. If the patient relapses, then surgery should be considered

   (b) propranolol gives symptomatic relief, particularly of tachycardia, palpitations, tremor, sweating and nervous-

Continued on p. 186

Continued.

ness. The usual dose is 80–120 mg/day in divided doses. It is used in the preoperative preparation of the patient (see below), in the control of a 'thyroid crisis' and in patients who need to have their own production of thyroid hormones monitored (e.g. following ^{131}I therapy).

2 Radioactive iodine treatment. Because of the slight risk of late malignancy, radioactive iodine is contraindicated in younger patients and is reserved for those with thyrotoxicosis over the age of 50 years. It is also used for recurrent thyrotoxicosis after thyroidectomy. The patient drinks radioactive iodine, which is concentrated in the thyroid, which thus undergoes self-destruction. A variable dose is required and it takes about 3 months to take effect. In that time propranolol is used to control symptoms. A second dose of radioactive iodine may be needed. Regular follow-up is required and at least 40% of patients become hypothyroid within 10 years, requiring replacement therapy.

3 Surgical treatment. This is subtotal thyroidectomy. It is indicated for patients:

  (a) with large goitres which are causing pressure symptoms or are unsightly
  (b) who relapse after one or two courses of drugs
  (c) with nodular goitre
  (d) who do not want the inconvenience of prolonged medical treatment
  (e) who are planning a pregnancy.

Summary of management of thyrotoxicosis

Patients under the age of 50 years are usually treated medically in the first instance. If they relapse following cessation of medical treatment, operation is indicated. Young patients developing thyrotoxicosis have a high relapse rate and many physicians refer patients under the age of 25 years for surgery as soon as they become euthyroid, rather than undertaking a trial of medical therapy.

Patients over the age of 50 years are usually treated with radioactive iodine.

Preoperative management

It is dangerous to operate on a patient who is actively thyrotoxic. Manipulation of the gland during operation produces considerably raised blood levels of T4 and this can result in a 'thyroid crisis' (see p. 188). A crisis is prevented by adequate preoperative preparation. Two methods are possible.

1 Antithyroid drugs. The patient is made euthyroid by using carbimazole or some other antithyroid agent that blocks the production of T4. This also causes the gland to become larger and more vascular. The treatment is therefore stopped 10 days before the operation is planned and changed to propanolol.

2 β-blockade. An alternative method of preoperative preparation is to give the patient large enough doses of propanolol to suppress the adrenergic toxic effects (40 mg 8-hourly, although more may be required). In this case the serum T4 remains raised, but is ineffectual in producing cardiac dysrhythmias, tachycardia or hyperpyrexia.

The advantage of the second method is that the gland does not become large and haemorrhagic and is therefore easier to operate on. In addition, the preparation is much more rapid than with carbimazole. With the latter a preparation of 2 or 3 months is required but with propranolol the patient can be made ready for surgery within a week or 10 days.

The drug should be given with the premedication and continued for a few days postoperatively, using reducing doses as the pulse stabilizes.

The vocal cords should be checked before the operation to make sure they are moving adequately.

The patient's serum must also be checked for antibodies as thyrotoxicity is not uncommon early in Hashimoto's disease and thyroidectomy may be contraindicated in this condition (see p. 183).

OPERATION: SUBTOTAL THYROIDECTOMY
The thyroid is exposed by a 'collar' incision. Care is taken to avoid damage to the recurrent laryngeal nerves and also the parathyroid glands. Seven-eighths of the thyroid gland is removed leaving remnants posteriorly on both sides of the trachea. The wound is drained with or without suction. A pressure bandage is usually applied over the wound.

Codes

Blood .... Group and save serum
GA/LA .... GA
Opn time .... 90–120 min
Stay .... 5–7 days
Drains out .... 24 h
Sutures out .... 3–4 days (clips 2–3 days)
Off work .... 4–6 weeks

Postoperative care

The patient has a very sore throat and usually has a desire to cough. Cough suppressant analgesics such as Omnopon or codeine are of value. Rarely the neck swells up rapidly due to haemorrhage, and there is a danger of compression of the trachea. In this case the wound may have to be reopened in the ward to avoid asphyxia. A pair of clip removers should be kept close to the bed. When the neck has been decompressed, the patient is returned to theatre to restore haemostasis.

Postoperative stridor may be due to laryngeal oedema and unconnected with contained haemorrhage. The patient must be returned to the theatre and reintubated by an experienced anaesthetist. Failure to reinsert the tube will necessitate tracheostomy. The intubated patient is nursed in intensive care for 12 h, given hydrocortisone or dextramethasone and can usually be extubated without problem.

The vocal cords should be routinely checked to ensure that the recurrent nerves have not been damaged.

Hypocalcaemia is an occasional complication of operations for thyrotoxicosis. This may be due to accidental removal of parathyroid glands but is more often due to calcium being mopped up by the skeleton after the decalcification associated with the thyrotoxic state. If the serum calcium does fall, tetany may occur (see p. 202).

Treatment of thyroid crisis

This is caused by a sudden surge of T4 and may occur if surgery is performed on inadequately prepared patients. It may also be seen if the postoperative dose of propranolol is omitted in patients prepared on this drug alone. Signs include delirium, anxiety, tachycardia, cardiac failure, hyperpyrexia, abdominal pain and diarrhoea. It may result in adrenal failure and coma.

It is treated by a slow infusion of propranolol (5–15 mg) followed by oral administration of 40 mg 8-hourly. Intra-venous fluids may be required and steroids may be given to cover adrenal failure. Chlorpromazine (100 mg i.v.) is useful.

Long-term follow-up
The patient should be reviewed regularly for signs of develop-ing myxoedema. The serum T3, T4 and TSH are measured regularly. The serum TSH is usually raised after partial thyroid-ectomy but this does not matter providing the serum T4 remains in the normal range.

Solitary thyroid nodule

Lesions presenting as solitary thyroid nodules can be classified as follows:

1 Benign:
  (a) cyst
  (b) adenoma
  (c) a discrete nodule in a nodular goitre.
2 Malignant, primary:
  (a) thyroid adenocarcinoma
  (b) malignant lymphoma
  (c) medullary carcinoma.
3 Malignant, secondary:
  (a) direct spread
  (b) indirect spread from:
    • breast
    • rectum
    • colon
    • hypernephroma
    • lung
    • lymphatic tumours.

Having decided that the lump is in the thyroid, determine whether the opposite lobe of the thyroid is also palpable and whether it is nodular. In this way you may be able to determine whether the nodule is truly solitary or part of a nodular goitre. The patient should also be fully examined to determine his thyroid status (as on p. 181).

All solitary nodules should be investigated by the following:
1 Fine-needle aspiration cytology. A fine-bore needle is posi-tioned in the tumour and cells aspirated. The smear produced is interpreted by an expert cytopathologist.

2 Chest X-ray. This is done to look for signs of pressure on the surrounding structures, particularly the trachea. A chest X-ray may show a retrosternal extension of the mass, or pulmonary metastases.

3 Thyroid hormones (T3, T4, TSH). These determine the patient's thyroid status.

4 Thyroid antibodies. To look for evidence of thyroiditis.

Management

Cystic lesions may be aspirated. Most solitary solid thyroid nodules will require surgical removal and histological examination in order to exclude thyroid malignancy. This usually involves a hemi-thyroidectomy. This will first be described, followed by some notes on the individual lesions presenting as a solitary thyroid nodule.

Preoperative management

As for subtotal thyroidectomy, the patient's vocal cords are examined to make sure there is no pre-existing paralysis. The patient is warned of the slight danger of a husky voice following the operation.

OPERATION: THYROID LOBECTOMY

The thyroid gland is explored through a 'collar' incision. The involved lobe is exposed and excised completely. In order to do this the recurrent laryngeal nerve must be exposed.

There are differing views as to what to do once the lobe has been removed. Some surgeons send it for frozen-section histology and may proceed to a full total thyroidectomy at the same operation if the lesion is malignant. Others will leave the contralateral lobe strictly alone and be prepared to come back and remove the other lobe later if necessary (see under management of individual thyroid carcinomas). The author's preference is for the second course.

Codes

Blood	Group and save serum
GA/LA	GA
Opn time	60–90 min
Stay	4–7 days
Drains out	24–48 h
Sutures out	3–4 days (clips 2–3 days)
Off work	4 weeks

Postoperative care

This is as for subtotal thyroidectomy and is described on p. 188. Hypocalcaemia and hypothyroidism are not a problem if the other lobe has been left intact.

OPERATION: TOTAL THYROIDECTOMY

In this procedure both lobes of the gland are removed. There is an increased danger of parathyroid deficiency postoperatively, although it is usually possible to leave at least one parathyroid on each side of the neck.

Codes

Blood	Group and save serum
GA/LA	GA
Opn time	2–3 h
Stay	5–7 days
Drains out	24–48 h
Sutures out	3–4 days (clips 2–3 days)
Off work	4–6 weeks

Postoperative care

The serum calcium is monitored daily and any hypoparathyroidism treated as on p. 202. The patient will require thyroid replacement therapy (200 µg/day of T4).

In the unlikely event of both recurrent laryngeal nerves being damaged at operation, the patient will develop severe stridor or complete airway obstruction. Emergency reintubation is required and a tracheostomy may be necessary.

Cysts and adenomas

Thyroid cyst

This is usually a degenerative part of a nodular goitre although true thyroid cysts do occur. A common complication is haemorrhage into the cyst. When this occurs, there is rapid enlargement and the lump may be painful. There is a possibility that such rapid enlargement may compress the trachea.

Recognizing the pattern

The patient is of any age and is euthyroid. There may be a history of rapid enlargement and pain.

Proving the diagnosis
The lump may be shown to be cystic on fine-needle aspiration.

Management
If the swelling is thought to be cystic and the rest of the gland is normal, some surgeons will aspirate the cyst. It tends to refill, however. Some carcinomas have cystic areas in them but cytology should identify these. We therefore tend to excise the cyst.

Thyroid adenomas
There are four types of thyroid adenoma. The names refer to the histological appearance. They are:
1 Papillary
2 Follicular
3 Embryonal
4 Hurtle cell.

A few adenomas are functioning and may even produce thyrotoxicosis (solitary hot nodule). Occasionally haemorrhage may occur into the tumour causing a rapid increase in size.

Management
The distinction from a carcinoma can only be made on histological examination. For this reason most adenomas are excised. If, however, the lesion shows as a 'hot' nodule on thyroid scanning, it may be possible to suppress it with T4 treatment. Otherwise the management is thyroid lobectomy as above.

Papillary adenomas are hard to differentiate from carcinoma and routine follow-up after excision is necessary.

Nodule of a nodular goitre
A solitary nodule often turns out to be part of a nodular goitre and not truly solitary. However, this may well be impossible to distinguish before operation and so the affected lobe has to be excised to be certain. If this is in fact the diagnosis, no further treatment is necessary.

Carcinoma of the thyroid
There are five types of primary thyroid malignancy:
1 Papillary adenocarcinoma
2 Follicular adenocarcinoma
3 Anaplastic carcinoma

4 Medullary carcinoma

5 Lymphoma.

Each has a characteristic pattern of behaviour and response to treatment.

> ## Management
>
> The tumour is excised by ipsilateral thyroid lobectomy as above. In the case of anaplastic carcinoma this may not be possible, in which case the lesion is biopsied. Descriptions of the individual types of thyroid carcinoma together with their management, are given below.
>
> Table 13 shows the main features of each type.

Papillary carcinoma

Papillary carcinoma is of low-grade malignancy and rarely fatal. It occurs in the younger age group, usually in children or young adults, and is more common in females. On histology there is hyperplastic epithelium in the follicles with very little colloid. The disease may be multifocal. It tends to spread to lymph nodes and these may appear before the primary growth is palpable. This was described in the past as a 'lateral aberrant thyroid'. There is an association with irradiation of the neck in childhood.

Treatment

Papillary carcinomas are hormone sensitive. Following thyroid lobectomy the patient is started on T4 and maintained on this therapy for life. Some surgeons perform a total thyroidectomy for this lesion because of its multifocal nature. Others adopt a 'wait and see' policy and remove the other lobe of the thyroid gland if there is evidence of further disease. Direct suppression is achieved with T4 100 μg/day. This tumour is usually not

Table 13 The features of various types of thyroid cancer.

Type	Age group	Response to hormone therapy	Response to deep X-ray	Response to ^{131}I	Spread
Papillary (paediatric)	Teenagers and 20s	++	−	− (10–20%)	Lymph nodes
Follicular (forties)	40–60	+	−	+	Bloodstream
Anaplastic (aged)	50–60	−	+	−	Local and lymphatics

sensitive to radioactive iodine therapy and if metastases occur to lymph nodes locally they are usually treated by limited block dissection.

Follicular carcinoma

This tends to occur in slightly older patients, often middle aged. Females are more affected than males. The growth spreads through the bloodstream and bony secondaries are common. The lesion may arise in a pre-existing nodular goitre. The tumour is radiosensitive.

Treatment

Radioactive iodine is the treatment of choice for secondary disease. Metastases will not, however, take up the iodine if the rest of the thyroid is present and the gland has to be ablated by radioactive iodine or excised before they can be treated. Metastases can then be detected and treated by further radio-active iodine scanning. Patients with follicular carcinoma are also maintained on T4 suppression therapy.

Anaplastic carcinoma

This aggressive carcinoma occurs in elderly patients, particularly in women. It grows rapidly and infiltrates the tissues in the neck. Compression of the trachea is common. Cervical lymph-adenopathy and recurrent nerve paresis are often apparent when the patient is first seen.

Treatment

Many anaplastic carcinomas are sensitive to radiotherapy and this is the treatment of choice, although there are special problems when the airway is compromised, as it frequently is. Treatment with radiotherapy causes further swelling of the gland and this can prove fatal. A recent advance has been to give the patient helium and oxygen to breathe during the initial radiotherapy and this can allow ventilation to continue. Otherwise a tracheostomy is required. This can sometimes be carried out at the initial biopsy operation.

Medullary carcinoma

This carcinoma arises in the parafollicular cells. It is of moderate malignancy and spreads to lymph nodes. It secretes calcitonin which can then be used as a tumour marker. There is a familial incidence and an association with adenomas elsewhere (see p. 202). Genetic screening is now available to detect the affected relatives of the index case. The patient may be of any age and the tumour has an equal sex incidence. In these respects it is different from other thyroid carcinomas. It is also much less common.

Treatment
Medullary carcinoma is treated by total thyroidectomy and block dissection of lymph nodes. Calcitonin can be regularly measured postoperatively to detect metastases.

Malignant lymphoma
There is much lymphatic tissue in the thyroid gland and lymphomas can arise there. They may also occur as secondaries from other sites. Lymphomas may occur in patients with Hashimoto's thyroiditis.

Treatment
They are treated in the same way as lymphomas elsewhere.

Thyroglossal cyst
The thyroid develops from the floor of the mouth. It migrates down from the foramen caecum of the tongue passing anterior to, and then behind, the hyoid bone, to eventually lie in the pretracheal space. As it descends it leaves a small canal connected to the tongue called the thyroglossal duct (Fig. 35a). Remnants of this duct may persist and give rise to a thyroglossal cyst.

The cyst lies in the midline anywhere between the chin and the thyroid isthmus. Fifty per cent lie over the hyoid bone. It may be connected to the tongue or the thyroid by fibrous remnants of the thyroglossal duct. Very occasionally these remain patent, forming either a sinus or a thyroglossal fistula.

Recognizing the pattern
The patient may be of any age, although the condition is commoner between the ages of 15 and 30 years. Women are more often affected.

The patient notices a painless lump in the neck. It may become infected, in which case it presents as a localized abscess which points to the skin.

On examination
There is a smooth, round, 1–3 cm diameter swelling lying in the midline of the neck, often near the hyoid bone. The skin

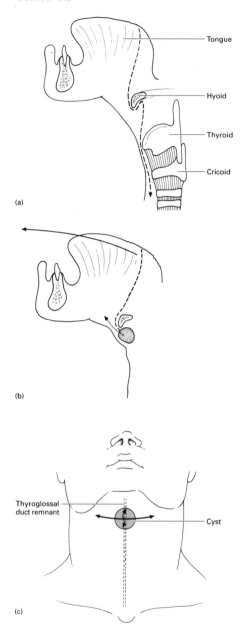

Fig. 35 (a) The descent of the thyroid — the track forms the thyroglossal duct. (b) As the tongue is protruded a thyroglossal cyst moves forward. (c) A thyroglossal cyst is more mobile from side to side than up and down.

moves over it unless it has been fixed by scarring following an episode of inflammation. The lump is of firm consistency and may fluctuate and transilluminate.

Ask the patient to open the mouth, steady the jaw and then protrude the tongue. Characteristically the cyst will move upwards (Fig. 35b). This may be easier to feel than see and is due to traction on the fibrous remnant of the thyroglossal duct. The cyst is more mobile from side to side than up and down (Fig. 35c). It may also move on swallowing, due to its attachment to the hyoid bone.

Palpate the base of the tongue for any thyroid tissue and look for any sinus opening to the skin (usually just above the thyroid isthmus).

Management

The treatment is to excise the cyst and any remnant of the thyroglossal duct. Because of the latter, the operation is more extensive than the patient will expect and he should be informed of this preoperatively.

OPERATION: EXCISION OF THYROGLOSSAL CYST

A transverse elliptical incision is made over the lump and the cyst is dissected out. The fibrous track running up towards the tongue is also excised and this should include removing the central portion of the body of the hyoid bone. Similarly any downward extensions are also removed.

Codes

Blood	Group and save
GA/LA	GA
Opn time	60–90 min
Stay	3–5 days
Drains out	48 h
Sutures out	4–5 days
Off work	2 weeks

Postoperative care

This is usually uncomplicated. If remnants of the track have been left behind, however, recurrent sepsis can occur.

4.2 Parathyroids

Hyperparathyroidism

The diagnosis and management of hyperparathyroidism rests on an understanding of the nature and physiology of the parathyroid glands and their secretion, parathormone. There are two glands on each side of the neck and they lie behind the thyroid gland. Each measures about $4 \times 2 \times 2$ mm. They consist of one main cell type, the 'chief cell', which has a 'water clear' appearance on microscopy when it is active.

Parathormone is an amino acid peptide hormone which regulates calcium metabolism. It has effects on the kidney, bone and gastrointestinal tract. Its secretion is controlled by the serum calcium level, being increased in hypocalcaemic states.

In the kidney it increases the reabsorption of filtered calcium, but the increased load of calcium results in an increased excretion of both calcium and phosphate. It also stimulates the production of the active metabolite of vitamin D.

In bone parathormone increases the number and osteolytic activity of osteoclasts and osteocytes, thereby mobilizing both calcium and phosphate. Vitamin D metabolites are necessary for this process.

In the gut parathormone indirectly increases calcium absorption by increasing the production of 1,25-dihydroxycholecalciferol (the active metabolite of vitamin D).

Hyperparathyroidism may be primary, secondary or tertiary.

Primary hyperparathyroidism

The parathyroid glands may become overactive and secrete excess parathormone causing hypercalcaemia.

This is due to one of the following:

1 A solitary adenoma (in 80% of cases of hyperparathyroidism)
2 More than one adenoma (2%)
3 Generalized hyperplasia of all four glands (16%)
4 Carcinoma (2%): this is locally invasive and may metastasize via the bloodstream. Recurrence after removal is common.

Secondary hyperparathyroidism

This occurs as a physiological response to chronic hypocalcaemia (e.g. chronic renal failure).

Tertiary hyperparathyroidism

Occasionally one of the glands involved in secondary hyperparathyroidism may develop an autonomous adenoma. This is tertiary hyperparathyroidism.

Recognizing the pattern

Primary hyperparathyroidism is more common in women than men and is usually seen after the age of 40 years. There may be a familial history of multiple endocrine neoplasia (see p. 202).

The majority of patients diagnosed are asymptomatic and discovered incidentally on biochemical analysis. When present the clinical features are very varied.

1 Renal stones. The patient presents with ureteric colic, haematuria or urinary tract infection. Three per cent of those with stones are shown to have primary hyperparathyroidism.

2 Renal disease. The kidneys are damaged by nephrocalcinosis, which predisposes to pyelonephritis and eventually chronic renal failure.

3 Bone involvement. This can cause vague rheumatic bone and joint pains. Pathological fracture is rare.

4 Hypercalcaemic symptoms, e.g. anorexia, weight loss, dyspepsia, polydipsia, polyuria, muscle weakness and tiredness. Hypertension and dyspnoea can occur.

5 Pancreatitis. There is a raised incidence of this condition with parathyroid overactivity.

6 Duodenal ulceration. This can occur in hyperparathyroidism and the latter is diagnosed when a serum calcium is measured as part of the general work-up.

On examination there is rarely anything to find. There may be corneal calcification adjacent to the corneoscleral margin. Bone disease can cause tenderness and swelling. It is very rare to feel an adenoma in the neck.

Proving the diagnosis

The following investigations may be undertaken:

1 Serum calcium. The specimen must be taken from a fasting patient with no cuff on the arm. Fifty per cent of the calcium is bound to albumin so a correction must be made if the albumin is low. The range of normality (which may vary slightly between laboratories) is 2.25–2.55 mmol/L.

2 Serum phosphate. This is low in primary disease but may be increased if there is any renal impairment.

3 Alkaline phosphatase. This is raised if there is significant bony disease.

4 Urinary calcium and phosphate clearance. The 24-h clearances of both calcium and phosphate are usually elevated but this is not consistent.

5 Parathormone assay. Parathormone can be measured by an immunoradioactive assay of intact parathormone (normal range 0.9–5.4 pmol/L). Patients with primary hyperparathyroidism occasionally have normal levels of parathormone, but this is still inappropriate in the presence of their high calcium levels. Hypercalcaemia from other causes will suppress parathormone production and the levels will be undetectable.

6 Radiology. There are characteristic bone changes due to excess of parathormone, particularly seen in the skull and hands. X-rays also help in the differential diagnosis, e.g. carcinoma of the bronchus seen on chest X-ray or myeloma seen on a skull X-ray.

7 Localization of an adenoma. It is now possible to cannulate the inferior thyroid veins selectively and measure the parathormone levels, a technique reserved for patients who have had a failed cervical exploration. This and proton emission scanning (PET) using Sestamibi (a modern radioisotope) are the most reliable methods of localization of a difficult adenoma.

Other causes of hypercalcaemia

Once hypercalcaemia has been detected, other causes of hypercalcaemia must be excluded. These include:

1 Carcinoma (bone metastases causing mobilization of calcium, or production of parathormone by a tumour).

2 Myeloma.

3 Vitamin D intoxication (due to excess intake of vitamin D-containing foods).

4 Milk — alkali syndrome (due to ingestion of milk and alkalis for indigestion).

5 Thyrotoxicosis.

6 Sarcoidosis.

7 Addison's disease.

8 Paget's disease or osteoporosis (where the patient is immobilized).

Management

The management of primary or tertiary hyperparathyroidism is surgical.

Preoperative management
Acute hyperparathyroidism. In this state the calcium level exceeds 3.75 mmol/L. The patient is dehydrated due to vomiting and polyuria and complains of headache, weakness and thirst. There may be tachycardia and low blood pressure, and eventually coma. An electrocardiogram (ECG) may show a short QT interval and evidence of dysrhythmia.

This condition must be treated before operation can be undertaken, primarily by correcting dehydration. A saline infusion is given and potassium may be required. Intravenous therapy should be monitored by central venous pressure measurement as the mortality is high. Intravenous calcium chelators are available (e.g. intravenous phosphate or disodium edetate). These should only be used in specialized centres as they are not without risk (e.g. intravenous phosphate can precipitate acute renal failure). If the calcium level still remains very high after rehydration, dialysis should be considered.

Vocal cord check. The vocal cord movements should be checked both before and after operation.

Arrange frozen section facilities. Immediate histology may be required during operation if there is doubt identifying parathyroid tissue.

Calcium estimations. It is worthwhile warning the laboratory that serial calcium estimations will be required postoperatively, particularly if this will be over a weekend.

OPERATION: EXPLORATION OF THE NECK FOR PARATHYROID ADENOMA
The neck is opened with a transverse skin crease incision and the thyroid is exposed as in subtotal thyroidectomy. The thyroid lobes are mobilized and retracted forwards. A methodical search is made for each parathyroid gland. If an adenoma is found it is removed and the diagnosis confirmed on frozen section. Further adenomas must also be excluded.

When all four glands are hyperplastic as in secondary hyperparathyroidism it is usual to remove three and a half glands, possibly reimplanting a remnant into a forearm muscle for ease of subsequent access. The other three removed glands may also be stored by cryopreservation.

If carcinoma is found, a radical local excision is performed.

Codes

Blood	Group and save
GA/LA	GA
Opn time	1–2 h
stay	2–3 days
Drains out	24 h
Sutures out	Clips or sutures 3–4 days
Off work	1–2 months

> *Postoperative care*
> As with thyroid surgery a pair of skin clip removers must be placed next to the bed in case acute haemorrhage should occur and cause tracheal compression.

Hypocalcaemia

This is common in the first 48 h after operation and may be transient due to bruising of the remaining parathyroids, or permanent if they have all been removed. Serum calcium levels must be taken each day for the first 3 days after operation. The clinical features of hypocalcaemia are tingling of the lips, fingers and toes, followed by the development of spasm of the hands and feet (tetany). Incipient tetany can be demonstrated by Trousseau's sign (if the patent is hypocalcaemic, carpal spasm develops within 2 min of inflating a blood pressure cuff on the arm above systolic pressure) or Chvostek's sign (tapping of the facial nerve in the cheek causes a twitch of the corner of the mouth and side of the nose). Overt tetany is shown by carpopedal spasm, when the hand is flexed at the metacarpophalangeal joints with straight fingers and the thumb strongly adducted. The foot and toes are plantar flexed.

Treatment of hypocalcaemia in the short term is with intravenous boluses of calcium gluconate (10% 10 mL). If the calcium level does not return to normal over the next few days, long-term treatment with vitamin D is required. Often large doses are needed and it may take a week before it begins to work. The newer synthetic analogues (e.g. 1α-hydroxycholecalciferol) work more quickly. Control can be difficult and often the levels need to be topped up with oral calcium preparations.

Multiple endocrine neoplasia

Parathyroid neoplasia (adenomas/hyperplasia) may be associated with neoplasia of other endocrine tissues that are characterized by the presence of amine precursor uptake and decarboxylation

(APUD) cells. The most frequently encountered endocrine tumours linked in this way are medullary carcinoma of the thyroid, phaeochromocytoma, and parathyroid adenoma (multiple endocrine neoplasia type IIA/Sipple's syndrome). The other principle syndrome is multiple endocrine neoplasia type 1 in which tumours may arise in APUD cells of the pituitary (e.g. prolactinoma), pancreas (insulinoma) and gastroduodenum (gastrinoma).

4.3 Adrenals, Benign Pancreatic Tumours

Adrenal tumours

The adrenal gland consists of an inner medulla and an outer cortex. The medulla originates from neuroectoderm and secretes catecholamines. The cortex develops from mesoderm and produces glucocorticoids, mineralocorticoids and some androgens and oestrogens.

Primary tumours may arise in both parts of the gland and can be benign or malignant. The adrenal gland is also occasionally a site for metastases, particularly from carcinoma of the breast or bronchus or from melanoma.

If the tumour is actively secreting hormones, specific treatment may be required before surgery can safely be undertaken. This section outlines the management of four conditions.

1 Phaeochromocytoma
2 Cushing's syndrome due to adrenal adenoma or carcinoma
3 Conn's syndrome due to adrenal adenoma or carcinoma
4 Adrenal carcinoma.

The initial diagnosis is usually made by the physicians, who then refer the patient for surgery. A detailed account of the presentation and investigation is therefore not included, the emphasis in this section being placed on surgical management.

Phaeochromocytoma

This is a tumour of chromaffin cells which secretes noradrenaline and adrenaline. There is a familial incidence and an association with medullary carcinoma of the thyroid, parathyroid adenomas and/or neurofibromatosis (multiple endocrine neoplasia type II A/B). It usually occurs as a single benign tumour in the adrenal gland. It is useful to remember that 10% are bilateral, 10% are malignant and 10% arise outside the adrenal gland. Tumours arising from chromaffin cells outside the adrenal gland only secrete noradrenaline.

The tumour causes hypertension which may be persistent or paroxysmal.

Recognizing the pattern

The patient may present with attacks of sweating, pallor, palpitations, angina, nausea and vomiting, abdominal pain, headache and nervousness.

Proving the diagnosis

The diagnosis is proved by finding high concentrations of catecholamine metabolites in the urine (metanephrine, normetanephrine and vanilylmandelic acid, VMA).

The tumour must be localized. An abdominal mass may be palpable or the blood pressure may rise during deep palpation in a particular site. If metanephrine (from adrenaline) is found in the urine then the tumour lies in the adrenal gland.

Various methods of localization are used. CT scanning is most frequently used to define tumour site and size. I^{131} MIBG (*m*-iodo benzyl guanidine) scintigraphy can locate active chromaffin tissue especially in secondary and ectopic phaeochromocytomas. T_2-weighted magnetic resonance imaging (MRI) is also helpful in difficult cases as is selective venous sampling.

Management

The tumour is treated by surgical removal. Traditionally this is by open operation through a laparotomy but endoscopic removal using a laparoscopic approach, or a retroperitoneal route is now possible, and results in a quicker less painful recovery.

Preoperative management

There is usually a degree of hypovolaemia in these patients due to prolonged vasoconstriction. A sudden drop in catecholamine levels as the tumour is removed may cause severe hypotension. The patient should be admitted 5 days before operation and given a- and b-blockers in an attempt to reverse this vasoconstriction and restore blood volume. The drugs used are the following:

1 Phentolamine (1 mg/kg orally or i.v.). One regime is to start with 10 mg 8-hourly and increase this dose until the blood pressure is controlled. Postural hypotension may occur.
2 Propranolol (40 mg 8-hourly orally).

An alternative is to use phenoxybenzamine and α-methyl paratyrosine.

The preoperative management must be discussed with the anaesthetist.

OPERATION: OPEN EXCISION OF AN ADRENAL PHAEOCHROMOCYTOMA

During operation there are two potential problems.
1 α- and β-blockade inhibits the sympathetic response to

Continued on p. 206

Continued.

hypovolaemia and so a central venous pressure (CVP) line is needed. A cardiac monitor and arterial line are also used.
2 Handling the tumour may cause a sudden surge in catecholamine levels which, despite the preoperative blockade, may cause a hypertensive crisis. A short-acting α-blocker, Phentolamine (5 mg i.v.), must be available to treat this. Propranolol (0.5–1 mg i.v.) or sodium nitroprusside (0.5–1.5 μg/kg/min i.v.) may be used.

The tumour is usually approached transabdominally and the whole adrenal gland removed, after the adrenal vein and multiple arteries are secured. This can be a difficult procedure, particularly in an obese patient. The sophistication and accuracy of preoperative investigation alerts the surgeon to possible bilateral or ectopic adrenal disease, which may also have to be removed.

Codes

Blood	4–6 units
GA/LA	GA
Opn time	2–3 h
Stay	About 2 weeks
Drains out	48 h
Sutures out	7 days
Off work	6 weeks

Postoperative care
A close watch must be kept on the CVP to detect any hypovolaemia. Volume loading to anticipate vascular dilatation secondary to the sudden withdrawal of catecholamines is essential. This is more appropriate than the use of pressor agents. Hypoglycaemia can also occur as a result of catecholamine withdrawal.

OPERATION: LAPAROSCOPIC ADRENALECTOMY
The gland may be approached transperitoneally or through the retroperitoneal tissues. A retroperitoneal space can be formed by placing cannulae in the flank and expanding the space using a balloon or dissection. The perirenal fascia is exposed and followed upwards to find the adrenal within its fascia. This is then mobilized and its vessels clipped and divided. The gland is removed.

Codes

Blood .... 4–6 units
GA/LA .... GA
Opn time .... 2–4 h
Stay .... 2–4 days
Drains out .... Nil
Sutures out .... Absorbable
Off work .... 2–4 weeks

> *Postoperative care*
> This is as for the open operation but the patient has much
> less pain and is therefore somewhat easier to manage and
> recovery is quicker.

Cushing's syndrome due to adrenal tumour

Cushing's syndrome is due to excess production of glucocorticoids. This is most commonly secondary to an abnormally
high adrenocorticotrophic hormone (ACTH) level, itself produced either by a pituitary adenoma or from an ectopic site (e.g.
carcinoma of the bronchus). In 20% of patients with Cushing's
syndrome there is a primary lesion in the adrenal gland, either
an adenoma or a carcinoma. Adenomas may be bilateral.

Recognizing the pattern

The patient characteristically gains weight and develops a bloated
appearance. The syndrome also consists of hypertension, hyperglycaemia and glycosuria, increased protein catabolism and a
predisposition to infection.

Proving the diagnosis

The diagnosis is proved by finding an elevated serum cortisol
with loss of the normal diurnal variation. There are increased
levels of cortisol metabolites in the urine. An adrenal primary
lesion is characterized by markedly depressed serum ACTH
levels. The tumour can be localized and assessed by CT scanning. When the lesion is over 6 cm in diameter arteriography,
venography or MRI scanning may identify vascular invasion
indicating malignancy and possible inoperability.

Management

The tumour is removed surgically.

Continued on p. 208

Continued.

Preoperative management
The production of adrenal hormones by tissue other than the tumour will be suppressed and the patient will be unable to respond to the stress of operation by increasing steroid secretion. Supplemental therapy must therefore be prescribed starting at the time of premedication. The usual dose is hydrocortisone 100 mg intravenously or intramuscularly.

OPERATION: ADRENALECTOMY FOR CUSHING'S SYNDROME
The tumour may either be approached anteriorly or postero-laterally. A posterolateral approach is used when the tumour site has been positively identified, particularly if it is large and on the right side and the other adrenal has been shown to be normal. This approach may involve opening the pleura, so it is necessary to warn the patient and the anaesthetist of this. A chest drain may be required postoperatively.

During the operation 100–300 mg of hydrocortisone is given intravenously.

The adrenalectomy can also be performed endoscopically as above.

Codes
Blood .... 4–6 units
GA/LA .... GA
Opn time .... 2–3 h
Stay .... 2–3 weeks
Drains out .... Chest 2 days, abdominal 2 days
Sutures out .... 10–14 days
Off work .... 2 months

Postoperative care
Steroid supplements must be continued. The usual regime is as follows.
Day 1: 100 mg hydrocortisone i.m. 8-hourly
Day 2: 50 mg hydrocortisone i.m. or orally 8-hourly
Day 3: 50 mg hydrocortisone i.m. or orally 12-hourly
Day 4: 25 mg hydrocortisone i.m. or orally 12-hourly.

After this the steroids may gradually be stopped in the hope that the other adrenal will start working. Occasionally a small dose of ACTH may be required. If, despite this, the other gland does not function, or if both glands have been removed at operation, replacement therapy will be required long term. This is as follows:

1 Hydrocortisone 20–30 mg/day in twice daily dosage, two-thirds given in the morning and one-third in the evening.
2 Fludrocortisone 0.1–0.2 mg/day in twice daily dosage, two-thirds given in the morning and one-third in the evening.

During the first 24–48 h the blood pressure should be measured half-hourly to detect evidence of steroid insufficiency. A close watch must be kept on the electrolytes and blood sugar. If any complications arise, the steroid supplements must be increased.

Cushingoid patients are more susceptible to postoperative complications such as poor wound healing, wound infection or haemorrhage, which is a compelling reason to consider the less traumatic endoscopic removal.

Conn's syndrome

This is due to excessive production of aldosterone by an adenoma of the zona glomerulosa cells of the adrenal gland. Occasionally it is due to bilateral hyperplasia. Carcinoma is a rare cause.

The syndrome is characterized by hypertension, renal damage, hypokalaemic alkalosis and muscle weakness.

Proving the diagnosis

Investigations show a high urinary potassium content despite a low serum potassium and a high serum bicarbonate. The serum aldosterone level is elevated.

Localization of the tumour is difficult as it is often small and may be multiple and bilateral. Radionucleotide imaging using radiolabelled cholesterol during dexamethasone suppression identifies functioning adrenocortical tissue and can detect tumours as small as 5 mm in diameter.

Management

The tumour must be removed.

Preoperative management

The body is potassium-depleted and this should be corrected before operation by a high-potassium, low-sodium diet. Spironolactone (200–400 mg/day) also helps. Steroid supplements as above should start with the premedication.

OPERATION: ADRENALECTOMY FOR CONN'S
SYNDROME

The best approach is probably laparoscopic or by an open
posterior route. An anterior approach can also be used. The
tumour is removed.

Hydrocortisone may be required during operation as
described above.

Codes

Blood	4–6 units
GA/LA	GA
Opn time	1–2 h
Stay	2–5 days
Drains out	Rarely required
Sutures out	7 days
Off work	6 weeks

Postoperative care
Replacement therapy may be required as above.

Adrenal carcinoma

Carcinoma may occasionally present with no evidence of endocrine disturbance. It is usually fast growing with rapid invasion
and early metastases. It presents with loin discomfort, weight
loss and possibly a palpable mass. It is localized with the aid of
CT, ultrasound or MRI scan.

Management

In view of the very poor prognosis any surgery is mainly
palliative. Some inoperable or recurrent disease responds to
chemotherapy using mitotane (*o,p'*-DDD, a derivative of the
insecticide DDT) Removal must be accompanied by steroid
supplements as outlined above.

For the operation note, codes and postoperative management, see under adrenalectomy for Cushing's syndrome,
p. 208.

Benign endocrine tumours of the pancreas

The most important benign tumours of the pancreas are those
derived from the islet cells. These are part of the APUD system
(see p. 203). An insulinoma is a tumour derived from the β cells
of the islets. It produces an excess of insulin. A gastrinoma is

derived from non-β cells and produces an excess of gastrin. The latter results in gastric hyperacidity and severe duodenal ulceration (Zollinger–Ellison syndrome).

Other tumours may secrete vasoactive intestinal peptide (VIP), causing diarrhoea and hypocalcaemia (Verner–Morrison syndrome), or glucagon, causing mild diabetes. Most of these tumours are benign and for convenience both benign and malignant forms are described here. They may be associated with other lesions in the APUD system.

Insulinoma

Ten per cent of β-cell tumours are multiple and 10% are malignant. Over 90% are situated in the pancreas, the remaining few being found in ectopic pancreatic tissue. The tumour is frequently less than 2 cm in diameter.

Recognizing the pattern

The patient is usually between the ages of 20 and 40 years. The excessive insulin production results in marked hypoglycaemia and the patient suffers from attacks of unconsciousness or strange behaviour and may become intensely hungry. He may gain a lot of weight.

Proving the diagnosis

This may be difficult. Patients are frequently misdiagnosed as having epilepsy or psychiatric disease. Whipple's triad is helpful when trying to make the diagnosis and states the following:

1 The attacks are induced by starvation or exercise.

2 Hypoglycaemia is present during an attack (blood glucose less than 2 mmol/L).

3 The episode is relieved by giving sugar orally or intravenously.

Once the possibility of this condition has been recognized the diagnosis can be confirmed by the following:

1 Measuring the plasma insulin levels by radioimmunoassay. The levels are inappropriately elevated in the presence of hypoglycaemia.

2 Fish insulin test. The patient is given an injection of fish insulin. This produces hypoglycaemia which would normally suppress the patient's own insulin production. In the presence of an insulinoma this suppression does not occur.

3 The actual tumour may occasionally be identified by the following:

   (a) abdominal CT scan or ultrasound (detection rate 40–50%)

(b) selective coeliac axis arteriography. An abnormal tumour 'blush' is seen in 60–70% of cases

(c) venous sampling. The portal vein is cannulated transhepatically and blood is sampled from various sites around the pancreas. The level of insulin is measured and can give an indication of the site of a tumour. The technique is not without hazard.

Management

The tumour is excised. Medical treatment can be used when the tumour is not found at operation or if there is a malignant tumour with metastases. Diazoxide (5 mg/kg daily in divided doses) suppresses insulin release and is effective in 50% of patients. Streptozotocin (1 g/m^2 body surface) can be used for malignant insulinomas. It is selectively toxic to malignant islet cells.

Preoperative management

Set up an intravenous infusion of 5–10% dextrose 12 h before the operation to maintain the blood sugar during the preoperative fast.

OPERATION: EXCISION OF AN INSULINOMA

A laparotomy is performed and the pancreas and surrounding tissues palpated and scanned with intraoperative ultrasound, to search for the tumour. When it is found, it is excised. If no tumour is found, the surgeon may elect to remove the body and tail of the pancreas in the hope that an impalpable tumour will be found on microscopy. Alternatively, the patient can be treated with diazoxide and re-explored after a period of time, when the tumour may be larger and easier to find. If a tumour is found, the rest of the pancreas must be palpated to exclude multiple adenomas. Blood sugar may be measured after enucleation. Persistent hypoglycaemia suggests that a second tumour is present.

Codes

Blood	2–4 units
GA/LA	GA
Opn time	2–3 h
Stay	7–14 days
Drains out	5–7 days
Sutures out	7 days
Off work	6 weeks

The remaining b cells may be suppressed by the chronic hypoglycaemia. When the tumour is removed, rebound hyperglycaemia may develop in the first 4–5 days and insulin therapy may be needed for a short period. There is also a danger of postoperative pancreatitis, and pancreatic sepsis and fistula formation are not uncommon. If a pancreatic fistula develops, the skin must be protected from autodigestion, using a barrier cream. The fistula will usually heal spontaneously in 2–3 weeks.

Zollinger–Ellison syndrome

In this condition there is excessive production of gastrin by a non-β cell adenoma often situated in the pancreas. The patient develops severe duodenal and gastric ulceration and his life may be threatened by recurrent haemorrhage or perforation. Thirty per cent of such tumours are malignant and 80% are multiple in the familial form (multiple endocrine neoplasia type I). Sixty per cent are malignant and solitary in the sporadic form.

Recognizing the pattern

The usual age at presentation is around 40 years and the condition is slightly more common in males. The symptoms and signs are those of an aggressive duodenal ulcer which is difficult to control (see p. 295). The condition should always be considered in patients who develop recurrent ulcers after adequate surgical treatment.

Proving the diagnosis

The diagnosis is proved by finding high serum gastrin levels in spite of a low gastric pH (which normally inhibits gastrin secretion).

The gastric function tests show a raised basal acid output (e.g. over 15 mmol/h). A barium meal and endoscopy show extensive ulceration and scarring.

Secretin or calcium administration produces an abnormal rise in serum gastrin. This rise is not seen with simple hyperplasia of the antral cells.

Methods of localizing the tumour are the same as those described above for insulinoma.

Management

This may be medical or surgical, and is still controversial. Symptoms may be relieved by cimetidine or ranitidine

Continued on p. 214

Continued.

(cimetidine 1–3 g daily) and more recently with proton-pump inhibitors (omeprazole 20–180 mg/day). This may be used either for short-term treatment before operation or in the long term.

In order to prevent ulcer formation total gastrectomy used to be performed. This is rarely required with medical treatment today. However, tumour enucleation or excision (distal pancreatectomy) are performed.

Many patients can now undergo curative resection following improved methods of early preoperative detection. The proportion may be as high as 40%. Complete tumour resection enhances survival over incomplete resection or medical management from 21 to 76%.

5 Breast Surgery

5.1 Breast Lumps and Benign Breast Conditions

Most women presenting to hospital breast clinics have benign breast conditions, including fibroadenomas, fibroadenosis, cysts, cyclical and non-cyclical mastalgia and nipple discharge.

Normal breast

Normal breast tissue is in continual change in response to the changing hormonal profiles during the menstrual cycle. There are 15–20 lobes in each breast. Each lobe is separated by fibrous tissue joining the pectoral fascia to the skin and thus supporting the breast (Cooper's ligaments). The secretory unit of the breast is the lobule. Each lobule consists of a variable number of acini, which drain into an intralobular duct. This links to extralobular ducts, which in turn form subsegmental, then segmental ducts (Fig. 36).

The lobule has a loose connective tissue, while the extralobular tissue has a denser fibrous structure. The rest of the breast is made up of adipose tissue with blood vessels and lymphatics.

Normal breast and the menstrual cycle

The breast undergoes minor changes during the menstrual cycle. The lobular stroma becomes oedematous under the influence

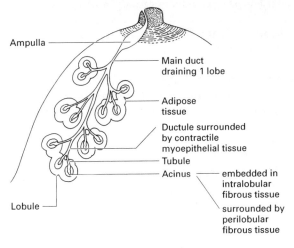

Fig. 36 A schematic diagram of the anatomy of a breast lobe — see text for a detailed description.

of oestrogens. There is mild proliferation of the acinar epithelium in the second half of the menstrual cycle, with programmed cell death (apoptosis) when hormone levels fall.

Changes in the breast with age

Following maturation during the teenage years, the female breast is composed of very variable proportions of fat and glandular tissue, contributing to considerable variations in size, shape and consistency. Varying degrees of asymmetry between left and right breast are not uncommon. The breast varies in consistency from softness to considerable nodularity, particularly palpable in the upper outer quadrants of the breast.

The fatty tissue tends to involute with age at a faster rate than the glandular tissue, a process which is often accelerated following childbirth and breast-feeding. This brings the underlying glandular tissue and natural lumpiness into greater prominence.

The responsiveness of the breast to the fluctuating endocrine environment often changes considerably in the late 30s and 40s, with mastalgia becoming much more common. Involutional and ageing changes also make breast cysts very common between 35 and 50 years. These cysts can sometimes be multifocal and very large (up to 50 ml).

The growing popularity of hormone replacement therapy may also alter the pattern of ageing of the female breast, and the pattern of presentation of benign breast disorders. For example, there may be a prolongation of the age range over which breast cysts and mastalgia may persist.

Assessment of symptomatic breast disorders

Objectives

1 To reach an accurate diagnosis as rapidly and cost-effectively as possible, so as to be able to reassure the patient with a benign breast lump or disorder.

2 To initiate treatment as rapidly as possible where malignancy is confirmed.

3 To avoid surgery where possible on benign breast lesions.

4 To use 'triple assessment' with the diagnostic triad wherever appropriate. This combines the skills of surgeons, radiologists and pathologists comprising:

   (a) clinical history and examination
   (b) imaging (ultrasound scan and/or mammography)
   (c) cytological or histological examination, usually from fine-

needle aspiration (FNA) cytology, or from devices to obtain cores of tissue.

Many breast units score each component of the triad on a scale of 1–5 (or –2 to +2), such that the higher the score, the stronger the indication for definitive treatment, thus:

- 1 or –2: completely normal
- 2 or –1: abnormal, definitely benign
- 3 or 0: abnormal, uncertain
- 4 or +1: probably malignant
- 5 or +2: definitely malignant.

With adequate organization and resources, it is often possible to achieve these objectives with a single hospital visit. This has become popularized as the 'one stop' clinic concept.

History

The following points may be helpful in reaching the diagnosis:

1 Age. Fibroadenomas and fibroadenosis are common below the age of 30 years, but cancers are uncommon.

2 Length of history. Determine how long the lump has been noticed. What was the relationship of its appearance to the menstrual cycle? Has it changed in size?

3 Pain. Was the lump painful and is it painful now?

4 Menstrual history. Remember that a premenopausal woman who has had a hysterectomy with ovarian conservation may still experience cyclical breast symptoms.

5 The presence of a lump. Has a lump been noticed and does it vary in size?

6 Nipple discharge (colour, volume, pattern, duration, frequency).

7 Pregnancy and breast-feeding. Has she had children and if so how old are they? This will tell you how old she was when she conceived them. There is some evidence to suggest that pregnancy in early life protects against malignancy. Were any children breast-fed or not and if so for how long?

8 Family history. A detailed family history will be helpful for epidemiological purposes and for risk assessment, in conjunction with specialist advice on screening and follow-up. Many breast units now run a family history clinic. Current information suggests that between 5 and 10% of breast cancer cases may have a genetic or familial component, with a predisposition to other epithelial and ovarian carcinomas.

9 Medication, particularly whether she has been on the pill or hormone replacement therapy. What is the form of administration (e.g. depot, oral)?

Examination

The patient must be examined in a good light, as changes in the contour of the breast are helpful in making a diagnosis.

1 Ask the patient to sit up first and observe both breasts looking for masses or dimpling of the skin. Ask her to indicate any lump.

2 If a lump is found, determine:
   (a) Shape
   (b) Size
   (c) Surface
   (d) Edge
   (e) Consistency
   (f) Fixity, and attachments.

Ask the patient to raise both elbows high in the air. Skin tethering due to a tumour may become visible. Attachment to the pectoral fascia is assessed by asking the patient to place her hand on her hip. Pressure on the hip causes contraction of the pectoral muscle and this will increase fixity of the lump if it is attached deeply.

3 Observe for breast erythema and oedema, and for arm lymphoedema.

4 Sit the patient comfortably at 45 degrees. Palpate each quadrant of each breast systematically. Start with the normal breast. Palpate with straight fingers, and avoid digging into the breast with the fingertips.

5 Look for evidence suggestive of metastatic spread. Make no assumptions! Palpable axillary nodes are sometimes reactive and not malignant. Examine the axillary and supraclavicular lymph nodes, the chest (for an effusion) and the abdomen (for hepatomegaly). The liver may be enlarged for many reasons other than for metastatic breast cancer (Fig. 37).

Self-examination

Women should be encouraged to assess their own breasts and told to report any new lumps which persist beyond menstruation, or which change in character.

Ultrasound scanning

Ultrasound examination of lumps and nodularity is an essential part of the assessment of breast disorders in women under the age of 40 years. It has a useful adjunctive diagnostic role in older women, where it can be used to guide FNA sampling. Its accuracy depends on the skill of the radiologist performing the examination. In trained hands it can be confidently used to distinguish cysts, tumours and benign nodularity. As the natural

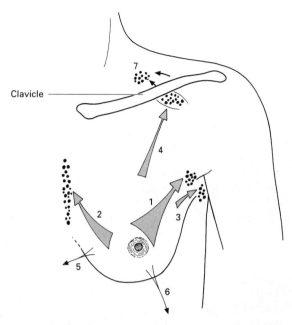

Fig. 37 The lymphatic drainage of the breast. 1, 2: Main routes of drainage, to the anterior axillary nodes and internal thoracic nodes. 3, 4: Minor routes; the axillary tail drains to the posterior axillary nodes and the upper and outer quadrant drains to the infraclavicular nodes. 5, 6: Potential routes of drainage, to the opposite breast, axilla and the extraperitoneal lymphatics of the anterior abdominal wall. 7: Routes 1, 3 and 4 drain ultimately to the supraclavicular nodes.

density of glandular tissue in the under 40s significantly reduces the sensitivity of mammography, ultrasound is usually the imaging investigation of choice in this age group.

Mammography

There are a number of reasons for performing mammography, including the assessment of symptomatic breasts, and the screening of asymptomatic women.

The features on a mammogram suggestive of cancer are as follows:

1 The general crab-like shape with disruption of the normal structure.

2 Microcalcification within the substance of the mass.

3 Thickening of the skin over the lesion due to early oedema.
There is a small false-negative and false-positive rate.

Symptomatic presentation

Mammography is a key part of the diagnostic triad in the over 40s age group. It is particularly useful in the detection and characterization of deep, radiodense and bilateral lesions. Single or biplanar views (oblique and craniocaudal) may be selected. The false-negative rate is significant (up to 10%), and some obviously palpable tumours do not show up on X-rays. It should thus not be used in isolation from FNA and skilled examination.

Breast screening

The introduction of a nationwide breast screening programme in the late 1980s, has had a major impact on the organization and provision of breast services in the UK. It allows for community-based mammographic screening of all women between the ages of 50 and 64 years at 3-yearly intervals, and sets strict criteria to ensure quality and cost-effectiveness. Patients with lesions diagnosed on screening are further assessed and treated in specialist referral centres.

FNA cytology

Where a lump is present, FNA will commonly be performed. Trained cytopathologists can interpret FNA samples with considerable accuracy when sufficient sample is provided. FNA is usually undertaken after imaging. Tissue distortion induced by bruising, a common event, may otherwise mislead the radiologist. Cell samples may be 'hot reported' from slide smears immediately, or stored in fixative solutions for later study. The accuracy of this method depends on the experience of the cytologist and the ability to produce an adequate sample.

To perform FNA, the lump is fixed between the thumb and forefinger. A 21-gauge needle attached to a 10-ml syringe is passed several times through the centre of the mass. The consistency of the lump to the needle may identify the 'gritty' feel of a carcinoma or the rubbery feel of normal glandular tissue. A cyst may immediately yield fluid.

Breast biopsy

A guiding principle of modern breast surgical practice is the avoidance of open surgery without a definitive diagnosis. FNA sampling is sometimes uninformative and Trucut-type biopsies may be helpful. With this technique a small cylinder of the lesion is excised using a Biopsy gun or Trucut needle. There is no good evidence to suggest that either aspiration or needle biopsy causes local spread of cancer.

Open surgical biopsy is occasionally necessary for symptomatic lumps, and usually for screen detected lesions.

OPERATION: BIOPSY OF BREAST LUMP
Open biopsies are usually undertaken under general anaesthetic. The lump must be marked preoperatively by the surgeon undertaking the procedure and confirmed by the patient. A periareolar incision often provides good access and excellent cosmesis. Good haemostasis within the biopsy cavity is necessary. The wound may also be vacuum drained.

Codes
Blood .... Not needed
GA/LA .... GA
Opn time .... 15–30 min
Stay .... Day case
Drains out .... Same day or within 24 h
Sutures out .... 7 days
Off work .... Less than 1 week

Postoperative care
An early outpatient appointment should be made for the discussion of results and removal of the suture.

Histology
Biopsy samples may be studied in two ways:
1 Paraffin section. The tissue is first embedded in wax and allowed to set before sections are cut and stained. The process takes about 2–3 days.
2 Frozen section. The fresh tissue is frozen hard and cut immediately. A histological diagnosis is usually available in about 15–20 min. The quality of such sections is slightly inferior to paraffin sections.

Requests for frozen-section diagnoses at the time of breast surgery are becoming increasingly uncommon. They do not allow informed planning with the patient of the treatment options in advance of surgery. It is also sometimes difficult to determine an accurate diagnosis on a frozen section.

Other investigations
The most useful predictor of metastatic potential of breast cancer is the presence of deposits of tumour in the regional

lymph nodes. A number of investigations (e.g. liver function tests, bone scan, skeletal survey, ultrasound scan of the liver) may indicate the presence of other metastases. However, it is not now considered efficient or cost-effective to undertake them as screening investigations in the absence of specific symptoms or indications.

Summary of the management of a breast lump

Figure 38 summarizes the steps in the management of a benign lump in the breast.

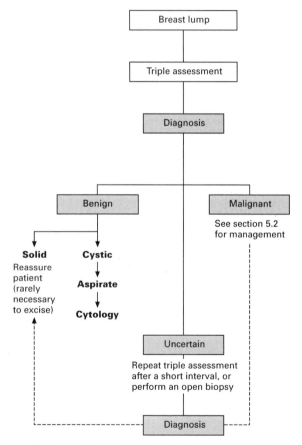

Fig. 38 A generally accepted scheme for the management of a breast lump. Note that all such schemas are only outlines of the management pattern and principles. Management may vary considerably according to specific circumstances and clinical judgement.

Benign mammary disorders

Terminology about benign breast disorders has in the past been very confusing. Most symptoms, even when severe, are simple manifestations of normal physiological change and occur in the absence of any pathology. Nodularity and mastalgia are separate conditions that can coexist. The inappropriate use of terms like mastitis (strictly implying infection or inflammation), or dysplasia (strictly implying premalignant change) can be misleading.

Benign mammary nodularity (fibrocystic change)

Fibrocystic change is the normal, nodular variant of glandular breast tissue. It represents a variation of the normal changes of hyperplasia and involution. It is usually symmetrical, but can be unilateral. It is most prominent in the upper, outer quadrant or axillary tail of the breast. It may or may not be associated with mastalgia (pain) and/or cyst development. It becomes more prominent with age, as the fatty tissue which gives the breast its fullness involutes.

Various terms are used to describe the changes that occur in the breast. Fibroadenosis is the prominence and the relative hypertrophy of the glandular–elements. The ductal epithelium can become hyperplastic (usual or regular ductal hyperplasia). An increase in the number of acini is known as adenosis. An increase in the interlobular fibrous tissue is known as fibrosis.

Women with marked nodularity are particularly difficult to assess by clinical examination, and may need to be followed up in a specialist clinic. Regular self-examination is helpful.

Recognizing the pattern

The patient has diffuse nodularity, particularly in the axillary tail. This may be either unilateral or bilateral, and may or may not be associated with breast cysts, discrete fibroadenomas or mastalgia. Women between 16 and 60 years of age may be affected. The nodularity may change with the menstrual cycle. There may be an associated history of premenstrual breast pain. There may be one or several areas of thickening in one or both breasts. The nodularity is diffuse and difficult to define. It is not fixed and there is no skin puckering. It may be tender.

Proving the diagnosis

This is done by conventional triple assessment.

Management of benign nodularity

Modern practice in the UK is conservative. It is geared towards the exclusion of malignancy, reassurance and avoidance of surgery. Scar nodularity can give rise to further anxiety later in life.

Fibroadenomas

Fibroadenomas may arise throughout adult life, either independently or in association with fibroadenosis. They are most common in the early adult years. They may be discreet or semidiscreet, and occur in a range of sizes, from a few millimetres to several centimetres.

In intracanalicular fibroadenomas, the stroma predominates and projects into the lumen of the ducts within the adenoma. In pericanalicular fibroadenomas, small, rounded islands of glands are encircled by whorls of stroma. The giant fibroadenoma (phyllodes tumour) is *not* a sarcoma. It may present as a large lobulated mass. Malignant change and local recurrence can occur with phyllode tumours.

Recognizing the pattern

The patient complains of a lump. Fibroadenomas may enlarge gradually. Their discovery may bring the patient rapidly to a doctor. Pain is rarely a feature. On examination the fibroadenoma is hard, discrete and mobile beneath the examining fingers.

Proving the diagnosis

Clinical examination and FNA cytology may be sufficient. Ultrasound scan and/or mammography may help in equivocal cases.

Treatment

Once the diagnosis has been made with confidence modern practice is to avoid surgery where possible, provided adequate imaging and cytology sources are available. Double and triple assessment has dramatically reduced the benign biopsy rate in specialist breast units in recent years. However, some women will still need to be reassured or relieved of symptoms by surgical removal of the fibroadenoma. If there is doubt histological confirmation is required.

Breast cysts

Breast cysts are a very common feature of breast involution and usually occur in the fifth decade. Acini may dilate and form cysts. The degenerating epithelial cells draw in fluid due to osmosis and quite large cysts may form rapidly.

Cysts may be single or multiple, unilateral or bilateral, and of various diameters from a few millimetres to several centimetres, with volumes of 0.5 to 50 ml. They usually present as a palpable lump, sometimes painful. The cyst fluid may be straw coloured, greenish or brownish. Blood in the cyst fluid is usually iatrogenic, although it may occasionally indicate a coexisting tumour. It is usually straightforward to aspirate cysts to dryness. Incidental small cysts noted on screening mammography can be left alone.

Recognizing the pattern

Breast cysts can occur at any age before the menopause. They may be recurrent, multiple and unilateral or bilateral. The lump usually appears and enlarges rapidly. It may be painful. Some cysts may regress spontaneously. On examination cysts are usually discrete, tense, smooth and rounded. The cyst may arise deep within the breast and may then be less well defined.

Proving the diagnosis

Triple assessment is appropriate where there is doubt. FNA proves the diagnosis. Cytology is not always essential for recurrent or multiple large cysts.

Management

Surgery is rarely necessary even if the same cyst fills repeatedly. Suspicion of a coexisting tumour is increased if FNA fails to produce complete resolution of the lump.

Follow-up is not essential, and common practice is to allow the patient an open access appointment if the cyst refills or if new cysts appear. Repeated presentation with cysts should not induce complacency. New lesions should be investigated.

The cyst fluid sample should be sent for cytology if:
1 The fluid aspirated contains 'old' blood
2 The mass does not disappear completely
3 The cyst refills.

Benign mastalgia

Mastalgia is a painful breast and may be cyclical or non-cyclical, and unilateral or bilateral. It varies considerably from one patient to another. There are no consistent histological changes in the breast. However, because it arises at an age when other changes such as the development of cysts are also common, it has attracted a number of misleading terms implying true pathology, for example mastitis, dysplasia and cystic mastopathy. The symptoms may occur in breasts of all consistencies, from the very soft to the very nodular.

Breast pain is very rarely due to carcinoma. It may be severe when caused by a breast abscess. Referred pain is rarely a cause of mastalgia.

Recognizing the pattern

Mastalgia usually arises in otherwise normal breasts in the 16–25 and 35–50 age groups. The onset, duration, severity and relief can be very variable. Symptoms usually do improve with time, although this may take weeks or months. The history is very variable in pattern and severity.

Cyclical pain
1 Worse at the time of periods
2 Awareness of breast swelling
3 Locally tender to touch.

Non-cyclical pain
1 Pain throughout or at random intervals during the menstrual cycle. Many women in this age group have undergone hysterectomies with ovarian preservation, and so cannot be precise about their cycle, although they remain susceptible to hormone-associated mastalgia
2 Otherwise as for cyclical mastalgia.

Proving the diagnosis

Imaging and cytology are rarely helpful except as a process of exclusion in nodular breasts.

Management

Most mastalgic pains will settle with time. Sympathetic support and reassurance are essential. A host of medical remedies have been proposed, of which most are ineffective. Evening primrose oil in its various formulations is sometimes of help. Endocrine manipulations such as danazol or bromocryptine are somewhat drastic and are rarely indicated, but may be effective in cases of disablingly severe and persistent pain.

Nipple discharge

Nipple discharge takes a variety of forms, and may be either physiological or pathological. Milky or serous discharge can persist for many months after cessation of breast-feeding. Most non-lactational presentations are minor physiological or involutional discharges of clear, milky, greenish or brownish discharge. Most are minor and self-limiting. One form which can be troublesome is mammary duct ectasia, in which ducts fill with degenerate epithelium, which is a thick green fluid.

Bloody discharge is suggestive of a duct papilloma or sometimes of a carcinoma.

Recognizing the pattern

Nipple discharges may occur at any time in the adult years. Physiological and duct ectasia discharges are frequently minor, intermittent, of low volume and persist for several months. Blood usually brings the patient much more rapidly to the clinic.

Proving the diagnosis

Smear cytology of the discharge may be helpful. The patient may be encouraged to express any fluid herself at the consultation. Mammography is usually necessary in the over 40s to exclude an underlying malignancy.

Management

Surgical intervention is very rarely indicated for physiological discharge and duct ectasia. In the case of persistent bleeding from a duct, with or without positive cytology, surgical biopsy by microdochectomy may be indicated.

The site of bleeding is noted and the patient is encouraged *not* to express fluid preoperatively. A microdochectomy is indicated where the discharge is from a single, defined duct. A subareolar resection of the ducts (mammodochectomy) is undertaken where a blood-stained discharge issues from several ducts or where the sites of the discharges have not been determined.

OPERATION: MICRODOCHECTOMY

At operation, a fine probe is passed down the involved duct, allowing its accurate excision either by an ellipsoid or a periareolar incision.

Codes

Blood	Nil
GA/LA	GA
Opn time	30 min
Stay	Day case
Drains	24 h where used
Sutures out	7 days
Off work	1–2 weeks

OPERATION: MAMMODOCHECTOMY
(SUBAREOLAR RESECTION)

In this case the nipple is again raised off the underlying tissues by a periareolar incision. The main ducts underneath the nipple are then excised as a block and sent for histology.

Codes

Blood	Nil
GA/LA	GA
Opn time	30–60 min
Stay	24 h
Drains out	24 h where used
Sutures out	5–7 days
Off work	1–2 weeks

Postoperative care

Bruising and haematoma may occur. Persistent and recurrent abscess formation may follow incomplete subareolar resection in particular.

Nipple inversion

Although not a pathology, this is a frequent cause of presentation. It may be unilateral or bilateral.

Most women develop nipple inversion naturally as part of the normal process of involution and postpartum change. The nipple is then often easily everted by gentle manipulation.

Recent change, or that associated with an underlying mass, may be caused by a tumour and is an indication for further investigation.

Mammary duct ectasia

The ducts are dilated and fill with foamy macrophages. The duct may rupture and cause a foreign body reaction. This reaction is characterized by the presence of plasma cells and is known as 'plasma cell mastitis'.

Recognizing the pattern

The patient is usually in her third to fifth decade. There is a history of discharge from one or more duct orifices.

On examination the lump may be palpable and tender, and there may be surrounding inflammation.

> **Management**
> This is usually conservative. The patient may be encouraged to express the fluid and to wear an absorbent pad or tissue within her bra. Sympathetic reassurance is essential.

Post-traumatic haematoma and fat necrosis

Bruising following traumatic injury to the breast may lead to residual organized scar tissue. Even when the history is clear, the examining surgeon cannot be certain whether the lesion is indeed scar tissue or a tumour arising *de novo*, and the lesion must be fully assessed. Beware the patient with cancer who claims a history of injury.

Recognizing the pattern

The patient will often give a history of trauma, although domestic violence may be concealed. On examination there may be bruising associated with an underlying lump.

> **Management**
> Usually conservative once a carcinoma has been excluded.

Galactocele

A galactocele is a milk-containing cyst which arises during late pregnancy or lactation. Ultrasound is helpful. Milk may be aspirated from the cyst. The cyst may recur, in which case repeated aspirations may be necessary.

Breast abscess

Breast abscesses commonly occur in the lactating breast, but can occur in non-lactating breasts throughout adult life.

Recognizing the pattern

The patient complains of a rapid onset of severe localized pain, which may be associated with a lump, erythema or discharge of pus. On examination there may be signs of inflammation with a hot, tender swelling of the infected area. This may become indurated or fluctuant.

Proving the diagnosis

Pus may be aspirated and sent for culture.

Management

Early bacterial infection may respond to antibiotics alone. In other cases, incision and drainage may be necessary.

OPERATION: DRAINAGE OF BREAST ABSCESS
The abscess is incised and curetted. Periareolar incisions give excellent long-term cosmesis. The wound is irrigated, and packed or drained.

Codes

Blood	Nil
GA/LA	GA
Opn time	15 min
Stay	1–2 days
Drains out	As determined by the size of the cavity and the rate of healing
Sutures out	Not applicable
Off work	According to circumstances

Postoperative care
Lactating mothers may continue feeding the baby from the opposite breast. Most wounds can be managed on an out-patient basis by district nursing staff.

Mammillary fistula

Occasionally, when an abscess has been incised or drained spontaneously, a fistula occurs between the skin and the duct, and continues to discharge. Treatment is to excise or lay open the fistula. The areola usually heals remarkably well.

Plastic surgery for benign disorders

Plastic surgery of the breast encompasses the various procedures which are undertaken primarily for cosmetic reasons, and which are thus driven by patient choice rather than mandated by disease. The major procedures may be classified as augmentation or reduction.

Breast augmentation

Augmentation may be unilateral (for congenital hypoplasia or atrophy) or bilateral. It may be used to correct significant asymmetry, or at the request of the patient for cosmetic enhancement. Augmentation is usually performed by insertion of one of a variety of expanders in the plane between the breast and the pectoral muscle, accessed through a fine inframammary incision.

Prosthetic augmentation can be complicated by early haemorrhage and infection, and later by trauma to the prosthesis, migration, leakage of contents and fibrous capsule formation. The presence of a prosthesis is a relative contraindication both to mammography and to FNA.

Breast reduction

Excessive unilateral or bilateral breast development relative to a woman's size and build can be a very disabling problem. Gross hypertrophy can occasionally follow lactation. A variety of breast reduction procedures have been developed. Resected breast tissue should be examined histologically after a reduction mammoplasty. Unexpected tumours and ductal carcinoma *in situ* (DCIS) are occasionally found.

5.2 Carcinoma of the Breast

Cancer of the breast is the most common malignant disease in women in the Western world. There is an incidence of approximately 24 000 tumours per year in the UK, and 15 000 deaths. Six per cent of women will develop the disease in the UK (50 per 100 000) per annum. Most carcinomas of the breast are invasive ductal carcinomas: histological subtypes include lobular and tubular tumours.

The natural history of established breast cancer is variable. Some tumours progress in a logical pattern from primary tumour to regional node metastases to distant metastases while others spread in a less predictable fashion. Axillary node status remains the best indicator of metastatic potential and adjuvant treatment.

Many biological factors are associated with poorer prognosis, and in particular the tumour grade, which correlates broadly with the degree of tumour differentiation. Unfortunately, there are no absolutely certain predictors of future behaviour which can be gleaned from study of the primary tumour. This unpredictability of behaviour has a major influence on the variety of treatments practised in different specialist breast units and on the many controversies which still surround the disease.

UK breast screening programme

The national programme has had a major impact upon clinical practice and upon the presentation of breast cancer. Women between 50 and 64 years are invited for community-based mammographic screening every 3 years. Some of these women have DCIS, a premalignant condition (see below), or small, impalpable invasive carcinomas. Films are reviewed by trained radiologists, who arrange the recall to multidisciplinary assessment clinics in specialist centres of all women with suspicious radiological abnormalities. A small proportion proceed to surgical biopsy, which may be radiologically guided in the case of impalpable lesions.

Ductal carcinoma *in situ*

DCIS is a premalignant condition which may be unifocal or widespread and which has come to prominence through screening programmes. Its propensity for microcalcification allows its early detection by mammography in many instances.

Management

The management of screen-detected breast cancer is shown in Fig. 39.

Localized DCIS may be fully excised by limited lumpectomy. Paradoxically, widespread DCIS may mandate a mastectomy to pre-empt the progression to invasive malignancy.

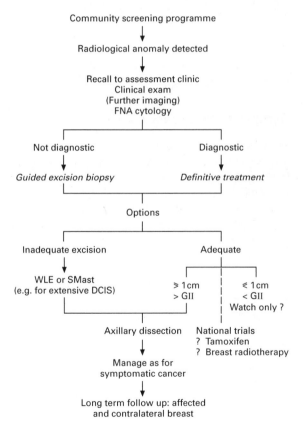

Fig. 39 The management of screen-detected breast cancer. (WLE, wide local excision; SMast, simple mastectomy.)

OPERATION: EXCISION OF THE SCREEN-
DETECTED TUMOUR
This is often performed as a day case. The patient will
usually be admitted on the day of surgery and will attend
the X-ray department for ultrasound scanning or wire localization of the lesion. The surgeon will aim to remove the
lesion through a small incision as suggested by the radiologist. The surgical specimen will be X-rayed immediately to
confirm excision of the radiological lesion.

Codes

Blood	Nil
GA/LA	GA
Opn time	45 min
Stay	Day case
Drains out	Where used 24–48 h
Sutures out	7 days
Off work	1 week

Symptomatic breast cancer

Recognizing the pattern

The incidence of cancer increases from the late teens, when it
is very rare, to old age. The tumour may present as:

1 A lump
2 With indrawing or other deformity of the nipple or skin
3 With pain (uncommonly)
4 With bloody discharge (uncommonly).

Women still present *de novo* (usually delayed through fear
rather than ignorance) with grossly advanced disease, including
huge masses with ulceration, erosion, oedema ('peau d'orange')
and erythema (inflammatory tumours). Involvement of axillary
and supraclavicular lymph nodes may be obvious.

The patient may find the lesion, or it may be noticed by a
partner or during a medical examination.

On examination. The lesion may be hard or soft and of any size.
Look for puckering of the skin over the lump. Where the primary treatment modality will be pharmacological, the size should
be carefully recorded at the first examination, to allow assessment of response.

Proving the diagnosis

The diagnosis is made on triple assessment, with percutaneous
or open biopsies occasionally necessary.

Table 14 The TNM classification of breast cancer.

Tumours	Nodes	Metastases
0 None	0 No nodes	0 No metastases
Tis = no tumour palpable		
1 0–2 cm, no skin fixation	1 Palpable mobile nodes (a) not significant (b) significant	1 Evidence of metastases
2 2–5 cm, skin distortion, no pectoral fixation	2 Palpable immobile axillary nodes	
3 5–10 cm ulceration, pectoral fixation oedema	3 Supraclavicular nodes	
4 >10 cm, skin involved, deep fixation		

Example: T_2N0M0 = a malignant mass less than 5 cm in diameter causing puckering of the skin on elevation of the arm but no other abnormalities found.

Management

Breast cancer is a complex and unpredictable disease. Treatment will be planned on an individual basis, taking into account many factors, including the patient's age and well being, the size and position of the tumour, and the patient's views.

Below the age of 70 years

The patient should have a chest X-ray and a careful examination carried out to look for axillary or other metastases. Generally patients below the age of 70 years judged to have operable tumours and with no overt evidence of metastases (including a clear chest X-ray) will be offered surgery. This will either be a wide local excision (WLE) of the primary tumour, or a simple mastectomy (SMast). Most units have a policy of axillary sampling or dissection (Ax. Dissn) to obtain sufficient lymph nodes to stage the disease. With histology available, the tumour can be staged according to the internationally recognized tumour node metastasis (TNM) system (Table 14).

Schematic illustrations of common treatment pathways for breast cancer are shown in Figs 40 and 41.

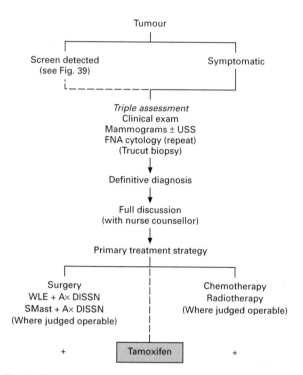

Fig. 40 The primary management of symptomatic breast cancer in the under 70s. A suggested scheme of management of a primary tumour (see also Fig. 38).

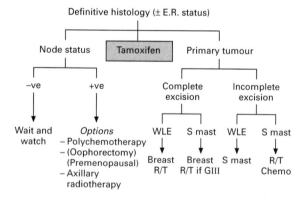

Fig. 41. The further management of breast cancer in the under 70s (see also Fig. 38). Note that extensive investigation is usually unnecessary in the absence of specific symptoms. Also, this diagram is for general guidance only. Treatment may differ considerably on the basis of individual and local circumstances.

Breast cancer in the over 70s

In the over 70s, primary treatment may be with tamoxifen or its analogues. Surgery is then reserved for those tumours which progress despite treatment when followed up for a number of months or years. The specific management will always be guided by an assessment of the woman's 'biological' age, circumstances and coexisting infirmities.

Paget's disease (carcinoma in the nipple)

Paget's disease is an eczematous, scaling plaque which appears around the nipple, caused by malignant cells infiltrating the epithelium of the areola. There is no connection with the underlying ductal carcinoma.

Recognizing the pattern

There is a red, scaly, weeping plaque involving part of the nipple and areola. There may be a lump beneath the areola.

Proving the diagnosis

The diagnosis of Paget's disease is proved on biopsy.

Management

The lesion is managed as an early carcinoma of the breast. Because the carcinoma is central, a simple mastectomy will often be necessary.

Surgery for breast cancer

Preoperative management

The consultant and breast counselling nurse should discuss the treatment plan with the patient. Breast radiotherapy is usually used as a postoperative adjunct to conservative surgery. The patient will need to consider this in making her choice. The breast and lesion will be marked preoperatively and checked by the surgeon.

OPERATION: WIDE LOCAL EXCISION

The lesion is removed together with a generous margin of surrounding tissue, influenced by the position and depth of the tumour and the shape and size of the breast. Deep closure often distorts the breast so vacuum drainage of the cavity is usually employed without deep sutures. Subsequent scar capsule formation and filling of the breast cavity with serous fluid often restores a degree of normal form to the surgically distorted breast. Subcuticular sutures usually produce a satisfactory cosmetic result with a fine narrow scar.

Codes

Blood 0

GA/LA .... GA

Opn time .... 30 min

Stay .... 48 h

Drains out .... 48 h

Sutures out .... 7–10 days

Off work .... 2–3 weeks

OPERATION: SIMPLE MASTECTOMY

Despite modern trends to conservative surgery, the simple mastectomy remains an important operation for central tumours, for those tumours that are large relative to the patient's breast size and for where radiotherapy is relatively contra-indicated. Mastectomy also reduces the risk of local recurrence compared to WLE and it remains the preferred operation by and for many women. The breast is excised, usually using a transverse elliptical incision to include the entire breast pad.

Codes

Blood .... Group and save

GA/LA .... GA

Opn time .... 45–60 min

Stay .... 5–7 days

Drains out .... 5–7 days

Sutures out .... 10–14 days

(or a buried subcuticular suture)

Off work .... 3–4 weeks

OPERATION: AXILLARY DISSECTION

This is an important adjunct to either wide local excision or simple mastectomy and is practised by most major units, with two principal objectives:

1 To obtain information on the metastatic potential of the tumour as a determinant of adjunctive therapy.

2 To remove malignant disease and thus to disrupt the pattern of spread.

Different surgeons dissect the axilla to differing degrees, recorded as level 1, 2 and 3 for the most radical dissections. Most adopt a level 1 approach, which yields a median of around eight lymph nodes per case in most series. Some units sample fewer nodes as a policy.

Axillary dissection is almost invariably followed by serous collections of fluid, which may require repeated needle aspiration for several weeks after removal of the surgical drains.

The axillary nodes may be sampled by extending the incision laterally, or through a separate incision. The surgeon aims to preserve the long thoracic nerve and the neurovascular bundle to the latissimus dorsi muscle.

Codes

Blood	Group and save
GA/LA	GA
Opn time	30 min
Stay	5–7 days
Drains out	3–5 days
Sutures out	7–10 days
Off work	3–4 weeks

OPERATION: RADICAL MASTECTOMY

This operation has largely been consigned to the history books. It is very deforming. The breast is excised *en bloc* with the sternal head of the pectoralis major and pectoralis minor. In the supraradical operation the chest is opened and the internal mammary chain of nodes is also removed. In Patey's operation, the pectoralis major muscle is left *in situ* but the pectoralis minor muscle is excised from beneath it, together with a full dissection of the axillary nodes.

Postoperative care

Serous collections commonly form beneath the skin flaps despite drainage. Axillary dissections usually lead to continued production of serous fluid for up to 3 weeks. It is usual practice to remove all drains at around 1 week, and to deal with further collections by percutaneous needle aspiration.

Other aspects of breast cancer care

Combined clinics

The treatment of breast cancer is multidisciplinary, and wherever possible, centres are being organized to facilitate communication between surgeons and oncologists, for example through combined treatment planning clinics.

Continued on p. 242

Continued.

Breast care (counselling) nurse

The breast care nurse plays an important part in the pre-, peri- and postoperative care, and psychological support. She will ensure that arrangements have been made for fitting an external prosthesis when the patient is discharged from hospital. In the early phase after mastectomy, patients may be issued with a lightweight external prosthesis, which may be replaced by a more permanent model after swelling has resolved and wound healing is complete.

Adjuvant radiotherapy

Adjuvant radiotherapy finds three general applications in breast cancer care. Details of technique, timing and dosage may vary from one unit to another.

Breast and chest wall

This is usually employed in the under 70s after WLE. In older women, tamoxifen treatment is often judged sufficient adjuvant treatment. It may also be used after simple mastectomy for aggressive, grade 3 poorly differentiated tumours or where there is doubt about surgical clearance at the deep margin of the breast.

Axilla

Some breast units perform limited node sampling (with radiotherapy in most cases). In other units, where more extensive node dissection is undertaken, postoperative radiotherapy is often not used. Where a nodal mass of tumour is judged inoperable, radiotherapy may be used. Axillary irradiation significantly increases the likelihood of arm lymphoedema.

Palliation

Radiotherapy may be used to palliate advanced local disease or bony metastases.

Adjuvant systemic chemotherapy

Drugs may be used singly or in combination, and the treatment may be intermittent or continuous. The agents commonly used are doxorubicin (Adriamycin), cyclophosphamide, methotrexate, 5-fluorouracil and vincristine. There is not yet complete agreement about the indications for postoperative chemotherapy. In general 'chemo', usually meaning serial courses of cytotoxic drugs in various combinations, is used in the following circumstances:

1 Where one or more axillary nodes are positive at primary surgery in the under 70s.

2 For grade III, histologically aggressive node-negative primary tumours in the under 70s.

3 For very large, advanced or inflammatory tumours at presentation.

4 For recurrent disease.

Chemotherapy does not guarantee cure. Meta-analysis of numerous clinical trials suggests that cytotoxic polychemotherapy reduces the overall risk of death by up to 14%. In premenopausal patients the reduction may be 20% or so. It may render an apparently locally inoperable tumour operable. Side-effects of these drugs may be severe, including bone marrow suppression, hair loss, nausea, diarrhoea and vomiting.

Endocrine treatment

Oestrogen receptors, tamoxifen and its analogues
Oestrogen receptor measurements are used in some breast units as predictors of response to tamoxifen therapy. Many primary breast cancers are receptor positive. Fewer metastases are oestrogen receptor positive. Most well-differentiated and lobular cancers are receptor positive.

Premenopausal women have a low rate of oestrogen receptor positive cancers. There is no definite indication for adjuvant tamoxifen in premenopausal patients outside clinical trials.

Hormone therapy is effective for many (perhaps 50–60%) oestrogen receptor positive tumours and also for some oestrogen receptor negative tumours (perhaps 10%). In post-menopausal women, tamoxifen reduces the chance of death by about 15%. Conversely, some patients fail to respond to hormonal treatment despite the presence of oestrogen receptors. Thus, in most units, tamoxifen is used empirically in virtually all postmenopausal women with invasive ductal tumours, regardless of oestrogen receptor status. It is continued until there is conclusive evidence of treatment failure, or for up to 5 years if there is a response.

The side-effects of oestrogens include withdrawal bleeding from the vagina. There may be a very small risk of endometrial cancer with prolonged tamoxifen treatment (> 5 years).

Continued on p. 244

Continued.

Oophorectomy

Meta-analysis of many trials shows that ovarian ablation may be as effective as polychemotherapy in survival terms. Ovarian ablation can be achieved by irradiation of the ovaries, or by ovarian removal (open or laparoscopic oophorectomy).

OPERATION: BILATERAL OOPHORECTOMY

A transverse lower abdominal incision (Pfannenstiel) is used. Alternatively, the same operation can be performed laparoscopically with a telescope in the umbilicus. Two other port sites are used, one of which will be slightly enlarged to remove the specimen.

In both approaches the opportunity is taken to look for evidence of other abdominal disease.

Codes

Blood	Group and save
GA/LA	GA
Opn time	1 h
Stay	Day case: 3 days
Drains out	24 h
Sutures out	7 days
Off work	Variable

Lymphoedema

Severe lymphoedema is less common since the demise of radical mastectomy and radical axillary radiotherapy. Modern axillary dissections are sometimes accompanied by milder degrees of lymphoedema, particularly after infection. Measures to reduce lymphoedema include the use of graded compression stockings, other forms of compression therapy and arm elevation. Some centres run lymphoedema clinics.

Management of advanced carcinoma

Cases of advanced primary disease may be referred directly for chemotherapy and/or radiotherapy. Women may be referred following surgery and when the histology results are available, for a variety of adjuvant treatment protocols in radiotherapy and chemotherapy.

Carcinoma of the breast typically metastasizes to the bone marrow, lungs, brain and liver. It may also recur locally despite seemingly adequate earlier treatment.

Many authorities now recommend that a widespread search for metastases should *not* be undertaken in the absence of symptoms at the time of presentation. The yield is very low, while the economic and emotional costs are very high. A chest X-ray is sufficient in most primary cases.

Metastatic spread and evidence of advanced disease may be revealed from a variety of investigations, which should only be used very selectively in response to specific symptoms. Possible tests include:

1 Liver function tests; alkaline phosphatase and alanine transaminase (ALT)
2 Serum calcium
3 Chest X-ray to look for any pulmonary deposits
4 Bone scan or skeletal survey by X-rays
5 Computed tomography may become increasingly useful in detecting metastases.

If evidence of more distant spread is found, the likelihood of long-term cure is remote, and management is then aimed at improving and sustaining the quality of life as far as is possible, and at preventing undue physical and emotional suffering. The early involvement of doctors and nurses specializing in palliative care may be helpful. A general scheme of the treatment options in advanced disease is shown in Fig. 42.

Continued on p. 246

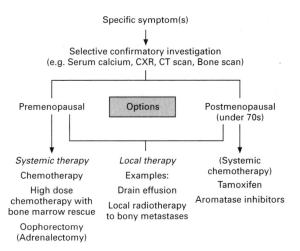

Fig. 42 The management of advanced breast cancer.

Continued.

Tools for palliative management
These include:
1 Palliative surgery (including fracture fixation)
2 Radiotherapy
3 Other hormonal manipulations.

Tamoxifen and its analogues — and aminoglutethamide and aromatase inhibitors, which impair steroid synthesis have —virtually replaced aggressive surgical procedures (bilateral adrenalectomy, hypophysectomy) to reduce oestrogen production.

OPERATION: BILATERAL ADRENALECTOMY
This is now rarely performed. The adrenals may either be exposed through bilateral loin incisions or through an upper abdominal transverse incision anteriorly (see pp. 205–206). The exposure is difficult, particularly on the right side, and ligation of the right suprarenal vein as it drains into the vena cava may be hazardous. The operation can also be performed endoscopically.

Terminal care
Advanced carcinoma of the breast requires positive management. It produces profound distress, fear and unpleasant physical symptoms. Analgesia should be given frequently and in sufficient doses to keep the patient out of pain. Hypercalcaemia may be managed by intravenous fluids and by osteoclast inhibitors such as pamidronate and etomidate. Corticosteroids and aspiration of the effusion can help breathlessness from a pleural effusion or lymphangitis carcinomatosa. Symptoms from hepatic metastases (e.g. pain and anorexia) may also respond to corticosteroids. Cerebral metastases may cause severe headache and focal neurological deficits and these may respond to dexamethasone or radiotherapy.

Plastic surgery of the cancerous breast
Most patients adapt satisfactorily to wearing an external prosthesis over the mastectomy scar. The prospective and actual loss of a breast can have profoundly depressive consequences for some women and their partners. Unilateral reconstruction can be beneficial and rewarding in selected

cases. However, immediate or delayed breast reconstruction should not be perceived to be, or offered as, a panacea to all psychological symptoms consequent upon the diagnosis of breast cancer.

There are a number of reasons why reconstruction may not be appropriate for a patient undergoing mastectomy or even WLE:

1 It involves additional surgical dissection and tissue trauma.

2 It introduces an additional range of complications.

3 It is difficult to achieve breast symmetry in all positions of arm and body movement, particularly with a large contralateral breast.

4 It is difficult to reproduce the natural ptosis of the more mature or postpartum breast.

5 Prostheses and postoperative scarring can make the assessment of new and recurrent breast cancer difficult in later years. FNA and mammography may be contraindicated in the presence of a prosthesis.

6 Immediate reconstruction may interfere with postoperative radiotherapy.

Where a patient is determined upon reconstruction, options include:

1 A silastic prosthesis or saline-inflatable implant placed either subcutaneously or under the pectoralis major.

2 A myocutaneous flap using lattisimus dorsi.

3 A transfer of the rectus abdominis myocutaneous flap (TRAM) with reconstruction of the abdominal wall defect.

5.3 Conditions of the Male Breast

The male breast is susceptible to many of the conditions of the female breast, including benign hypertrophy and less commonly, DCIS and invasive cancer.

Gynaecomastia

This is hypertrophy of the male breast. It may occur on one or both sides. There are many causes, the most important of which are listed in Table 15.

Recognizing the pattern

The condition is most commonly seen at puberty, in the 20s (and also affects users and abusers of anabolic steroids), in the 30s (testicular tumours), in the elderly and obese (idiopathic) and in men undergoing endocrine treatment for prostate cancer.

The presenting complaint is of unilateral or bilateral swelling beneath the nipple. There may be some discomfort. It may be discovered as part of more widespread disease, e.g. cirrhosis. It is important to take a careful drug history.

Table 15 Causes of gynaecomastia.

Physiological
neonatal
pubertal

Idiopathic

Hormonal
decreased androgens: hypogonadism
oestrogen therapy
tumour: testis, adrenal and liver
misuse of anabolic steroids

Cirrhosis

Hyperthyroidism

Drugs
digoxin
spironolactone
cimetidine

On examination the breast pad is enlarged. Tenderness is common. Inspect the testes for a tumour and look for evidence of liver failure or hyperthyroidism.

Management
Pubertal gynaecomastia usually settles within months. The patient should be reassured. If it causes persisting embarrassment, a subareolar mastectomy may be carried out. The management of other forms of gynaecomastia depends on the cause.

OPERATION: SUBAREOLAR MASTECTOMY FOR GYNAECOMASTIA
A semicircular incision is made around the edge of the areola and the nipple raised as a skin flap. The enlarged breast tissue is separated from the skin and underlying muscle, and removed through the central incision. The wound is drained using suction. The excised breast pad should be sent for histology.

Codes

Blood	Group and save
GA/LA	GA
Opn time	30–60 min
Stay	2 days
Drains out	2 days
Sutures out	7–10 days
Off work	1–2 weeks

Postoperative care
Removal of the breast pad leaves a large subcutaneous space which tends to fill with blood and serum. It is important to maintain suction drainage and external pressure to minimize troublesome haematoma formation. Day-case surgery can be inappropriate.

Carcinoma of the male breast
Approximately 0.6–1% of breast malignancies occur in men. There is an association with Klinefelter's syndrome.

Recognizing the pattern
The patient may notice a lump beneath the areola. Bloody discharge may rarely occur from the nipple.

On examination there is a lump within the breast pad, which is usually painless. There may be palpable, involved, axillary lymph nodes.

Proving the diagnosis

FNA or excision biopsy are diagnostic.

Management

Early carcinoma may be treated as in the female patient by mastectomy and/or radiotherapy and/or chemotherapy. The role of tamoxifen is uncertain. Orchidectomy may produce remission of advanced disease.

6 Chest Surgery

6.1 Chest Drainage and Thoracotomy

Chest drains

The indications for chest drainage are as follows:

1 A pneumothorax
2 A pleural effusion — serous fluid or pus
3 Haemothorax
4 To prevent the collection of fluid or air, e.g. after thoracotomy.

The procedure of insertion is described in some detail, as it is something most housesurgeons will have to do.

OPERATION: INSERTING A CHEST DRAIN
Make sure that all the equipment you require is ready before you start. This includes the following:

1 Local anaesthetic (1 or 2% Xylocaine).
2 Skin preparation.
3 A suitable tube drain (e.g. 20–26 Charrière gauge 'Argyle'), preferably with a radio-opaque line in it.
4 Stitches. It is useful to use materials of different colours. Stitches needed for:
    (a) holding the drain in
    (b) later closure of the skin.
5 The underwater seal drain with saline in it.
6 Straight artery forceps.
7 Available wall suction and a suitable connection for it.
8 A tube clamp.

The procedure should be done in the treatment room or theatre if possible.

The drain is usually inserted in the fourth or fifth intercostal space in the mid-axillary line, or in the second space anteriorly.

Position of the patient. He should be sitting up, and can either lean forward over a suitably placed bed table with his arms folded in front of the body (for a posterior or lateral approach), or lie back on pillows (for an anterior approach).

If you are about to drain an effusion check the presence of fluid by inserting a 19-gauge needle on a syringe at your chosen site. It can be helpful to mark the skin before scrubbing up.

Continued on p. 254

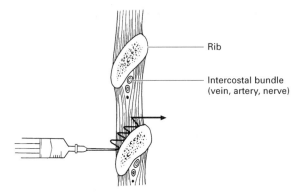

Rib

Intercostal bundle
(vein, artery, nerve)

Fig. 43 Avoiding damage to the intercostal bundle when entering the pleural cavity.

Continued.

1 Clean the skin.
2 Inject local anaesthetic, infiltrating the underlying tissues down to the parietal pleura. The presence of fluid can also be checked during this manoeuvre.
3 Incise the skin with a sharp, pointed scalpel and cut down on to the rib below the intercostal space chosen for the drain. Move upwards to enter just above the rib (Fig. 43) and enlarge and deepen the hole by inserting closed artery forceps into the pleura, thus creating a track for the drain. You may then enter a gloved finger into the pleural space to ensure that the tract is wide enough to accommodate the drain without having to push hard. Your finger will also confirm that you are in the pleural cavity and exclude the presence of viscera that could be damaged. There may be an egress of air or blood.
4 Put in two sutures:
   (a) a 2/0 nylon across the incision. This is left loose for tying to close the wound when the drain is removed
   (b) a 0 silk purse string for securing the drain.
5 Remove and discard the trochar and mount the tip of the chest drain tube onto a long curved artery forceps (Roberts). Introduce the chest drain into the track you have created and use the Roberts to angle its direction into the appropriate spot. Be sure that you put the chest drain in far enough.
6 Connect the drain to the underwater seal as shown in Fig. 44.
7 Tie it in securely and check that the meniscus is fluctuating.

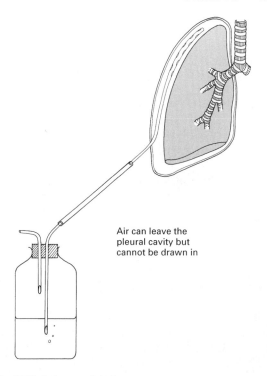

Air can leave the
pleural cavity but
cannot be drawn in

Fig. 44 Underwater seal drainage.

8 Suction should be applied to the venting tube of the bottle whenever significant drainage of fluid or air is expected. For preference use wall suction providing a high volume at low pressure. A Roberts pump is inadequate. 7–13 KPa of suction are applied.

Use of suction
Suction is applied to the chest drain to maintain a negative pressure (relative to atmospheric pressure) within the hemithorax. Suction is needed if there is an air leak from the lung into the pleural space as this prevents the lung expanding. If there is any degree of obstruction of an air leak by flaps of pleura on the lung surface or chest wall, a tension pneumothorax may build up.

Once a lung has collapsed its compliance (which is normally slightly less than that of the chest wall) will increase, often dramatically. This will tend to cause the lung to remain collapsed if suction is not applied.

Continued on p. 256

Continued.

Postoperative care

1 Check the position of the tube and the expansion of the lung by an early chest X-ray. This should be repeated daily.

2 Position of the bottle. The water seal must at all times be kept below the patient, ideally on the floor. If it is lifted up above the patient, the water may siphon into the patient's chest. Everyone, including the patient, nurses, auxiliaries and ward cleaners, must be told this.

3 Moving the patient. Have two clamps next to the patient to double clamp the tube when a change of position is required. One clamp may give way. Be certain these clamps are removed again once the move is over. **Never clamp a bubbling drain**.

4 Checking patency. The tube can be seen to be patent, and therefore draining, by observing the meniscus fluctuate on breathing or coughing. The swing reflects changes in pressure in the pleural sac and will remain high if the lung compliance is high.

5 Re-expansion of the lung. This is encouraged by early ambulation and breathing exercises. When the fluctuation of the meniscus in the tube becomes small, the lung is fully expanded and compliance returns to normal. If there is no 'swing' on the meniscus, the tube is blocked and is performing no useful function. Take a chest X-ray. If the lung is expanded, then the tube may be removed. This is done in two ways. After lung puncture or following spontaneous pneumothorax, it is usual to leave the clamped tube *in situ* for 24 h, then X-ray again. If the lung is still expanded, then the tube is removed. In other circumstances this practice is unnecessary provided:

   (a) there is absolutely no air leak present, nor has there been for a minimum of 24 h

   (b) there is a minimal or non-existent 'swing' of the meniscus within the drain.

Here the tube may simply be removed.

6 Removal of chest drain. Ask the patient to breathe in and then hold his breath (i.e. to do a Valsalva manoeuvre). In this way no air is sucked into the pleural space as the tube is removed. When the tube comes out, tie the skin closure stitch.

Some common problems with chest drainage

Tube bubbling on suction
1 There is a continuing air leak from the lung, or a major airway
2 The drain has slipped out and exposed one of the side holes
3 A fault or a leak somewhere in the circuit.

No bubbling on suction, but the lung is still partially or wholly collapsed
1 Tube blocked
2 Tube in incorrect space
3 Tube kinked or clamped by bed wheel or other item placed on top of it.

Breathlessness
1 Pneumothorax (?tension pneumothorax)
2 Pneumothorax on the opposite side of the chest
3 Haemothorax
4 Haemopericardium.

Thoracotomy
A thoracotomy maybe performed on a general surgical unit and you should be familiar with the pre- and postoperative care that this entails.

Preoperative management
Explain to the patient that he will have one or two tubes draining the chest postoperatively and tell him why (see p. 258). It will be important that he breathes fully and coughs adequately and to do this he must be given adequate analgesia.
One of the three following major incisions may be used.

OPERATION: POSTEROLATERAL THORACOTOMY
This may be used for access to the lung, oesophagus or descending aorta. The patient is placed in a prone or lateral position. The fifth, sixth or seventh intercostal space is opened.

Continued on p. 258

Continued.

OPERATION: ANTERIOR THORACOTOMY

This approach may be used for access to the heart, pericardium or anterior aspect of the lung for biopsy. The patient lies obliquely with the side to be opened uppermost. Access is usually gained through the fifth space.

OPERATION: MEDIAN STERNOTOMY

This is the best approach for the heart, pericardium, great vessels and anterior mediastinal structures. The patient lies supine and the sternum is split longitudinally with a reciprocating saw.

During closure, after the procedure has been completed, chest drains are inserted. There are usually two — one at the apex and one at the base. They are brought out through separate stab incisions, usually through the seventh or eighth space.

The chest drains are attached to underwater seal drainage.

Codes

Blood	4 or more units
GA/LA	GA
Opn time	Depends on indication for thoracotomy
Stay	7–10 days (except for oesophagectomy, see pp. 279–281)
Drains out	When air and fluid loss stops and there is no significant 'swing' on the fluid level or the drainage tube
Sutures out	7–10 days unless absorbable
Off work	2–6 weeks depending on procedure

Postoperative care

It is most important that the patient has sufficient analgesia to breathe adequately and cough. This may be achieved either by intercostal nerve blocks with long-acting anaesthetic (e.g. Marcain), a thoracic epidural (which requires careful nursing) or parenteral opiate drugs.

The management of the chest drain has already been described.

Thoracoscopic surgery

An increasing number of intrathoracic techniques are now being carried out thoracoscopically. The lung on the side of the

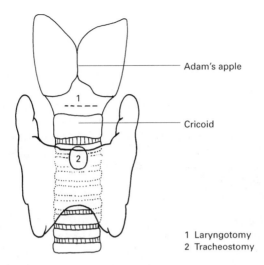

Fig. 45 Sites for laryngotomy and tracheostomy.

lesion is collapsed using a double-lumen endotracheal tube. An endoscope attached to a video camera is introduced through a suitable intercostal space, and instruments through other ports.

Lung resections, oesophageal operations and even cardiac procedures are now being done by these techniques. The advantage lies with the more rapid and less painful recovery achieved by avoiding an open thoracotomy.

Tracheostomy

Tracheostomy is indicated in three situations.

1 Upper airways obstruction, e.g.
  (a) impacted foreign body
  (b) laryngeal oedema due to epiglottitis, angioneurotic oedema of the tongue or spreading infection of the floor of the mouth (Ludwig's angina)
  (c) severe facial injury
  (d) facial burns
  (e) assault with direct laryngeal injury.
2 Conditions requiring prolonged ventilation.
3 In severe respiratory disease, to decrease the dead space and allow regular direct suction of the airways.

In an emergency situation the simplest and fastest method of establishing an airway is through the cricothyroid membrane (laryngotomy). Tracheostomy is, however, the method of choice when there is rather less urgency (Fig. 45).

OPERATION: LARYNGOTOMY

Hold the head still and make a transverse stab incision over the cricothyroid membrane (palpable in the space between the thyroid and cricoid cartilage) using any available knife blade or, if necessary, a 14-gauge intravenous needle. Stay in the midline and continue backwards until air is heard hissing in and out. The cricothyroid membrane has now been pierced. Insert a sterile laryngotomy tube if available or else any tube which will help keep the hole open. Once breathing has been restored, the procedure can be completed tidily.

OPERATION: TRACHEOSTOMY

The patient is positioned supine on the table with the neck extended. A 3 cm transverse incision is made two fingerbreadths above the sternal notch. The strap muscles are separated in the midline and retracted sideways. The thyroid isthmus is either retracted or divided and sutured. When all bleeding has been controlled, a 1 cm disc is excised or an ∩-shaped flap is made in the trachea over the third or fourth ring and a tracheostomy tube is inserted and secured. The skin is loosely sutured around the tube.

Codes

Blood 0
GA/LA .... LA/GA
Opn time .... 30–45 min
Stay .... Dependent upon the underlying condition
Drains out .... Nil
Sutures out .... 7 days
Off work .... Variable

Postoperative care

A spare tube, introducer, retractor and sucker should be available by the patient's bed. The airways must be aspirated regularly to remove retained secretions. The inspired air must be humidified to prevent the secretions becoming too viscid.

7 Upper Gastrointestinal Surgery

7.1 Oesophageal problems
Dysphagia
Impacted foreign body
Oesophageal perforation
Acute caustic stricture
Chronic benign stricture
Oesophageal achalasia
Pharyngeal pouch
Plummer–Vinson syndrome
Barrett's oesophagus
Carcinoma of the oesophagus

7.2 Stomach and duodenum
Abdominal pain
Gastroduodenal disease
Carcinoma of the stomach
Postgastrectomy syndromes

7.3 Central abdominal pain
Acute appendicitis
Mesenteric adenitis
Intestinal obstruction
Meckel's diverticulum
Ischaemic bowel
Intussusception in adults
Small bowel tumours

7.1 Oesophageal Problems

Dysphagia

Dysphagia is defined as difficulty in swallowing. A list of common causes of dysphagia is shown in Table 16.

Recognizing the pattern

The characteristic clinical patterns of various conditions are given in the subsequent pages but certain points in the history and examination are helpful in reaching a diagnosis.

1 Onset. Dysphagia due to a foreign body is sudden in onset whereas that due to carcinoma may develop more slowly with a final obstruction. With achalasia and benign stricture, the symptoms develop over several years, and are often accompanied by pain.

Table 16 Causes of dysphagia.

Arising within the oesophagus
Chronic benign stricture
Carcinoma of the oesophagus
Foreign body
Achalasia and other dysmotility states
Oesophageal perforation
Acute caustic stricture
Pharyngeal pouch
Plummer–Vinson syndrome
Oesophageal candidiasis

Compressing the oesophagus from outside
Bronchial carcinoma
Thoracic aneurysm
Enlarged left atrium
Enlarged mediastinal lymph nodes
Large retrosternal goitre

Pseudo/general conditions
Bulbar palsy
Myasthenia
Hysteria
Anxiety state

---

2 Site. Food sticking in the pharynx suggests a high lesion such as a pharyngeal pouch or carcinoma. Generally speaking, the level at which the patient feels the dysphagia is at or above the lesion, rarely below.

3 Progression. Carcinoma produces a progressive dysphagia which varies greatly in rate of development but ultimately becomes complete. Other conditions such as benign stricture and achalasia progress very slowly.

4 Severity. Is the dysphagia for fluids or solids? This gives an indication of how tight the stricture is.

5 Pain. Benign stricture is usually associated with a history of heartburn, whereas achalasia may be painless. It is often accompanied by a severe epigastric pain radiating to the throat and jaw, which can be difficult to differentiate from angina. Carcinoma of the oesophagus may progress to produce a constant central chest or epigastric pain. Oesophageal pain is commonly referred between the shoulder blades in the back.

6 Regurgitation. A long-standing history of reflux is characteristic of a hiatus hernia. Patients may begin to regurgitate oesophageal contents from any tight obstructive lesion once oesophageal stasis develops. This symptom is often associated with the onset of paroxysms of coughing at night due to tracheal aspirations.

7 Systemic symptoms. A history of weight loss suggests carcinoma, although it can follow long-standing obstruction due to other causes. Patients with a neurological cause may have a past history of stroke or symptoms from other neurological deficits. Non-steroidal anti-inflammatory drugs and potassium preparations may cause benign strictures when given for other conditions such as arthritis or heart failure.

On examination look carefully for cervical or other lymphadenopathy (spreading from a lesion in the chest), and for hepatomegaly or an abdominal mass. A neurological examination may give a clue to the presence of more generalized neurological disease.

Proving the diagnosis

Every patient with mechanical dysphagia should have a barium swallow and oesophagoscopy.

The barium swallow may demonstrate the site and length of the oesophageal narrowing. It will show if it is extrinsic or intrinsic and reveal any features of malignancy.

Oesophageal physiology studies

All patients with symptoms referable to the oesophagus who do not have carcinoma should undergo three tests.

1 24-h oesophageal pH. This is the most accurate method of documenting gastro-oesophageal reflux.

2 Oesophageal manometry. This technique demonstrates normal or abnormal peristalsis and muscle tone.

3 Video barium swallow. Recording the passage of barium in moving pictures gives more accurate information on the act of swallowing.

Oesophagoscopy is carried out with either a flexible fibroscope or a rigid instrument and is described below.

Routine blood tests should look for anaemia, a raised erythrocyte sedimentation rate (ESR), and abnormal liver function tests (low plasma proteins and abnormal clotting). Any regurgitated fluid may be tested for acid. A plain chest X-ray may reveal a fluid level behind the heart, evidence of aspiration or a mediastinal mass.

OPERATION: FIBROSCOPY

A fibroscope is a flexible instrument with a tip that may be angled in four directions. The tip has a light beam, a suction channel and a channel for biopsy forceps or a brush. The patient is sedated and lignocaine spray used to anaesthetize the throat. The instrument is then passed down the oesophagus. The examination may be combined with examination of the stomach and duodenum (oesophagogastroduodenoscopy). An oesophageal stricture can be biopsied, and also dilated as described on p. 272.

Codes

Blood	0
GA/LA	LA
Opn time	30 min
Stay	Day case
Drains out	0
Sutures out	0
Off work	1–2 days

OPERATION: RIGID OESOPHAGOSCOPY

This is performed with the patient anaesthetized, intubated and relaxed. A sandbag is placed underneath the shoulders. An assistant controls the position of the head and neck.

Continued on p. 266

Continued.

Under direct vision with the head and neck flexed, the rigid oesophago-scope is introduced. A scale on the instrument measures the distance of the tip from the incisor teeth. As the tube is advanced the head and neck are gradually extended. The cardia of the stomach is seen at about 40 cm. A stricture can be dilated under direct vision (see p. 272).

Codes

Blood 0
GA/LA .... GA
Opn time .... 30 min
Stay .... 24–48 h
Drains out 0
Sutures out 0
Off work .... 48 h

Whichever method is used, the cause of the dysphagia can be directly visualized and if it is within the oesophagus a biopsy is taken. Any gastric reflux or oesophagitis may also be noted.

Postoperative care

Both these procedures carry the risk of oesophageal perforation. The patient requires close observation postoperatively.

1 Admit for 24 h after rigid endoscopy.
2 Do not allow anything by mouth for 2–4 h or until fully awake and in control of airway.
3 Monitor pulse, blood pressure, temperature.
4 Perform a chest X-ray after the procedure to look for mediastinal air or surgical emphysema in the neck.
5 If there is pain or pyrexia when the patient attempts to swallow or if surgical emphysema develops in the neck, an urgent barium swallow should be performed to look for a perforation.

Management

The further management of lesions in the oesophagus is discussed below. The treatment of an oesophageal perforation is dealt with on p. 268. Lesions causing dysphagia which are outside the oesophagus or which are neurological are not discussed further here but are listed in Table 16 (p. 263).

Impacted foreign body

This can occur either in a normal oesophagus or at the site of a carcinoma or a stricture. In a normal oesophagus there are three sites of narrowing.

1 At the level of the cricopharyngeus.

2 Where the oesophagus passes behind the left main bronchus with the arch of the aorta crossing its left side.

3 At the level of the diaphragm.

These three positions are, respectively, at about 15, 25 and 40 cm from the incisor teeth.

Recognizing the pattern

The patient notices that something has stuck in the back of the throat resulting in acute difficulty in swallowing. There is pain which is increased by any attempt to swallow. The patient will notice excessive salivation.

On examination the patient is distressed and retching. Occasionally there may be signs of perforation or mediastinitis (surgical emphysema, tachycardia and fever).

Proving the diagnosis

The foreign body may occasionally be seen on plain chest X-ray if it is radio-opaque. It may be demonstrated on a barium swallow. An oesophagoscopy should always be undertaken, preferably using the rigid endoscope.

Management

The primary treatment is oesophagoscopy (see p. 265) with removal of the foreign body.

Postoperative care

The patient must be admitted for observation (see p. 266). A chest X-ray is performed to detect signs of perforation. If the foreign body was swallowed deliberately, then a psychiatric assessment may be advisable.

If the foreign body passes on into the stomach, the management is conservative. An X-ray is taken to establish its position and the patient is reassured that foreign bodies usually pass through the gastrointestinal tract. In the unlikely event of the gut being perforated lower down (causing abdominal pain and peritonism), a laparotomy will be necessary.

Oesophageal perforation

A common cause of oesophageal perforation is injury during oesophagoscopy or other oesophageal instrumentation. The site of the rupture is usually through Killian's dehiscence above the cricopharyngeus or just above the stricture. Perforation may be due to a crushing injury against osteoarthritic cervical vertebrae or may follow biopsy, dilatation of a stricture or removal of a sharp foreign body.

Spontaneous rupture or tearing may occur as a result of excessive vomiting. This is called Boerhaave's syndrome. Spreading mediastinitis and collapse due to septicaemic shock often follows perforation. The mortality is high if the condition is not treated within 12 h. The mortality in the absence of operation is 80% after 48 h.

Recognizing the pattern

A history of violent or prolonged vomiting may be obtained. A high index of suspicion should always be present after any endoscopy. The patient is distressed and experiences severe pain at a site related to the level of the perforation. The pain is worse on attempted swallowing even of saliva. There may also be dyspnoea if the pleural space is involved (pneumothorax and/or pleural effusion).

On examination there may be little to find in the early stages. Once mediastinitis has developed, the patient may be shocked and pyrexial with a tachycardia. Palpation of the neck may reveal crepitation beneath the skin. This is due to air leaking from the oesophagus into the tissues of the neck (surgical emphysema). If the cervical oesophagus is perforated, there is localized tenderness and an abscess can form very quickly (24–36 h).

Proving the diagnosis

1 A chest X-ray (normal and overpenetrated) may demonstrate surgical emphysema in the mediastinum. It may also show widening of the mediastinum. Look for a pleural effusion or pneumothorax.
2 An urgent barium swallow usually, but not always, demonstrates the perforation. A lateral decubitus film on the side of the pleural effusion may reveal an otherwise undetected leak of barium.

Management

If the leak is small and contained within the mediastinum and there are no pleural effusions or pneumothorax, the patient may be treated conservatively. That means nothing to eat or drink for 10 days and intravenous antibiotics with regular observation and close nursing care. If the patient's condition deteriorates then surgical intervention may become necessary. This involves exploration and repair of the tear under antibiotic cover. This should be done immediately on diagnosis to minimize the degree of mediastinal contamination.

Preoperative management
The patient is started on intravenous broad-spectrum antibiotics, e.g. metronidazole (1 g 8-hourly) and a third-generation cephalosporin.

OPERATION: REPAIR OF OESOPHAGEAL PERFORATION
This must also ensure that there is no distal obstruction.

Perforation of the cervical oesophagus. The upper oesophagus is approached through the neck. The incision is made anterior to the left sternocleidomastoid and the carotid sheath is retracted laterally. The tear is oversewn and the wound drained. This may be much more difficult than anticipated and should not be attempted by a surgeon without experience.

Codes
Blood .... Group and save
GA/LA .... GA
Opn time .... 1–2 h
Stay .... 7–10 days
Drains out .... Withdraw slowly after 5 days
Sutures out .... 5–7 days
Off work .... 6–8 weeks

Perforation of the middle or lower oesophagus. A thoracotomy is performed (see p. 257). A tear in the middle third of the oesophagus is approached from the right side. One in the lower third is approached through a lower left thoracotomy. The tear is usually oversewn. Occasionally, if it is very ragged, that part of the oesophagus is excised and the stomach brought up to bridge the gap. If there is a distal stricture this should be dealt with appropriately.

Postoperative care
The postoperative care is as for an oesophagectomy (see p. 280).

Acute caustic stricture

Ingestion of strong acid or alkali may be an accident or an attempted suicide. It causes a chemical burn of the oesophageal mucosa. The three sites mentioned above where foreign bodies commonly impact are also the sites commonly involved in caustic burns. The stomach may be involved. There is oedema, congestion and ulceration which can lead to acute obstruction. This is followed by fibrosis with stricture formation.

Recognizing the pattern

The patient may be of any age or sex, although accidental ingestion of caustic fluids is common in children.

The history is one of severe pain which is continuous and increased by any attempt at swallowing. Find out the nature of the fluid swallowed and estimate the volume. The need for treatment is urgent and further enquiry as to motive can be carried out when the patient has recovered.

On examination there may be signs of oropharyngeal inflammation. Look for evidence of circulatory collapse.

Management

Give immediate, strong, intravenous opiate analgesia. As soon as the patient has calmed down, wash away any remaining fluid with mouthwashes. The patient should swallow some water if possible. If the nature of the fluid is known, neutralize it (Table 17).

Do not attempt to wash out the stomach or provoke vomiting because the oesophagus is easily perforated. Check

Table 17 Agents causing stricture and their neutralizers.

Common agents causing stricture	Neutralizing agent
Bleach	Sodium thiosulphate
Sodium hydroxide/sodium carbonate (lye)	Dilute acetic acid or citric acid
Other inorganic bases	Dilute acetic acid or citric acid
Mineral acids	Magnesium hydroxide or sodium bicarbonate
Paraquat	Fuller's earth
Phenol or organic solvents	Liquid paraffin, olive oil or castor oil

the airway. If the oropharynx has been badly burned a tracheostomy may be required.

The oesophagus itself must be rested and the patient may be given fluid either intravenously or via a gastrostomy. Some centres initiate early treatment with steroids (hydrocortisone 200 mg, 4–6-hourly i.v.) and antibiotics and there is some evidence that this decreases the incidence of stricture formation. The patient must then be observed very carefully for evidence of oesophageal perforation. He or she will already be in pain, but signs of fluid in the chest, a developing pyrexia and the development of surgical emphysema may indicate that this complication has occurred. Regular chest X-rays should also be carried out.

Following this, the patient is observed for evidence of stricture development. In some centres the patient is asked to swallow a fine tube or guide wire as any resulting stricture is often tortuous and a wire greatly assists the passing of oesophageal dilators. Fibroscopy may then be performed (see p. 265) with the help of the guide wire to assess the extent of damage. Early endoscopy is fraught with danger as the oesophagus is easily damaged.

Should oesophageal dilatation be required, it is usually started 3–4 weeks after the incident. Long-term management may require resection of the stricture.

Remember to check for and manage any systemic manifestations of poisoning, e.g. renal failure (see relevant medical texts).

Chronic benign stricture

Recurrent gastro-oesophageal reflux, either acid (gastric) or alkaline (duodenal) will inflame the oesophagus and can result in a circumferential stricture. This is commonly secondary to a hiatus hernia but often occurs in the absence of a demonstrable hernia. Other causes include reflux in pregnancy, non-steroidal anti-inflammatory agents and potassium preparations.

Recognizing the pattern

The patient is most frequently middle aged or elderly, more commonly female than male, but can be any age and either sex.

There may be a long history of reflux oesophagitis with a more recent onset of dysphagia, the food sticking at the lower sternal level. If the obstruction is severe there is usually regurgitation of food immediately after swallowing and there may be episodes of aspiration of gastric contents into the chest associated with paroxysms of coughing, especially at night.

On examination there is usually very little to find.

Proving the diagnosis

Barium swallow demonstrates the stricture. The stricture is seen on oesophagoscopy (see p. 265). It is important to biopsy the lesion to exclude carcinoma. Malignant change can occur in a previously benign chronic stricture. Biopsy must never precede dilatation, as the weakening caused by biopsy will encourage perforation.

Management

Initial management is oesophagoscopy and dilatation of the stricture, followed by the use of acid suppressants and mucosal protective preparations for 6–8 weeks prior to review.

OPERATION: DILATATION OF OESOPHAGEAL STRICTURE

This may be carried out through a fibroscope or a rigid oesophagoscope (p. 265). Using a fibroscope a guide wire is passed through the stricture and bougies are then threaded down over the guide wire and the stricture dilated. A rigid oesophagoscope is wide enough to allow bougies to be passed directly through the instrument to dilate the stricture. A variety of dilators is available.

Codes

Blood	0
GA/LA	GA
Opn time	30 min
Stay	24 h, variable
Drains out	0
Sutures out	0
Off work	2–3 days, variable

Postoperative care

The main potential complication is perforation of the oesophagus. Postoperative management is described on p. 266. Further long-term management of the underlying cause will be necessary.

Oesophageal achalasia

Achalasia is a condition affecting the whole oesophagus in which the main feature is failure of relaxation of the circular muscles at the lower end of the oesophagus. The muscles hypertrophy and the oesophagus then dilates above the achalasia. The condition is thought to be due to neuromuscular incoordination and the histology shows a partial or complete loss of the myenteric plexus of nerves. The body of the oesophagus loses normal peristalsis.

Recognizing the pattern

The patient is typically aged 30–40 years old and the condition is slightly more common in females.

The history is one of gradual and slowly progressive dysphagia coming on over several years often preceded by spasms of epigastric pain radiating to the throat. Regurgitation of stagnant, undigested food occurs together with foul belching. Aspiration often takes place at night when the patient lies down, and it results in a fit of coughing. This is referred to as nocturnal asthma. Recurrent chest infections due to aspiration pneumonia are common. There may be loss of weight.

On examination there may be signs of chronic chest infection and possibly loss of weight.

Proving the diagnosis

1 Chest X-ray. The mediastinum may be widened with a fluid level behind the heart. This represents the dilated oesophagus. There may also be evidence of pneumonitis. None of these may be present however, particularly in the early stages.

2 Barium swallow. There is dilatation and tortuosity of the oesophagus, which tapers down to a narrow lower segment of achalasia.

3 Oesophagoscopy (p. 265). This may reveal a grossly dilated oesophagus containing a pool of stagnant undigested food. Biopsy shows no evidence of malignant disease.

Management

Mild achalasia may be treated by amyl nitrite and anticholinergics. However, the definitive management is balloon dilatation or surgical division of the longitudinal and circular muscle. The majority of patients are now treated initially by balloon dilatation via a flexible endoscopy.

OPERATION: HELLER'S OPERATION

The lower oesophagus is exposed by a thoracic approach. The muscle coats of the oesophagus are incised for at least 5 cm above the constriction, and no further than 1.5 cm on to the stomach below the gastro-oesophageal junction. This allows the mucosa to bulge through. The mucosa is not opened. This operation can now be done using thoracoscopic or laparoscopic techniques. This has the advantage of avoiding the considerable pain due to a thoracotomy.

Codes

Blood	2 units
GA/LA	GA
Opn time	Open 40–60 min; endoscopic 60–90 min
Stay	Open 7–10 days; endoscopic 3–4 days
Drains out	24 h
Sutures out	Open 7 days; endoscopic absorbable
Off work	Open 1 month; endoscopic 2 weeks

Postoperative care

Oral fluids are reintroduced after about 12–24 h and, providing there is no pain on swallowing, they may be gradually increased. Once free fluids are established, a light diet and then more solid food can be given providing swallowing is satisfactory. A normal diet can usually be established 1–2 days postoperatively.

The earliest complication that may occur after this procedure is a leaking oesophagus. Incomplete myotomy may result in persistent dysphagia. This may respond to dilatation but, if not, reoperation is required. Late complications include reflux oesophagitis and stricture formation and, rarely, oesophageal diverticulum.

Pharyngeal pouch

This is a rare cause of dysphagia due to a pulsion diverticulum occurring as a result of cricopharyngeal muscle spasm. It is described on p. 149.

Plummer–Vinson syndrome

This syndrome consists of:

1 Iron deficiency anaemia

2 Dysphagia due to a postcricoid web in the oesophagus.
It was described by Plummer and Vinson in 1921, and by Paterson and Kelly 2 years earlier.

There is hyperplasia of the squamous epithelium with hyperkeratosis in the mucosa of the upper oesophagus associated with patches of desquamation. This can lead to the formation of a web, which usually lies anteriorly.

Recognizing the pattern
The patient is typically a woman aged between 40 and 50 years.

The history is one of high dysphagia, the patient complaining that food appears to stick in the back of the throat. This may be associated with retching and a choking sensation. There may be symptoms of anaemia.

On examination the patient is usually anaemic with spoon-shaped nails (koilonychia), smooth tongue and angular stomatitis. He or she may also occasionally have a palpable spleen.

Proving the diagnosis
1 A barium meal shows a narrowing of the upper oesophagus due to a web-like fold in the anterior wall.
2 A full blood count shows anaemia with a hypochromic, microcytic picture.
3 Oesophagoscopy shows a friable web across the lumen of the oesophagus.
4 Biopsy of the bone marrow shows absent iron stores.

Management
The web is dilated at the time of oesophagoscopy. The condition is premalignant and so it must be biopsied.

Postoperative care
The patient is treated with iron therapy and vitamin supplements. Provided the anaemia is corrected, the condition does not usually recur. Occasionally a blood transfusion is required.

If the biopsy shows malignant cells, then the lesion is treated as a postcricoid carcinoma (see p. 276).

Barrett's oesophagus
This is a term that describes changes consisting of replacement of the normal squamous epithelial lining of the oesophagus proximal to the lower oesophageal sphincter by a mixture of columnar epithelial cell types. It appears deep red, as opposed to the pink colour of the normal squamous lining. There is a malignant predisposition (8–15%). As a result of altered sen-

sation within the Barrett's segment gastro–oesophageal reflux may be painless but is just as damaging. An early antireflux procedure is essential in all patients.

Carcinoma of the oesophagus

The oesophagus is lined by stratified squamous epithelium down to the lowest 2–3 cm.

In the proximal third of the oesophagus almost all cancers are squamous cell in origin.

In the middle third squamous cell types are also the most common except where columnar epithelium extends up to this level as in a Barrett's oesophagus.

In the lower third squamous cell tumours historically pre-dominate in a ratio of 7 : 3. Adenocarcinomas are, however, increasingly reported, probably associated with chronic gastro-oesophageal reflux and the change to a columnar cell epithelium associated with this. Many tumours are of mixed cell origin and small cell carcinomas can occur at this site.

Predisposing factors include oesophageal achalasia, a long-standing benign stricture and the Plummer–Vinson syndrome mentioned above. It is more common in smokers. There is an environmental factor involved and the condition occurs more commonly in certain areas (e.g. Brittany, Normandy and Transkei).

The tumour typically spreads by submucosal invasion along the oesophagus. Lymphatic spread is either to the supraclavicu-lar, subdiaphragmatic or mediastinal nodes. The oesophagus lies near other vital structures in the mediastinum, which may be involved by local invasion. For these reasons the prognosis is usually poor.

Recognizing the pattern

The patient is usually over the age of 60 years. The incidence in younger people is showing a disturbing increase. Lower-third carcinomas are more common in males than females. The sex incidence for carcinomas of the middle and upper thirds is equal. Postcricoid carcinoma is more common in females.

The patient typically presents with a short history of progres-sive dysphagia. This initially affects solids only, but gradually increases until even swallowing liquids becomes a problem. Retrosternal pain may occur but is usually a late symptom. There may be regurgitation of food or fluids, or blood-stained vomiting. There is frequently a history of significant weight loss.

On examination the patient is often cachectic. Look for

palpable nodes and an enlarged liver. Often, however, there are no abnormal signs.

Proving the diagnosis

1 Barium swallow. A carcinoma of the oesophagus has a characteristic appearance consisting of a narrowing of the lumen, which has an irregular, craggy, pitted surface and raised, rolled edges. The length of the narrowed lumen is used in staging (see below).

2 Oesophagoscopy and biopsy. The carcinoma may be seen either as a malignant ulcer, a papillary growth or an irregular stricture. A biopsy must be taken to confirm the diagnosis.

3 Oesophageal lavage and cytology. A cytological diagnosis of carcinoma may be made from cells picked up from oesophageal washings.

Management

The first step is to assess the degree of spread and the patient's general condition. This can be done as follows:

1 Haemoglobin and ESR. The patient may be anaemic.

2 Liver function tests. These may suggest the presence of metastases (elevated bilirubin and alkaline phosphatase) or show evidence of malnutrition (hypoproteinaemia).

3 The length of narrowing demonstrated by barium swallow: 90% of tumours have involved regional lymph nodes when the narrowed segment is more than 5 cm long.

4 Chest X-ray with or without bronchoscopy. This will show involvement of the trachea and bronchi with resultant risk of tracheobronchial fistula.

5 Lymph node biopsy. Any enlarged cervical nodes should be biopsied before major surgery is contemplated.

6 Computed tomography (CT). This may give a picture of the degree of mediastinal involvement.

As a result of these investigations it should be possible to determine whether the tumour is potentially curable by local resection or not, and whether the patient is fit for major surgery.

Forms of therapy

This carcinoma may be treated by one of the following methods:

1 Surgical resection

2 Radiotherapy and/or chemotherapy

3 Palliation — intubation or bypass.

Squamous cell carcinoma can be treated by either surgery or radiotherapy. Adenocarcinoma is not sensitive to radiotherapy.

Surgical resection

Curative resection can only be realistically expected for growths confined to the oesophagus with no evidence of lymphatic or mediastinal spread. Of the patients considered operable, two-thirds will be found to have more extensive tumours at the time of operation. Because of the likely presence of submucosal invasion, curative resection requires wide excision of the oesophagus above and below the growth.

OPERATIONS FOR OESOPHAGEAL CARCINOMA

The type of operation performed depends on the site of the growth (Fig. 46). Three types of curative procedure will be described (Fig. 47).

1 Pharyngolaryngo–oesophagectomy
2 Total oesophagectomy
3 Oesophagogastrectomy.

> *Preoperative management*
> The patient may require a supplemented diet or even intravenous nutrition to correct malnutrition. Oesophageal washouts are needed for lower segment growths. The mouth should also be cleaned. Some centres give prophylactic antibiotics.

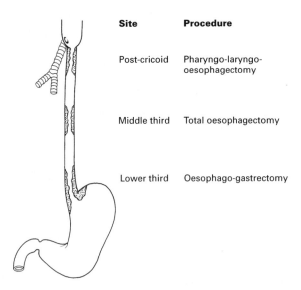

Site	Procedure
Post-cricoid	Pharyngo-laryngo-oesophagectomy
Middle third	Total oesophagectomy
Lower third	Oesophago-gastrectomy

Fig. 46 Carcinoma of the oesophagus: the sites of origin and the relevant surgical procedures.

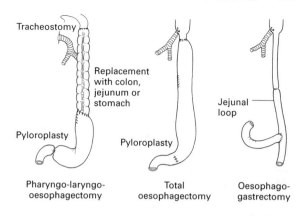

Fig. 47 Operations for carcinoma of oesophagus.

OPERATION: PHARYNGOLARYNGO-
OESOPHAGECTOMY (FOR UPPER THIRD
TUMOURS ONLY)

In this operation it is necessary to resect the larynx as well
as the oesophagus. A permanent tracheostomy is therefore
inevitable. Continuity is restored by suturing the fundus of
the stomach up to the lower pharynx in the neck, or by
interposing a loop of colon or jejunum as a conduit. This
conduit may be brought up inside the chest (retrosternally
or prevertebrally) or subcutaneously in front of the sternum.
The intrathoracic part of the operation may be performed
endoscopically.

Codes
Blood .... 10 units
GA/LA .... GA
Opn time .... About 5 h
Stay .... 10–14 days
Drains out .... Pleura 48 h; neck anasto-
mosis 7 days; mediastinum
3–5 days
Sutures out .... 7 days
Off work .... 2–3 months

OPERATION: TOTAL OESOPHAGECTOMY

This operation is performed for carcinoma of the mid-
oesophagus. Through an abdominal incision the stomach is

Continued on p. 280

Continued.

mobilized and the degree of spread assessed. If the lesion is operable, the chest is opened through a right thoracotomy incision. The tumour is removed with a wide margin of normal oesophagus and either the stomach is brought up into the chest for anastomosis with the oesophageal stump (Ivor Lewis operation), or a piece of jejunum or large bowel is brought up on its vascular pedicle to act as a conduit.

Codes

Blood	6 units
GA/LA	GA
Opn time	3–4 h
Stay	10–14 days
Drains out	Neck anastomosis 7 days; chest/ pleura 48 h; mediastinum 3–5 days
Sutures out	7 days
Off work	3 months

OPERATION: OESOPHAGOGASTRECTOMY

This operation is performed for carcinomas of the oesophago-gastric junction and lower oesophagus. The stomach and lower oesophagus are mobilized and the liver palpated. If the tumour is considered resectable, the chest is then opened along the eighth rib (left thoracoabdominal incision) and the lower oesophagus including the tumour, all or part of the stomach, the spleen and the omentum are removed. The continuity of the oesophagus is usually restored by anastomosis either to the stomach remnant or, if all the stomach is resected, to a loop of jejunum.

Codes

Blood	6 units
GA/LA	GA
Opn time	3–4 h
Stay	21–28 days
Drains out	Chest 5 days; anastomosis 7 days
Sutures out	7–10 days
Off work	2–3 months

Postoperative care

A thoracic epidural should be set up for pain control. If the chest has been opened the routine care of a thoracotomy is appropriate (pp. 257–259). A chest X-ray should be performed daily for the first few days. Patients who have had a thoracotomy and resection are usually nursed in intensive care.

The major postoperative complication of all these procedures is pulmonary aspiration. Leakage of the anastomosis occurs in 5–7% of cases. This is more debilitating if it drains via the pleural cavity. Hence anastomoses in the neck may be safer. Further management is then as follows:

1 Feeding. Most surgeons introduce fluids on the second to third postoperative day and soft solids as soon as fluids are tolerated orally, usually by 4–5 days. Some surgeons routinely perform a gastrostomy or enterostomy and use this to feed the patient once he has recovered from his abdominal ileus. Alternatively, a nasogastric tube may be passed through the anasto-mosis into the jejunum and feeding instituted through this after 4 or 5 days.

2 A barium swallow may be performed 6 or 7 days after the operation to look for signs of a leak if the surgeon is uncertain of the anastomosis.

3 If the barium swallow shows a small, insignificant leak, in the absence of other signs (i.e. fever, tachycardia or pleural effusion), the patient continues to have nothing by mouth until the leak has healed. Nutrition is maintained either as above or intravenously. Re-exploration and resuture of the anastomosis are required, if the leak is significant.

Chest infection associated with pulmonary collapse may occur. The patient should have good analgesia and physiotherapy to resolve this.

Some patients will experience recurrent dysphagia. Some may need oesophageal dilatation, but others with early recurrence at the anastomosis or in local lymph nodes will need an oesophageal stent.

Radiotherapy

At present this is used for squamous cell carcinoma in patients unfit for surgery or patients with a carcinoma involving the oesophagus in the neck. Radiotherapy is also effective for palliative treatment of dysphagia in some cases.

Complications include oesophageal disruption and leak, leucopenia, pulmonary fibrosis and spinal cord damage, all of which are rare with modern techniques.

Palliation

Many patients with oesophageal carcinoma will be found to have inoperable tumours and will require some form of symptomatic relief. The most significant symptom is dysphagia. This may be relieved by:

1 Intubation of the tumour
2 Extra-anatomical bypass of the tumour
3 Radiotherapy.

OPERATION: INTUBATION OF CARCINOMA OF THE OESOPHAGUS

This procedure involves implanting a tube within the stricture to maintain sufficient lumen for a liquid and semi-solid diet. Such tubes may block and become dislodged. The imbibing of fizzy drinks whilst eating helps to keep the tube clear. There are many different types of tube in use. Most can now be introduced perorally with radiological control.

Celestin tube. This has an olive-shaped head. A flexible pilot bougie is passed through the stricture under direct vision and into the stomach and recovered through a high gastrotomy. The Celestin tube fits on the end of the bougie and can then be pulled down the oesophagus into position. The tube is cut to the required length and may be sutured to the stomach wall. Recently the development of a specifically adapted introducer has enabled this tube to be inserted from above and thus avoiding a gastrotomy (Nottingham introducer, Fig. 48). Celestin tubes are rarely used nowadays and only for patients found to be inoperable at laparotomy.

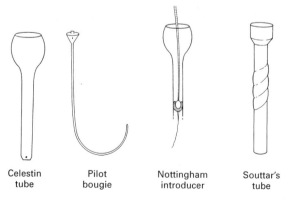

| Celestin tube | Pilot bougie | Nottingham introducer | Souttar's tube |

Fig. 48 The Celestin and Souttar tubes.

Codes

Blood	Group and save serum
GA/LA	GA
Opn time	30–60 min
Stay	3–5 days
Drains out	0
Sutures out	0
Off work	Variable

Souttar's tube (Fig. 48). A metal guide wire is first passed through the growth using an oesophagoscope. Bougies can be introduced to dilate the stricture. The tube is then pushed down over the guide wire or a bougie and impacted into the structure.

Codes

Blood	0
GA/LA	GA
Opn time	30–60 min
Stay	3–5 days
Drains out	0
Sutures out	0
Off work	Variable

Mousseau–Barbin tube. A bougie is passed through the stricture in either direction, access to the stomach being gained through a gastrotomy made in the stomach during a laparotomy. The tube has a long, thin end like a nasogastric tube and this is then pulled down via the patient's mouth, through the tumour and into the stomach. The surgeon then pulls the main tube down to impact it in the growth. The tube beneath the growth is then excised and the lower end of the prosthesis may be sutured to the lesser curve of the stomach (Fig. 49).

Codes

Blood	Group and save serum
GA/LA	GA
Opn time	30–60 min
Stay	7–10 days
Drains out	0
Sutures out	7 days
Off work	Variable

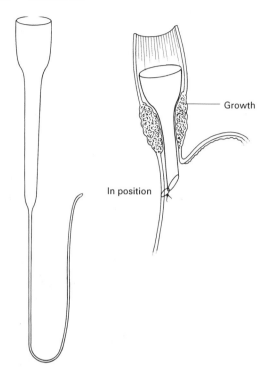

Fig. 49 Mousseau–Barbin tube.

Postoperative care
The patient must be instructed about diet and told to swallow only well-masticated soft food with plenty of fluids. Fizzy drinks are effective in flushing and cleaning the tube. It is useful to show the patient an identical tube to the one that has been inserted.

Expandable stents. The most frequently used stents are expandable metal stents that may be covered or uncovered. Covered stents are particularly useful for patients with tracheo-oesophageal fistulae. All can be inserted under radiological control and many patients can be discharged within 48 h.

OPERATION: SURGICAL BYPASS
If the tumour is found to be unresectable at operation, some form of bypass procedure can often be performed. This may involve bringing up a loop of jejunum, stomach or colon and suturing it to the oesophagus, leaving the growth *in situ*.

Palliative radiotherapy
Radiotherapy can also be used to relieve dysphagia.

In some patients the appropriate form of treatment is to provide adequate analgesia and symptomatic relief only.

7.2 Stomach and Duodenum

Abdominal pain

When a patient presents with abdominal pain the site of pain gives a primary clue as to the organ involved (Fig. 50). In this book abdominal conditions are grouped according to the site where the pain typically presents. Disease states may of course present in other ways apart from pain (e.g. haematemesis, jaundice, change in bowel habit, etc.) and the more important of these are included as seems appropriate in relation to other conditions discussed.

Important conditions presenting with upper abdominal pain, together with their complications and management, are dealt with on the following pages.

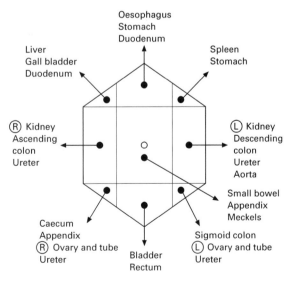

Fig. 50 Typical sites of presentation of visceral pain from different organs.

5 Carcinoma of the stomach (p. 308)
6 Carcinoma of the pancreas (p. 356)
7 Pancreatitis (p. 360).

Less commonly, upper abdominal pain may arise from disease in the liver, spleen or diaphragm. Examples discussed in this book are as follows:

1 Hepatic abscess (p. 72)
2 Hepatic metastases, secondary to malignant disease from many sites
3 Subphrenic abscess (p. 70)
4 Ruptured spleen (p. 658)
5 Liver injury (p. 656).

Gastroduodenal disease

Hiatus hernia

Two main types of hiatus hernia are recognized (Fig. 51). In the sliding variety (Fig. 51a) the gastro–oesophageal angle is straightened out and the junction between the oesophageal mucosa and gastric mucosa slides up into the chest. The main symptoms are due to reflux of gastric contents into the oesophagus. In the rolling variety (Fig. 51b) there is a large hiatus and the fundus of the stomach tends to roll up next to the oesophagus, forming a paraoesophageal hernia. In this type of hernia there is a danger of strangulation of the herniated part of the stomach. The two main types of hiatus hernia may be combined.

Recognizing the pattern

Hiatus hernia and reflux may occur in any age group in either sex. Typically, however, the patient is a middle-aged, overweight female.

In reflux oesophagitis the patient develops symptoms of heartburn and reflux of acid or food. Heartburn is an epigastric or low retrosternal burning pain, which may radiate to the back, neck or even down the arms. The symptoms are worse on bending forward or lying flat at night. Symptoms often come on when the patient has recently gained weight and are common in the last trimester of pregnancy.

With strangulation of a rolling hernia the patient complains of a sudden onset of very severe constricting lower chest and upper abdominal pain. The symptoms mimic those of a myocardial infarction.

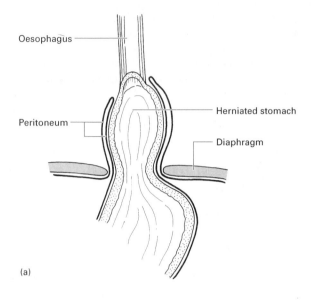

Oesophagus

Peritoneum

Herniated stomach

Diaphragm

(a)

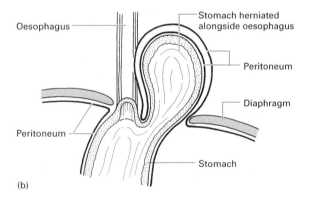

Oesophagus

Stomach herniated alongside oesophagus

Peritoneum

Diaphragm

Peritoneum

Stomach

(b)

Fig. 51 (a) Sliding hiatus hernia. (b) Rolling hiatus hernia.

Proving the diagnosis

The diagnosis of hiatus hernia is proved by performing a barium swallow and meal, or by fibroscopy. A chest X-ray may also show signs of aspiration pneumonia. In recent years, the diagnosis of gastro-oesophageal reflux disease is mainly by endoscopy, oesophageal manometry and pH studies. Ambulatory outpatient pH measurement is the gold standard investigation for reflux disease.

Management

The initial management of a hiatus hernia is usually conservative. The most important thing is for the patient to lose weight. Symptoms will often abate when even a few pounds of weight have been shed. In addition to advice about this, the patient is given a combination of antacids, alginates, a histamine receptor type 2 (H_2) blocker such as cimetidine, or a proton-pump inhibitor such as omeprazole. Prokinetic drugs such as metoclopramide, domperidone and cisapride may also be helpful.

Operation is indicated when the medical treatment fails to control symptoms or when complications such as ulceration of the oesophagus, stricture formation or haemorrhage occur. Patients with a rolling hernia who have had a possible episode of strangulation should always have an operation.

Preoperative management

Patients should be advised to stop smoking and to lose as much weight as possible. The surgeon may elect to perform the operation either through the chest or through the abdomen and you should find out which approach is intended.

OPERATION: OPEN REPAIR OF HIATUS HERNIA
AND NISSEN'S FUNDOPLICATION

The oesophageal hiatus is approached either through an incision in the bed of the eighth rib or through a vertical

Continued on p. 290

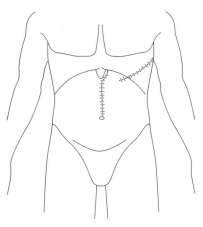

Fig. 52 Choice of incision for open repair of hiatus hernia.

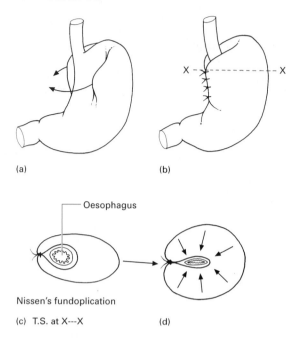

(a)   (b)

Oesophagus

Nissen's fundoplication

(c) T.S. at X---X   (d)

Fig. 53 (a, b) Nissen's fundoplication. A pouch from the anterior and posterior gastric fundus is pulled forwards (and to the patient's right) around the oesophagus. (c, d) Antireflux mechanism after Nissen's fundoplication. Raised intragastric pressure occludes the enclosed portion of the oesophagus.

Continued.

incision in the epigastrium (see Fig. 52). Any rolling hernia is reduced into the abdomen and the oesophageal hiatus is narrowed by inserting sutures into the crura posterior to the oesophagus. An antireflux procedure is then undertaken. The most popular is Nissen's procedure (Fig. 53).

Codes

Blood .... 2 units
GA/LA .... GA
Opn time .... 90–120 min
Stay .... 7–10 days
Drains out .... Abdomen 0; chest 24 h
Sutures out .... 7 days
Off work .... 6–8 weeks

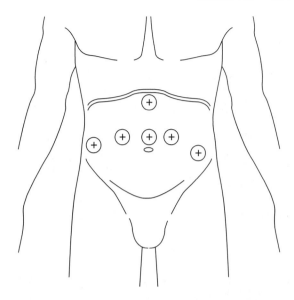

Fig. 54 Possible port sites for laparoscopic Nissen's fundoplication.

OPERATION: LAPAROSCOPIC NISSEN'S
FUNDOPLICATION (see Fig. 54)
The same procedure can be performed laparoscopically. The oesophagus is mobilized and encircled with a rubber sling. The crural defect is repaired with non-absorbable sutures. The short gastric vessels between the spleen and stomach are often divided and the fundus wrapped around the oesophagus. The wrap is secured with interrupted sutures.

Codes
Blood .... 2 units
GA/LA .... GA
Opn time .... 2–3 h
Stay .... 2–5 days
Drains out 0
Sutures out .... Absorbable
Off work .... 3 weeks

Postoperative care
The patient usually has a nasogastric tube for 24–48 h after the open operation and fluids are gradually introduced.

Continued on p. 292

Continued.

Patients can drink within hours of the laparoscopic procedure. Both groups often complain of dysphagia during the first few days and even weeks after the operation. They should keep to a fairly liquid diet and drink plenty of water with meals until the symptoms settle. Occasionally the patient may also suffer from the 'gas bloat syndrome'. Air is trapped in the stomach and cannot be belched upwards because of the antireflux procedure. Symptoms are often associated with air swallowing and the patient should try and avoid this habit.

Peptic ulcers

Peptic ulcers are becoming rarer but are of two types — those in the stomach and those in the duodenum. Although both present with pain after eating, they are two rather different conditions with different pathogeneses. They will be dealt with separately.

Gastric ulcer

Recognizing the pattern

The patient is typically middle aged or elderly, debilitated and thin, and complains of poor appetite, loss of weight and pain that comes on immediately after eating. The pain may be relieved by lying flat (when the gastric contents fall back into the fundus of the stomach and away from the ulcer on the lesser curve) and also by antacids. He may also present with haematemesis or melaena.

On examination there may be tenderness in the left hypochondrium.

Proving the diagnosis

The diagnosis may be proved by doing a barium meal, in which case the ulcer is seen as a niche projecting from the lesser curve of the stomach. All patients with a suspected gastric ulcer should, however, have an endoscopy in order that the ulcer may be biopsied, as there is a danger that the ulcer may be malignant (see carcinoma of the stomach, p. 308).

Management

The management of a gastric ulcer is medical, with antacids and mucosal protectives such as bismuth chelate (DeNol

5 ml 6-hourly in water before meals). Non-steroidal anti-inflammatory drugs should be discontinued and *Helicobacter pylori* irradication therapy instituted if tests for it are positive. One regimen for the irradication of *H. pylori* is omeprazole 20 mg for 1 week, and 2 weeks of clarithromycin, metronidazole or amoxycillin. The main danger of treating a gastric ulcer medically is that a malignancy may be overlooked. It is therefore essential to monitor healing by repeated endoscopy. If the ulcer fails to heal completely, then operation is indicated. Operation is also indicated if there is malignant change in the biopsy or if the patient suffers from repeated haematemesis or perforation of the ulcer.

The surgeon will usually wish to resect a gastric ulcer either locally or as part of a partial gastrectomy. Partial gastrectomy is the method of choice. Some surgeons also treat benign gastric ulcers with a highly selective vagotomy together with excision of the ulcer. The vagotomy operations will be dealt with in more detail under duodenal ulcer (p. 298).

Preoperative management
Patients with a gastric ulcer frequently have a severe gastritis and there may be gastric stasis. Attempts should be made to get the stomach as clean as possible before operation by instituting a liquid diet for at least 24 h before surgery and possibly by washing out the stomach if stasis is severe. We also give prophylactic antibiotics when the stomach is being opened (e.g. cefotaxime).

OPERATION: PARTIAL GASTRECTOMY
In a partial gastrectomy the pylorus, the antrum and the lesser curve containing the gastric ulcer are resected. Two major types of reconstruction are then possible. In the Billroth I reconstruction the upper stomach is reanastomosed to the cut end of the duodenum (Fig. 55). In the Billroth II (Pólya) type of anastomosis, the duodenal stump is closed and the proximal end of the stomach is anastomosed to a loop of jejunum. This loop may be brought up either in front of (antecolic) or behind the colon (retrocolic), the latter passing through an artificial hole in the mesocolon (as in a gastrojejunostomy, see Fig. 57, p. 298).

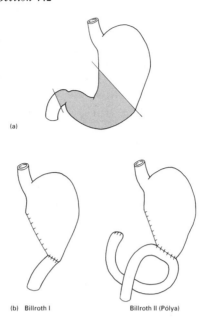

(a)

(b) Billroth I   Billroth II (Pólya)

Fig. 55 Two types of partial gastrectomy (the terms refer to the type of reconstruction). (a) Resection. (b) Reconstruction.

Codes

Blood	4 units
GA/LA	GA
Opn time	2–3 h
Stay	7–10 days
Drains out	3–6 days
Sutures out	7 days
Off work	6 weeks

Postoperative care

The stomach must be kept empty until adequate gastric emptying occurs. This is achieved by hourly aspiration of the nasogastric tube. Provided this is draining satisfactorily the patient can be given 30 mL of water to drink each hour. This keeps the mouth and throat more comfortable and has a beneficial 'washing' action on the stomach. A Billroth I gastrectomy takes longer to start emptying than a Billroth II because the stoma is smaller.

The onset of gastric emptying is noted when the gastric aspirate diminishes and the patient begins to pass flatus per rectum. At this point oral fluids can be increased and the nasogastric tube removed. The intravenous drip is removed shortly afterwards.

Complications. Postoperative anastomotic bleeding may occur in the first few hours after surgery or again at 7–10 days. This usually settles. Adequate blood replacement must be available and occasionally it is necessary to stem the bleeding endoscopically, or even to take the patient back to theatre.

Persistently high gastric aspirates after a gastrectomy are frequently due to the nasogastric tube passing through the anastomosis into the duodenum. The first step is therefore to shorten the nasogastric tube. If there is no sign of gastric emptying by a week or more after the operation, then a barium meal may be indicated to ascertain the cause. There may be narrowing of the anastomosis, which will settle as the oedema resolves. Patience on the part of the doctor and the patient is usually rewarded. Metoclopramide (10 mg 8-hourly) can be helpful in assisting gastric emptying.

Once gastric emptying has been established, a light diet can be introduced and the patient's recovery thereafter is usually uncomplicated.

Late sequelae of gastrectomy include symptoms of bilious vomiting, dumping and diarrhoea. These are dealt with on p. 311. Patients may also develop anaemia due to vitamin B_{12} or iron deficiency. Patients who have had a gastrectomy should usually be put on iron and vitamin B_{12} injections for the rest of their lives.

Duodenal ulcer

The condition is associated with gastric hyperacidity. The ulcer in the duodenum usually heals with treatment which lowers gastric acidity, such as antacids, H_2-blockers and proton-pump inhibitors.

Recognizing the pattern

The patient is usually young and the condition is more common in males than in females. Unlike gastric ulcer patients, those with a duodenal ulcer tend to be overweight, as eating helps to ease the pain. Duodenal ulcers are more common in smokers.

The pain is situated in the epigastrium and may radiate through to the small of the back. It comes on 1–2 h after meals and also when the patient is hungry. It has a tendency to wake the patient up in the early hours of the morning when acidity is high and the stomach is empty.

There may also be 'periodicity' with periods (often weeks) when the ulcer is active and painful, followed by periods (often months) of inactivity and absent symptoms. Characteristically duodenal ulcers are worse in the autumn and spring and better in the summer months.

If the ulcer is chronic, the patient may develop the symptoms of perforation (see p. 300) or of fibrosis and gastric outlet obstruction (pyloric stenosis, p. 302) or the ulcer may erode a vessel and present with haematemesis and melaena (p. 304).

On examination there is tenderness to the right of and above the umbilicus, deep in the abdomen.

Proving the diagnosis

The diagnosis is proved either on a barium meal or on fibroscopy. The presence or absence of pyloric stenosis should also be noted on these investigations.

Gastric acid function studies, such as the pentagastrin and insulin stress test will show that the stomach is producing acid at a high normal or above normal rate but they are rarely used in practice.

Management

The initial management of an acute duodenal ulcer is medical. Patients are also advised to stop smoking and are taken off non-steroidal anti-inflammatory drugs. Treatment is with full dosage of H_2-blockers (e.g. cimetidine 200 mg t.d.s. after food and 400 mg *nocte*, or ranitidine 150 mg 12-hourly) for 1 month. Irradication therapy for *H. pylori* should be instituted if tests are positive.

The indications for surgery are failed medical management or the onset of complications.

Medical management may fail due to the following factors:

1 The patient continues to have pain whilst on H_2-blockers or proton-pump inhibitor (omeprazole). This is rare.

2 The symptoms recur as soon as the dosage is lowered or the drug stopped.

3 The symptoms recur after a period of weeks or months of treatment but are rapidly brought under control by further treatment. When this has been going on for more than 3 years, surgery should be considered.

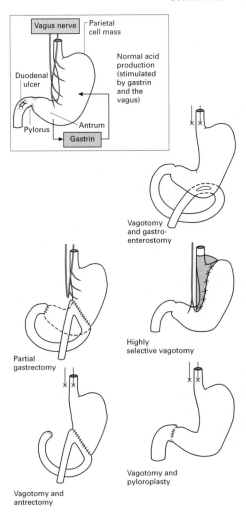

Fig. 56 Operations to lower gastric acidity.

Surgical management

Surgery is always indicated when the patient perforates a duodenal ulcer or if he has developed outlet stenosis. The management of haematemesis is described on p. 305.

Several procedures are available which satisfactorily lower the gastric acid output either by removing the antrum (gastrin mechanism) or part of the parietal cell mass, or by dividing the vagus nerves. These procedures are illustrated in Fig. 56 and include the following:

Continued on p. 298

Continued.

1 Partial gastrectomy
2 Truncal vagotomy and drainage (either pyloroplasty or gastroenterostomy)
3 Truncal vagotomy and antrectomy
4 Highly selective vagotomy (parietal cell vagotomy).

Modern surgical practice tends to favour highly selective vagotomy because of the absence of side-effects.

Preoperative management

Many duodenal ulcer patients are heavy smokers and they should be warned that continued smoking is liable to give them severe postoperative chest problems. They should be given chest physiotherapy before the operation.

OPERATION: TRUNCAL VAGOTOMY AND DRAINAGE

The trunks of the vagus nerve are cut as they enter the abdomen through the oesophageal hiatus. Total vagal

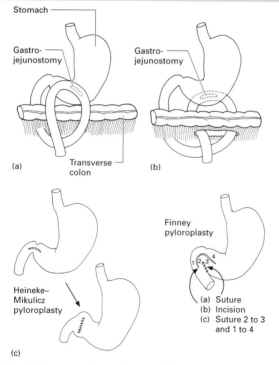

Fig. 57 (a) An antecolic anterior gastrojejunostomy. (b) A retrocolic posterior gastrojejunostomy. (c) Two types of pyloroplasty.

denervation of the stomach results in gastric stasis and because of this a drainage procedure is necessary. Various types of pyloroplasty and gastrojejunostomy are shown in Fig. 57. This operation can be performed laparoscopically.

Codes

Blood .... Group and save serum
GA/LA .... GA
Opn time .... 60–90 min
Stay .... 7 days
Drains out .... 5 days (if used)
Sutures out .... 7 days
Off work .... 6 weeks

OPERATION: TRUNCAL VAGOTOMY AND ANTRECTOMY

The distal part of the stomach, which produces gastrin, is excised together with the pylorus. The stomach is usually reconstituted using a Billroth I procedure (see Gastric ulcer, p. 292). The trunks of the vagal nerves are also divided. This operation is usually reserved for disease that has recurred after previous surgery.

Codes

Blood .... 4 units
GA/LA .... GA
Opn time .... About 2 h
Stay .... 7–10 days
Drains out .... 3–6 days
Sutures out .... 7 days
Off work .... 6 weeks

OPERATION: OPEN HIGHLY SELECTIVE VAGOTOMY

Only the nerve fibres supplying the parietal cells in the body and fundus of the stomach are cut. The fibres supplying the antrum remain intact. In this operation, gastric emptying is almost normal and no drainage procedure is necessary. The procedure has the advantage of being free of the side-effects of diarrhoea, dumping and bilious vomiting. It can be performed laparoscopically but is tedious. It has been made easier by the advent of the ultrasonic harmonic scalpel that facilitates coagulation and division of the gastric vessels.

Codes

	Open HSV	Laparoscopic HSV
Blood	Group and save	Group and save serum
GA/LA	GA	GA
Opn time	90–150 min	2–4 h
Stay	5–7 days	2–3 days
Drains out	0	0
Sutures out	7 days	Absorbable
Off work	6 weeks	2–3 weeks

Postoperative care

The postoperative care of patients who have had a truncal vagotomy and antrectomy or truncal vagotomy and drainage is similar to that for patients who have had a partial gastrectomy (p. 294).

The postoperative care of highly selective vagotomy patients is usually very straightforward. The only major complication to be aware of is lesser-curve necrosis and this occurs in about 0.3% of patients. The patient suddenly deteriorates about 48 h after the operation and shows signs of increasing peritonitis. It may be difficult to diagnose the perforation because there is already air under the diaphragm on a straight abdominal X-ray. A limited barium meal will show the defect, however, and if in doubt a laparotomy is advisable.

Many patients complain of dysphagia after vagotomy. This is always transient. The patient should be advised to stick to soft, semi-liquid foods until the dysphagia improves. The symptom has usually disappeared by about 6 weeks after the operation. It is worthwhile warning patients about this symptom and explaining that it is due to the fact that the operation takes place around the lower oesophagus and that the difficulty in swallowing will settle as the operation site heals.

Perforated peptic ulcer

Either gastric or duodenal ulcers may perforate, although perforation of the latter is more common. As gastric ulcers are frequently posterior, they may perforate into the lesser sac. Anterior duodenal ulcers perforate direct into the main peritoneal cavity.

Recognizing the pattern

The typical pattern of symptoms suggesting gastric or duodenal ulcer has already been described. Not infrequently, however,

patients present with a perforation without much in the way of
past history of indigestion. There is a sudden, defined onset of
severe epigastric pain. The patient frequently remembers the
precise time of onset (e.g. 'just as the nine o'clock news was
beginning'). The pain rapidly spreads first to the right iliac fossa
and later all over the abdomen. When a gastric ulcer perforates
into the lesser sac, the symptoms are much more localized until
gastric contents leak out of the foramen of Winslow, giving rise
to a right-sided peritonitis. This picture can be confused with
acute appendicitis.

On examination there is typically marked tenderness over the
whole of the abdomen with 'board-like rigidity'. Percussion of
the liver may reveal absent liver dullness. This sign is due to
gas lying between the liver and the anterior abdominal wall.

Proving the diagnosis

The diagnosis is proved by doing an erect chest X-ray together
with a supine and erect abdominal X-ray. Gas may be seen
under the diaphragm.

Management

The management of an acute perforation is usually surgical.
It is, however, possible on occasion to manage these lesions
conservatively.

1 A nasogastric tube is positioned in the stomach and regularly aspirated. It is essential that the stomach is kept empty.
2 Adequate intravenous fluid replacement is given. These
patients have usually lost a lot of fluid into the peritoneal
cavity and are markedly dehydrated. A urinary catheter is
essential for adequate resuscitation. A central venous pressure (CVP) line may also be needed when large amounts of
fluid have to be given, especially in the elderly patient with
cardiac disease. Fluid requirement in excess of 2 L is not
uncommon.
3 The patient is given broad-spectrum antibiotic cover.

OPERATION: FOR PERFORATED PEPTIC ULCER
The abdomen is opened through a vertical incision. Deep
sutures are placed through the oedematous tissue around the
perforation and a patch of omentum sewn over to close the
defect (Fig. 58). If the perforation is less than 8 h old, a
definitive ulcer curing operation may be performed at the

Continued on p. 302

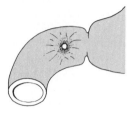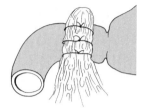

Fig. 58 Oversewing a perforated duodenal ulcer.

Continued.

same time. The peritoneum is carefully washed out and all food residue removed. Drains are placed at the site of the perforation and in the subphrenic spaces if there is extensive contamination.

This procedure is not difficult to do laparoscopically providing the surgeon is experienced in endoscopic suturing.

Codes

	Open	Laparoscopic
Blood	Group and save serum	Group and save serum
GA/LA	GA	GA
Opn time	1 h	60–90 min
Stay	If uncomplicated 5 days	If uncomplicated 48 h
Drains out	3–5 days	48 h
Sutures out	7 days	Absorbable
Off work	Variable, 4–6 weeks	4 weeks

Postoperative care
The main problem is of persistent intra-abdominal sepsis either in the subphrenic regions or in the pelvis. This may delay recovery. The management of intra-abdominal abscesses is dealt with on pp. 70–74.

Pyloric stenosis

The condition known as 'pyloric stenosis' in adults is usually, in fact, a duodenal stenosis secondary to scarring from a chronic duodenal ulcer (pyloric stenosis in babies is dealt with on pp. 614–15).

Recognizing the pattern

Pyloric stenosis can arise in any patient with a duodenal ulcer and the developing obstruction is usually heralded by the onset of vomiting. Characteristically this is copious and contains food ingested a day or two previously. In long-standing pyloric stenosis the patient may become very ill with lassitude and loss of weight. In some elderly patients there is very little history of previous indigestion until the stenosis develops.

If the vomiting has been prolonged the patient is dehydrated and weak. There may be tenderness over the duodenal region. The characteristic sign is a 'succussion splash'. A stethoscope is placed over the stomach and the patient gently shaken from side to side. Food can be heard splashing in the stomach several hours after the previous meal.

Proving the diagnosis

The diagnosis is proved either radiologically or by fibroscopy. The grossly distended stomach may be visible on a plain abdominal X-ray. If contrast studies are needed either very dilute barium or gastrografin should be used. On fibroscopy the stenosed duodenum is usually seen and the fibroscope cannot be made to pass through it. The food residue in the stomach makes the view difficult.

Management

Pyloric stenosis is one of the absolute indications for surgery in duodenal ulcer. Before surgery is undertaken, electrolyte and nutritional disturbances must be corrected. Several days of conservative management may be needed to achieve this. Prolonged loss of gastric vomitus leads to a metabolic alkalosis with a low serum potassium. Adequate intravenous therapy including potassium and chloride ions must therefore be given. A nasogastric tube is passed and the stomach kept empty. Intravenous cimetidine can also be given. Not infrequently the stomach begins to empty again with this management. Nevertheless, once obstruction has developed it is likely to recur and surgical treatment should be undertaken.

OPERATION: FOR PYLORIC STENOSIS

The most common procedure performed is a truncal vagotomy and pyloroplasty or gastroenterostomy. Some surgeons prefer to perform a highly selective vagotomy and in this case the stenosis is dealt with either by a duodenoplasty or by dilatation. In a duodenoplasty the stenosis in the

Continued on p. 304

Continued.

duodenum is incised longitudinally and sewn up vertically, thus widening the area. These manoeuvres allow the pylorus to be retained and thus obviate the development of problems related to abnormal gastric emptying after a drainage procedure (pp. 313–317).

Codes

Blood .... 2 units
GA/LA .... GA
Opn time .... 1–2 h
Stay .... 7–10 days
Drains out .... 3–5 days
Sutures out .... 7 days
Off work .... 4–6 weeks

Postoperative care
See p. 300.

Haematemesis and melaena

Haematemesis and melaena are due to bleeding from the upper gastrointestinal tract. Bleeding from the lower gastrointestinal tract is discussed under 'rectal' bleeding (p. 380). Upper gastrointestinal haemorrhage may be from the following sites:

1 The pharynx: e.g. vomiting of swallowed blood from a nasal haemorrhage.

2 The oesophagus: oesophagitis with ulceration secondary to hiatus hernia, oesophageal varices secondary to portal hypertension.

3 The stomach:

  (a) gastritis — biliary, drug-induced or alcoholic
  (b) gastric ulcer
  (c) benign tumours, e.g. leiomyoma
  (d) carcinoma
  (e) Mallory–Weiss tear.

4 The duodenum: duodenal ulcer.

The shocked patient vomiting blood is a common and dramatic surgical emergency. A houseman's training can be severely tested in these circumstances and the condition will be dealt with in some detail here. The patients are usually managed in coordination with the gastroenterology physicians.

A suggested scheme of management is as follows:

1 Initial assessment

2 Resuscitation

3 Secondary assessment
4 Further management.

Initial assessment
An assessment must be made of the following.

Amount of blood lost by the patient
This is assessed by an estimate from the history, state of the patient's blood pressure, pulse, peripheral circulation and level of consciousness. After a sudden bleed a patient who is unconscious with a minimal blood pressure, a rapid, thin pulse and cold clammy extremities has probably lost 1.5–2 L of blood. A patient who is conscious but mildly shocked, with a low blood pressure and a tachycardia, may have lost about 1 L. Signs of shock are not usually present when the patient has lost less than 500 mL.

Rate of bleeding
How rapidly is the patient bleeding? Is the history of a true massive single haematemesis or a more prolonged loss of blood? A patient who has had a massive haematemesis is likely to have another one that may prove fatal. Further assessment of the rate of blood loss is made after regular monitoring and resuscitation has been instituted. Response to resuscitation is a key feature in assessing the amount and rate of blood loss.

General condition
The age and general fitness of the patient will give an indication as to how much blood loss he can stand.

At the end of this initial assessment you should have a good idea as to how serious the situation is and how immediate the following steps must be.

Resuscitation
Insert two large-bore intravenous needles (14-gauge if possible). Take blood for cross-matching. Six to eight units should be cross-matched and blood sent for haemoglobin and packed cell volume estimation. Set up an intravenous infusion.

Types of intravenous fluid
For the patient who is not suffering from shock, set up an infusion of 500 cm^3 of normal saline over 4 h, thus maintaining intravenous access until blood arrives or in case the situation deteriorates rapidly.

For the shocked patient, any suitable intravenous infusion (e.g. normal saline) is better than nothing. Colloidal solutions (e.g. dextran or Haemaccel) are better than electrolyte solutions. Whole blood is better than colloid solutions, although it may not be available in the early stages.

Amount of intravenous fluid
Infuse sufficient to rapidly restore the blood pressure to an acceptable level (e.g. systolic blood pressure up to 100–120). In elderly or decrepit patients a CVP line may be essential during this process, to avoid overloading the patient and precipitating heart failure.

Install a urinary catheter
The urinary output per hour is a good indication of the perfusion of the central organs during shock.

Institute regular monitoring
For example, quarter-hourly pulse and blood pressure, CVP levels and hourly urine output.

After the initial assessment and resuscitation the situation should be coming under control. You must then push on rapidly with the next phase.

Secondary assessment
A full history should be taken either from the patient or from relatives, looking for symptoms suggestive of the causative pathology. Note particularly any indigestion, heartburn or reflux, abdominal pain, alcohol intake or recent use of drugs, especially non-steroidal anti-inflammatory drugs.

A general assessment of the patient's health must also be undertaken. Unless this is done, there are likely to be large gaps in the patient's record and these may become important as management continues. You should also review the parameters measured so far and revise your assessment of the rate of bleeding.

Fibroscopy should be undertaken to confirm your provisional diagnosis.

Further management
Most patients with upper gastrointestinal haemorrhage are controlled by conservative means, including the following:
1 Blood replacement
2 Sedation and bed rest

3 Antacid or other relevant medical therapy
4 Endoscopic injection therapy to stop bleeding.

The patient should therefore be admitted and kept under close observation.

If bleeding continues or recurs, then further management is usually surgical and depends on the causative lesion as below.

Bleeding peptic ulcer

The surgeon should be informed of any patient with gastrointestinal bleeding and called upon to see anyone who has:

1 Lost in excess of 6 units of blood
2 Had a massive haematemesis
3 Rebled during adequate medical management
4 Endoscopic evidence of high risk of bleeding, e.g. visible or bleeding vessel in the ulcer base.

Elderly patients are more likely to continue bleeding than younger ones because their arteries tend to be arteriosclerotic and less able to contract down.

OPERATION: FOR BLEEDING PEPTIC ULCER

A bleeding gastric ulcer is usually treated by emergency partial gastrectomy. The ulcer may be adherent posteriorly to the pancreas and may have eroded the splenic artery. In that case massive blood loss may be encountered. At least 10 units should be cross-matched for a posterior bleeding gastric ulcer.

A bleeding duodenal ulcer is usually treated by a vagotomy and pyloroplasty with under-running of the ulcer. Some surgeons prefer partial gastrectomy with excision of the duodenal ulcer. Surgeons who favour highly selective vagotomy may perform this procedure as an emergency and open the duodenum by a longitudinal incision to under-run the ulcer.

Postoperative care

In general, this is as described in the previous sections (p. 300). However, there is an increased risk of recurrent haemorrhage and the patient must be carefully monitored for this.

Mallory–Weiss tear

This lesion is a tear of the gastro–oesophageal junction occurring during an episode of vomiting. The patient often gives a history of vomiting at the end of which blood is noted. The condition is diagnosed on endoscopy and usually settles with conservative management. If laparotomy is required, the stomach is emptied and the bleeding point oversewn.

Acute gastritis
This is a frequent source of gastric haemorrhage. There may be a history of drug ingestion, particularly of drugs used in the management of arthritis, such as phenylbutazone, indomethacin, steroids and aspirin compounds. Acute gastritis can also occur in septicaemia.

Management
In most cases the condition settles with adequate medical therapy and withdrawal of the offending drug. In some cases, however, bleeding continues unabated and in that case operation becomes mandatory. There is no agreed surgical policy for dealing with this diffuse gastric condition. The majority of surgeons would probably perform a partial gastrectomy of the Pólya type.

Oesophagitis
The management of oesophagitis and hiatus hernia is dealt with on p. 287. Bleeding from these lesions usually settles with conservative management.

Oesophageal varices
These are dealt with in detail on p. 347.

Carcinoma of the stomach
Adenocarcinoma of the stomach is thought occasionally to arise on the basis of a previous gastritis or benign gastric ulcer. The macroscopic appearance varies from an ulcer to a cauliflower growth or the more diffuse 'leather-bottle stomach'. The latter is due to diffuse spread of malignant cells along the submucosal layer of the stomach. Carcinoma of the stomach is more common in those of blood group A.

Sixty-four per cent of growths are situated in the prepyloric region. Spread is by direct invasion into neighbouring organs, through the lymphatics and in the blood. Transcoelomic spread may give rise to peritoneal secondaries and secondaries in the ovary (Krukenberg's tumour).

Recognizing the pattern

The patient is typically aged between 40 and 60 years and the condition is more common in males.

There may or may not be a preceding history of indigestion due to a gastric ulcer. The patient begins to suffer from symptoms of nausea, anorexia and epigastric pain. The pain is initially worse after meals but later becomes continuous and starts to keep him awake at night. He also begins to lose weight.

On examination there may be a mass palpable in the left hypochondrium. Signs of spread of the disease should be looked for, including enlarged supraclavicular nodes in the neck (Troisier's sign) and enlargement of the liver. The patient is usually cachectic and may be jaundiced.

Carcinoma of the stomach may also present with haematemesis and melaena.

Proving the diagnosis

The diagnosis is demonstrated on a barium meal which shows an irregular craggy filling defect in the stomach. A fibroscopy is mandatory and a biopsy will confirm the diagnosis. Very small gastric carcinomas may be picked up on fibroscopy and these are the lesions which are most amenable to treatment.

Management

Patients with carcinoma of the stomach are frequently debilitated and both the haemoglobin and serum albumin must be checked before surgery is contemplated. Carcinoma of the stomach carries a poor prognosis and the only method of management that has any success is surgical removal of the lesion. Where surgical cure is impossible (e.g. where there are already distant metastases), operation is only indicated to relieve local symptoms such as persistent pain or obstruction with vomiting. 5-fluorouracil occasionally provides effective palliation for carcinoma of the stomach.

The surgical management is to excise the tumour and the local lymph nodes if a cure is to be attempted. Either a subtotal or total gastrectomy may be required in order to achieve adequate clearance of the tumour. The latter may be carried out through the abdomen alone, or through a thoracoabdominal incision. The extent of the resection is based on the stage, site of tumour and the lymph nodes involved.

Continued on p. 310

Continued.

Preoperative management

As with all cases of malignant disease, both the patient and his relatives will need careful counselling. The patient may require transfusion of blood or intravenous feeding for several days before the operation. If he is able to take oral fluids satisfactorily, then a high nutrition oral diet should be instituted. Adequate vitamins should be given including vitamin C.

If there is gastric outlet obstruction and stasis, the patient should be put on clear fluids for 48 h and the stomach washed out preoperatively.

OPERATION: GASTRECTOMIES FOR CANCER
(see also gastric ulcer, p.292)

Gastrectomies for cancer are classified according to how radical they are.

R1: includes resection of the lymph nodes along the greater and lesser curve of the stomach. The majority of resections undertaken in the UK are R1 gastrectomies.

R2: also includes resection of lymph nodes along the main arteries of the stomach, splenic (splenectomy) and retro-pancreatic nodes (distal pancreatectomy).

R3: also may include clearance of lymph nodes in the porta hepatis, middle colic nodes (transverse colectomy), retro-pancreatic nodes (subtotal pancreatectomy or Whipple), around the root of the mesentery and hepatic lobectomy.

OPERATION: TOTAL GASTRECTOMY

In this operation the whole of the stomach is removed, usually for a cancer on the lesser curve or the body. The oesophagus is anastomosed either to a loop of jejunum (with closure of the duodenal stump) or, rarely, directly to the duodenal stump. The oesophagojejunal anastomosis is vulnerable and leaks are common. Because of this, the surgeon may pass a nasogastric tube down through the anastomosis into the proximal jejunum.

Codes

Blood	4–6 units
GA/LA	GA
Opn time	3–5 h
Stay	2–3 weeks
Drains out	7 days
Sutures out	7–10 days
Off work	6–9 weeks

OPERATION: THORACOABDOMINAL
GASTRECTOMY

This operation is undertaken where the carcinoma of the stomach involves the lower oesophagus. In this case an oblique incision is extended up along the bed of the eighth rib and the chest opened. The anastomosis to the oesophagus is then carried out inside the chest.

Codes

Blood .... 4–6 units
GA/LA .... GA
Opn time .... 3–5 h
Stay .... 2–4 weeks
Drains out .... Pleural 2 days; anastomotic
                                          5–7 days; abdominal drain 7 days
Sutures out .... 7–10 days
Off work .... 8–12 weeks

Postoperative care

The patient is given no fluids at all by mouth for 7 days, at the end of which a limited barium swallow is performed. If the anastomosis is intact, oral feeding can recommence. If it is not, then the patient can be fed either through the nasogastric tube or intravenously. Intravenous feeding may in any case be continued throughout the early postoperative period.

Postgastrectomy syndromes

These are becoming rare as the number of gastric resections for benign disease diminishes. They include the following:

1 Bilious vomiting
2 Dumping
3 Diarrhoea (e.g. postvagotomy diarrhoea).

A fourth problem is recurrent pain, which may be due to the dumping syndrome, recurrent peptic ulcer disease, intestinal obstruction due to adhesions, gastritis due to *Helicobacter* infection or other new pathology.

Bilious vomiting

This is vomiting of pure bile and occurs in up to 10% of patients following a gastrectomy. The cause is not clearly understood but it can follow any operation in which the pylorus has been removed or bypassed. It is more common after a Pólya type II reconstruction or after a gastroenterostomy. The symptom is associated with a marked 'biliary gastritis' visible on endoscopy.

It may be associated with symptoms of abdominal pain and dumping.

Recognizing the pattern

The history is of intermittent sudden attacks of vomiting 15–30 min after a meal. The vomit typically consists of pure bile with no food. This may be preceded by epigastric cramping pain, which is relieved by the vomiting.

Management

Bilious vomiting is more common immediately after a gastric operation and tends to settle as time passes. It is therefore worthwhile exhibiting patience. The patient should be reassured that the symptoms usually settle.

Medical management includes substances which help to bind bile salts such as hydrotalcite (Altacite). Metoclopramide (Maxolon) may also be of value.

If the symptoms persist some form of bile diversion or gastric reconstruction procedure is required.

OPERATION: GASTRIC RECONSTRUCTION FOR BILIOUS VOMITING

If the original procedure was a truncal vagotomy and gastro-enterostomy (see p. 297), the gastroenterostomy can be closed, providing a year has elapsed since the vagotomy was performed. Similarly, a pyloroplasty can be taken down and reconstructed.

Bile diversion is best achieved by converting the standard enterostomy loop to a Roux-en-Y procedure (see Fig. 59).

This results in the bile entering the intestine well away from the stomach.

Codes

Blood	2 units
GA/LA	GA
Opn time	About 2 h
Stay	7 days
Drains out	2–5 days
Sutures out	7 days
Off work	4–6 weeks

Postoperative care

There are no special problems after these procedures. Oral fluids can be reintroduced as soon as the stomach is seen to be emptying (as evidenced by diminished gastric aspirate and passage of flatus).

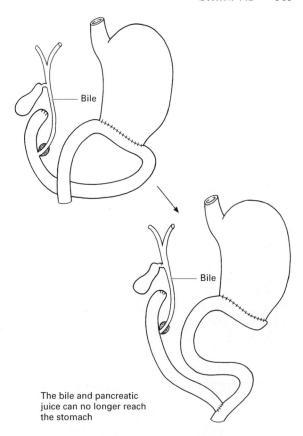

The bile and pancreatic
juice can no longer reach
the stomach

Fig. 59 Roux-en-Y conversion for biliary gastritis.

Dumping

This consists of abdominal distension and colic, and vasomotor
disturbance occurring after meals. It is seen after a gastrectomy
or a drainage procedure. There are two types.

Early dumping

This is due to rapid emptying of the stomach, a high osmotic
load in the small bowel and an increased splanchnic blood flow
resulting in a fluid shift from the vascular compartment to the
bowel lumen. This is precipitated particularly by hot, sweet or
bulky meals taken with fluid.

Late dumping

This is due to a reactive hypoglycaemia caused by increased
insulin output in response to the earlier hyperglycaemia. The
hyperglycaemia itself follows rapid gastric emptying.

Recognizing the pattern

Dumping is more common in women. Early dumping starts immediately after a meal and consists of attacks of sweating, flushing, tachycardia, palpitations, epigastric fullness, nausea and occasionally colicky abdominal pain, vomiting and diarrhoea.

Late dumping starts 1–2 h after meals and consists of faintness accompanied by sweating, tremor and nausea.

Proving the diagnosis

The diagnosis of dumping is made on the history. Hypoglycaemia may be confirmed by measuring the blood sugar during an attack.

Management

The symptoms are difficult to treat and are best managed by persuading the patient to modify his intake of food so as to minimize the rapid gastric emptying of foodstuffs. Patients with dumping must have the causes explained to them and should be reassured that the condition usually settles with time. After 6 months only 1–2% of patients are still affected.

Early dumping can be prevented by small, dry meals, with a diet consisting of fat and protein and restricted carbohydrate. Drinks should be taken between and not during meals. Late dumping is made worse by exercise after a meal so susceptible patients should rest for an hour after eating.

Severe persistent dumping can be treated by closing a gastroenterostomy or pyloroplasty as above, or by inserting a short reversed segment of jejunum just beyond the pylorus.

Diarrhoea

Truncal vagotomy not only decreases gastric secretion and motility, thereby delaying stomach emptying, but also affects the rest of the bowel to a variable extent. Up to 50% of patients after a truncal vagotomy suffer some increase in bowel habit and 5% need treatment for this. The diarrhoea is typically 'episodic'. That is to say, the patient has normal bowel actions most of the time but is then suddenly struck with episodes of urgency and looseness. The mechanism is uncertain and several factors may be responsible. The rapid emptying of the stomach which follows the accompanying gastric drainage procedure results in hyperosmolar contents arriving in the small bowel lumen. As the bowel rapidly dilutes this, vigorous peristalsis ensues, producing some of the symptoms of early dumping and also diarrhoea. There may also be a direct effect of loss of vagal influence on the small bowel and on the biliary tract. Diarrhoea is not seen following a highly selective vagotomy.

Recognizing the pattern

The patient complains of an increase in bowel habit, which in severe cases may consist of attacks of uncontrollable watery diarrhoea. These attacks are episodic and unpredictable.

Management

The diarrhoea sometimes responds to codeine phosphate (45–120 mg daily in three to six divided doses), diphenoxylate (Lomotil) or loperamide (Imodium). A short course of neomycin or phthalyl sulphathiazole occasionally provides long-lasting relief. For severe cases reoperation and insertion of a 10 cm reversed segment of jejunum at the gastric outlet or 100 cm down the jejunum can relieve the symptoms.

7.3 Central Abdominal Pain

Acute appendicitis

This is the commonest surgical emergency in this country. The appendix has a narrow lumen and there is a rich collection of lymphatic tissue in the submucosa. Obstruction of the lumen can follow impaction of a faecalith or swelling of the submucosal lymphatic tissue. Once this occurs, a vicious circle ensues with further swelling and obstruction, blockage of blood supply, infection and ischaemia of the distal appendix.

Recognizing the pattern

Acute appendicitis can occur at any age, although it is particularly common between the ages of 10 and 30 years.

The typical history is of central abdominal colic associated with nausea and vomiting. After a few hours the colic subsides and the pain settles in the right iliac fossa. At this stage the pain is worse on movement (walking, coughing).

The patient looks unwell and is flushed. There is often a fetor. The tongue is furred and the patient has a low-grade pyrexia, typically of 37.5°C (99.5°F). The fever is very rarely above 38.0°C (100.4°F) in the early stages of the disease. There is also a tachycardia.

Examination of the abdomen discloses marked tenderness in the right iliac fossa with guarding and rebound. By careful palpation it is usually possible to delineate a constant line of tenderness over the site of the appendix.

This localized tenderness is the single most important factor in making the diagnosis. Rectal examination may also disclose tenderness high up on the right side, especially if the appendix is in a pelvic position.

The clinical picture of appendicitis does, of course, vary widely and the presentation may be particularly confusing in the very young and the very old. A localized line of tenderness, together with signs of peritonitis, will indicate the need for operative exploration.

Proving the diagnosis

Surprisingly there are no absolute tests to prove or disprove the diagnosis of acute appendicitis. If the suspicion is strong enough, a laparoscopy or laparotomy must be performed in order to exclude the disease.

Management

Preoperative management

The patient must be adequately rehydrated before operation and the value of giving preoperative antibiotics with the premedication has been demonstrated. A metronidazole suppository is effective.

If the history is very long (e.g. 7 days) and if the pain is settling it may be justified to treat the condition conservatively. In these cases an appendix mass may be palpable in the right iliac fossa. The patient is observed to be sure the mass settles and an 'interval appendicectomy' is planned 2–3 months later.

OPERATION: OPEN APPENDICECTOMY

The abdomen is opened through a grid-iron incision situated in the right iliac fossa. The appendix lies under McBurney's point, which is on a line between the anterior superior iliac spine and the umbilicus, two-thirds of the way from the umbilicus. The incision is best made almost horizontally in Langer's lines (see Fig. 60). The muscles of the abdominal wall are split in the line of their fibres (grid-iron incision) and the peritoneum opened. The presence or absence of peritoneal fluid is noted and a swab taken. The upper part of the caecum is grasped and pulled out of the

Continued on p. 318

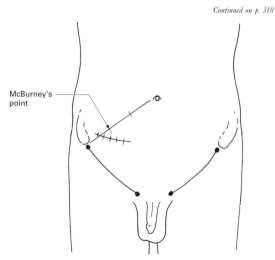

McBurney's point

Fig. 60 Appendicectomy: the incision is made just below McBurney's point, horizontally parallel to Langer's skin lines.

Continued.

wound towards the patient's feet. After completing this manoeuvre, the caecum is then pulled upward towards the patient's head and the appendix is thus delivered. It may be necessary to free adhesions in order to achieve this. With a retrocaecal appendix it is necessary to mobilize the lower pole of the caecum by dividing the peritoneum laterally. The appendix stump is crushed and tied with catgut. The appendicular vessels are tied and the appendix is removed. Many surgeons invert the appendix stump into the caecal wall using a purse-string or 'Z' suture. The terminal 100 cm of small bowel is gently examined to see if there is a coincident Meckel's diver-ticulum. A drain is inserted into the peritoneum if there is pus at the appendix site. The wound may also be drained.

Codes

Blood	0
GA/LA	GA
Opn time	15–20 min
Stay	4–5 days in absence of residual sepsis
Drains out	3–5 days
Sutures out	5–7 days
Off work	1 month

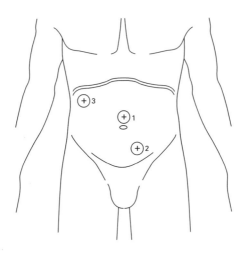

Fig. 61 Possible port sites for laparoscopic appendicectomy.

OPERATION: LAPAROSCOPIC APPENDICECTOMY
(see Fig. 61)

Ports are placed in the abdomen and a full initial laparoscopy is performed before the appendix is visualized. It is usually necessary to insert another port and atraumatic graspers to move the bowel around. If the appendix is normal it can be left alone though some surgeons prefer to remove it. If it is inflamed it is freed as in the open procedure mobilizing the caecum if necessary. The artery is clipped and the appendix stump is divided between ligatures. The stump is not usually inverted. The appendix is removed through a 10–12 mm port. This approach is particularly suitable for patients having an interval appendicectomy after the sepsis has all settled down.

Codes

Blood	0
GA/LA	GA
Opn time	30–60 min
Stay	1–3 days in the absence of residual sepsis
Drains out	2–3 days
Sutures out	Absorbable
Off work	2 weeks

Postoperative care

The postoperative ileus after the open operation is usually short-lived and fluids can be reintroduced orally after about 24 h. Thereafter the postoperative recovery is usually uneventful. A careful watch must be kept for developing sepsis in the wound or in the pelvis. The temperature chart is the best guide to this (see p. 66).

The wound must be inspected before the patient leaves hospital and a rectal examination should also be done. Surgeons vary widely in their use of antibiotics in and around the time of an appendicectomy. If antibiotics are given postoperatively, it has to be remembered that abscess formation may be delayed and the patient and his doctor should be warned of this.

A patient managed laparoscopically has the same danger of residual sepsis as one managed by open operation and must be warned of this if they leave hospital early. They should come back if they develop increasing pain or a fever.

For the management of wound abscess and pelvic abscess, see pp. 66 and 73.

Mesenteric adenitis

The mesenteric lymph nodes may become inflamed as part of a general infection or a gastroenteritis. The importance of the condition lies in differentiating it from acute appendicitis.

Recognizing the pattern

The patient is usually under the age of 30 years.

The complaint is of abdominal pain. This may be generalized or localized, possibly in the right iliac fossa. There may be symptoms of diarrhoea and/or vomiting, or of a recent upper respiratory tract infection.

On examination the tenderness tends to be moderate with little guarding or rebound, and poorly localized. The patient may be pyrexial, often with a fever above 37.5°C.

Proving the diagnosis

A laparotomy may be indicated to exclude acute appendicitis. In that case the appendix is normal and large inflamed fleshy lymph nodes are seen in the mesentery. Otherwise the diagnosis is clinical and there are no specific confirmatory tests.

Management

If appendicitis can be excluded, the management is conservative and the patient can be allowed home.

Intestinal obstruction

The bowel may become obstructed from a variety of causes anywhere along its length. The obstruction may be mechanical or adynamic (localized or generalized paralytic ileus).

Mechanical causes are usefully divided into those which compress the bowel from the outside, those which arise within the wall of the bowel and obstruct the lumen, and those which arise within the lumen (Table 18). Paralytic ileus is described on p. 42.

Recognizing the pattern

The patient can be of any age from a newborn baby, who complains of colicky central abdominal pains, onwards.

Some time after the onset of the colic, the patient begins to vomit and there is total constipation. The intervals between the waves of colic give some idea of the site of the obstruction. Higher obstruction is associated with a short interval between bouts of pain whereas obstruction of the ileum has longer intervals. Vomiting also occurs earlier in high intestinal obstruction.

Table 18 Mechanical causes of intestinal obstruction.

Outside the bowel	
Adhesions or bands	p. 322
Volvulus	p. 322
Invasion by neighbouring malignant growths	
Strangulated hernia, etc.	p. 322
In the bowel wall	
Tumours	pp. 326, 384
Infarction	p. 324
Congenital atresia	pp. 603–613
Hirschsprung's disease	p. 610
Inflammatory bowel disease	pp. 373, 375
Diverticulitis	p. 397
In the lumen	
Impacted faeces	p. 37
Bolus obstruction	
Gall stone ileus	p. 331
Intussusception	pp. 325, 615
Large polyps	p. 382

The three symptoms of abdominal pain, vomiting and absolute constipation are almost diagnostic of intestinal obstruction.

The patient may be dehydrated due to fluid losses into the intestine and vomiting, and there may be visible peristalsis under the abdominal wall. The degree and site of abdominal distension varies with the level of obstruction. The distended loops of obstructed small bowel are often tender on palpation. On auscultation there are hyperactive high–pitched bowel sounds.

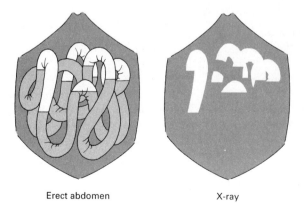

Erect abdomen   X-ray

Fig. 62 Fluid levels in obstructed small bowel.

Proving the diagnosis

The diagnosis is proved by performing a supine and erect abdominal X-ray, which shows the presence of distended loops of small bowel together with fluid levels (see Fig. 62). If the colon is obstructed the caecum will also be distended.

Management

The initial management of small bowel obstruction is to replenish the fluid loss and keep the bowel empty by nasogastric suction. In many cases this will relieve the condition. Indications for operation are failure of conservative treatment after 48–72 h, or a general deterioration in the patient's condition and the onset of abdominal tenderness and a tachycardia. These latter signs may indicate that part of the bowel is becoming ischaemic.

OPERATION: FOR INTESTINAL OBSTRUCTION

The procedure undertaken depends on the underlying cause.

1 Intestinal adhesions. The adhesions are divided and loops of bowel mobilized so as to free the obstruction. Occasionally it is necessary to resect a damaged segment of small bowel.

2 Volvulus. The volvulus is untwisted and the viability of the bowel checked. The surgeon may wait to see whether a dubious segment of bowel regains its colour satisfactorily after a period.

3 Strangulated hernia. The hernia is repaired and the bowel dealt with as above.

Codes

Blood	2 units
GA/LA	GA
Opn time	Variable, depends on cause
Stay	Variable, 1–2 weeks
Drains out	Nasogastric tube out when flatus passed; other drains according to general principles (see p. 119)
Sutures out	7–10 days
Off work	Variable

Other causes of intestinal obstruction are dealt with in other sections (see Table 18).

Meckel's diverticulum

This lesion is a remnant of the attachment of the small bowel to the embryological yolk sac. It arises from the antemesenteric border somewhere along the distal 100 cm of small bowel. The diverticulum may contain remnants of all types of intestinal mucosa (including acid-secreting gastric mucosa).

Recognizing the pattern

The patient may be of any age, although problems from a Meckel's diverticulum are more common in children.

The lesion may remain asymptomatic for the whole of the patient's life. If it does cause trouble, however, the presentation is in one of three ways.

1 The picture of acute appendicitis. This is due to obstruction of the lumen of the diverticulum in exactly the same way as the appendix becomes obstructed. This presentation is not common as the diverticulum usually has a wide neck.

2 The picture of intestinal obstruction. This is often due to the fact that the Meckel's diverticulum is associated with a band running up to the umbilicus and this may obstruct other loops of bowel.

3 Intestinal bleeding. If the diverticulum contains gastric mucosa a peptic ulcer may arise in the adjacent ileum. This bleeds and the patient passes fresh blood per rectum. This is perhaps the most common presentation of a Meckel's diverticulum in children.

Proving the diagnosis

This is difficult and frequently a laparotomy is necessary. An attempt should be made to define the diverticulum using radioactive technetium scanning, but this is not always reliable. The lesion may be demonstrated on a barium meal and 'follow-through', or even a barium enema, but again the investigation is unreliable. For this reason, if there is a strong suspicion that a Meckel's diverticulum might be present, a laparotomy is undertaken.

Management

OPERATION: FOR MECKEL'S DIVERTICULUM
The diverticulum is resected and the small bowel closed. If there is an ulcer in the ileum, this segment of ileum is resected together with the diverticulum. The appendix may be taken out in the same operation to avoid diagnostic confusion later. This operation can also be performed laparoscopically and is very similar to laparoscopic appendicectomy (see p. 318).

Codes

Blood ....0 (babies may require 1 unit)
GA/LA ....GA
Opn time ....1 h
Stay ....5–7 days
Drains out 0
Sutures out ....7 days
Off work ....3–4 weeks

Ischaemic bowel

Ischaemic bowel may arise either secondary to some of the causes of intestinal obstruction, or as a primary condition from interruption of the arterial or venous blood supply. This is usually due to an embolus from the heart or great vessels or due to thrombosis. Bowel infarction is a life-threatening condition and early laparotomy is mandatory. In this section primary ischaemia of the bowel will be considered. A more recent cause of intestinal necrosis is gas gangrene of the small intestine occurring in neutropenic patients while under treatment for leukaemia.

Recognizing the pattern

The patient is usually elderly and may have other signs of cardiac or vascular disease.

The patient complains of a sudden onset of abdominal pain which rapidly becomes very severe. The patient becomes very distressed and shocked. There may be a history of recent myocardial infarction or dysrhythmia.

On examination the signs may not seem to coincide with the severity of the patient's pain. There is usually some localized tenderness but not a lot in the way of guarding or rebound tenderness in the early stages. Rectal examination may reveal blood. The patient may be in atrial fibrillation.

Proving the diagnosis

The most important point to remember is the possibility of bowel ischaemia in undiagnosed severe abdominal pain. Straight abdominal X-ray may show a slightly dilated loop of bowel with thickened walls. The serum amylase should be measured to exclude pancreatitis. Remember that mesenteric infarction can cause a slightly elevated level (600–900 Somogyi units).

Management

Preoperative management

Before laparotomy, resuscitation may be required to treat shock. Broad-spectrum parenteral antibiotics must be given.

OPERATION: LAPAROTOMY FOR ISCHAEMIC BOWEL

At operation the ischaemic loop of bowel is identified. Various causes may be found. The ischaemia may be secondary to a volvulus or band causing obstruction of the mesenteric vessels. In this case treatment of the cause may result in adequate perfusion of the ischaemic segment.

Another possible cause is embolism or thrombosis of one of the major arteries supplying the bowel. If the bowel is still potentially viable, an embolectomy or bypass operation may be performed to restore the blood supply. Any bowel that fails to recover must be resected. Occasionally where there is a long loop of ischaemic bowel and viability is dubious, it may be permissible to close the abdomen and take a second look after 24–36 h to determine the viability of the bowel.

Codes

Blood	2 units
GA/LA	GA
Opn time	1–2 h
Stay	7–10 days
Drains out	0
Sutures out	7 days
Off work	Variable; at least 4 weeks but usually affected by the patient's general condition

Postoperative care

The patient is given intravenous fluids and nasogastric suction until flatus is passed, and bowel function restored.

Intussusception in adults

Intussusceptions are much commoner in children and are dealt with on p. 615. The management in the adult is very similar, although open operation through a vertical incision, and not reduction by barium enema, is the method of choice. This is because there is almost always a causative lesion in an adult, such as a polyp or a leiomyoma, which forms the head of the intussusception. This will need to be resected.

Small bowel tumours

Small bowel tumours are rare. Benign tumours include adenomas, lipomas and leiomyomas. They may bleed, causing melaena and anaemia, and they can cause intussusception. Multiple hamartomatous polyps of the small bowel occur in association with melanin pigmentation of the lips and oral mucosa as part of the Peutz–Jeghers syndrome. Malignant change is rare.

Primary malignant tumours include lymphosarcoma, spindle cell sarcoma and carcinoma. Again they present with symptoms of bleeding (melaena and anaemia), intestinal obstruction or general carcinomatosis. The bowel wall may perforate, causing acute peritonitis.

Carcinoid tumour is a malignant growth of the Kulchitsky cells (argentaffin cells, amine precursor uptake and decarboxylation system). Sixty-five per cent arise in the appendix and 25% in the ileum. Other primary sites include the rest of the gut and, very rarely, the bronchus, testis and ovary. The tumour may excrete serotonin and kinins (and possibly prostaglandins and histamine), resulting in the carcinoid syndrome. The main features of this are flushing attacks (precipitated by alcohol), diarrhoea, episodic bronchospasm and pulmonary stenosis. This only occurs once there are metastases in the liver, because hormones from the primary in the gut are detoxified in the hepatic circulation.

Proving the diagnosis

Small bowel tumours are often only found at laparotomy (e.g. for intussusception or bleeding). Occasionally, a barium meal may reveal a lesion in the duodenum or upper jejunum. Carcinoid syndrome is proved by demonstrating elevated levels of 5-hydroxyindole-acetic acid (5-HIAA, the breakdown product of serotonin) in the urine (normal range is 2–20 mg in 24 h). In this case a CT scan will show evidence of secondaries in the liver.

Management

Benign tumours are resected if they are causing symptoms of bleeding or obstruction. Malignant tumours are treated by wide excision including the local mesenteric nodes.

Metastases in the liver are often found at operation. Partial hepatectomy may be considered for metastases although the tumour is very slow growing and the patient may be managed conservatively for many years. Drugs used to control the carcinoid syndrome include methysergide, antihistamines and α-methyldopa. Another alternative is selective embolization or infusion of 5-fluorouracil in the hepatic artery.

OPERATIONS

1 See Right hemicolectomy, p. 385.

8 Hepatobiliary, Pancreatic and Splenic Surgery

8.1 Hepatobiliary Disease

Gall stones

Gall stones precipitate from bile concentrated in the gall bladder. They may be formed from cholesterol or from bile pigment though most stones are mixed. Ten per cent of gall stones are radio-opaque due to the presence of calcium salts.

Stones tend to obstruct the gall bladder or bile duct. Rarely a large gall stone may ulcerate through the gall bladder wall and enter the gut. The stone may then cause intestinal obstruction (gall stone ileus).

Recognizing the pattern

Gall stones are particularly common in the typical fat, fertile female in her 40s. However, they do also occur in other age groups and in men.

The typical symptoms are of two types.

1 Flatulent dyspepsia. This consists of epigastric fullness and distension coming on an hour or two after meals and particularly after fatty food. Often the patient has subconsciously decided to keep off fats and therefore does not give a positive history of fat intolerance. The dyspepsia commonly occurs in the evenings.

2 Gall bladder 'colic' is probably due to obstruction of the outlet of the gall bladder. It is a much more severe pain also coming on after fatty meals. The pain is situated in the epigastrium or the right hypochondrium and radiates around the costal margin to the right shoulder blade. It lasts a few hours and usually results in the patient seeking medical advice. It settles with an injection of pethidine but there may be soreness under the right hypochondrium for several days. This is worse on coughing or moving.

If the contents of the gall bladder become secondarily infected (acute cholecystitis), the patient can become very unwell with rigors, anorexia, nausea and vomiting.

On examination the patient may have a fever. There is tenderness maximal beneath the right ninth costal cartilage over the gall bladder. If the examining hand is placed 2–3 finger-breadths below the costal margin and the patient is asked to inspire deeply, he feels a sharp pain as the gall bladder descends on to the palpating hand (Murphy's sign).

Proving the diagnosis

During an acute attack there may be mild derangement of liver function tests. The presence of gall stones is confirmed by an ultrasound scan and once the acute attack is over they may also be demonstrated on an oral cholecystogram. A HIDA scan may show non-filling of the gall bladder during an acute attack (HIDA ia an imino diacetic acid derivative, excreted by the hepatocytes into the bile).

Management

Gall stones can sometimes be dissolved by medical treatment or removed percutaneously. These methods share the disadvantage of stone recurrence due to disease in the gall bladder wall. This disease also carries a small but definite long-term risk of malignancy. Shattering the stones by lithotripsy has been tried but the fragments have to pass and can cause jaundice or pancreatitis.

The definitive management of gall stones is therefore removal of the gall bladder. This is now usually carried out laparoscopically.

Acute cholecystitis

Acute cholecystitis is usually managed conservatively with bed rest and antibiotics (e.g. a parenteral cephalosporin). Some surgeons prefer to perform cholecystectomy as an emergency during the acute attack. The gall bladder is usually easy to remove in the early stages (48 h) as it is surrounded by oedema.

Obstructive jaundice due to gall stones

The management of obstructive jaundice is dealt with on p. 337. If the jaundice is known to be associated with gall stones, it is given the chance to settle and a cholecystectomy is performed later. The patient should be given an antibiotic which is effective in bile (e.g. ampicillin or a cephalosporin) to treat associated cholangitis. It is also important to maintain adequate hydration, as there is a danger of associated renal failure. If it fails to settle an emergency laparoscopic cholecystectomy and exploration of the bile duct or an endoscopic sphincterotomy (ES) is performed.

OPERATION: LAPAROSCOPIC
CHOLECYSTECTOMY

The gall bladder area is visualized on a video screen connected to a camera on a laparoscope. Operative manoeuvres

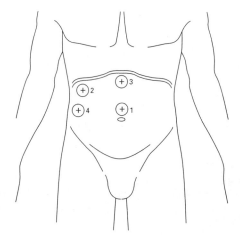

Fig. 63 Port sites for laparoscopic cholecystectomy.

are carried out through secondary laparoscopic ports (Fig. 63). The cystic duct and artery are clipped and divided and the gall bladder removed. A cholangiogram can also be performed. The main abdominal incision is therefore avoided in favour of three or more stab wounds for the laparoscopic cannulae.

OPERATION: LAPAROSCOPIC CHOLECYSTECTOMY AND EXPLORATION OF THE BILE DUCT

Although many surgeons will resort to open operation or ES when stones are found in the bile duct, it is possible to deal with these laparoscopically. A wire (Dormia) basket is introduced into the bile duct percutaneously via the cystic duct. Stones can be grasped under X-ray control and extracted. If the stone is too large to retrieve through the cystic duct the bile duct can be opened and later closed with sutures over a T-tube. The duct can also be inspected and stones retrieved under vision using a choledochoscope passed through a port. If stones are removed through the cystic duct the recovery is the same as for a simple cholecystectomy.

Codes
Blood .... Group and save serum
GA/LA .... GA

Opn time .... 1–2 h (with CBD
                                               exploration 2–3 h)
Stay .... 24–48 h
Drains out .... 0 (48 h after CBD
                                               exploration: T-tube 7 days)
Sutures out .... Absorbable
Off work .... 1–2 weeks (3–4 weeks if
                                               preoperative jaundice)

Postoperative care
The patient suffers very little pain and can usually resume
drinking and eating within a few hours after operation. Recovery is remarkably rapid and the patient can return to full
activity 1–2 weeks after surgery.

OPERATION: OPEN CHOLECYSTECTOMY AND
EXPLORATION OF COMMON BILE DUCT (CBD)
The open operation is usually carried out through a vertical
or an oblique (Kocher's) incision. An operative cholangiogram may be performed and the X-ray department must
be warned of this. The cholangiogram demonstrates the
presence or absence of stones in the CBD. Before the operation starts the patient must be positioned carefully on the
table so that the X-ray plate is beneath the patient's biliary
tree. If there are no stones in the duct, the cystic artery and
duct are ligated and the gall bladder is removed. A drain may
be placed down to the gall bladder bed.
   If stones are demonstrated in the CBD, the duct is opened
and the stones removed. The surgeon may wish to inspect
the duct using a choledochoscope. Occasionally a stone
impacted in the ampulla of Vater cannot be removed through
an incision in the CBD and in this case the duodenum may
be opened and a sphincterotomy performed. The stone can
then be removed through the widened ampulla of Vater. The
CBD is closed over a T-tube, which is brought out to the
surface (see p. 122).

Codes
Blood .... Group and save serum
GA/LA .... GA
Opn time .... 1 h (+ CBD exploration
                                               90–120 min)

Stay	7–10 days
Drains out	Drain 2–5 days, T-tube 7–10 days (see below)
Sutures out	7 days
Off work	4–6 weeks

> *Postoperative care*
> Oral fluids are given after 36 h or so when the patient's ileus recovers. If the CBD has been explored, a T-tube cholangiogram is performed after a week. This is to exclude the presence of further retained stones before the T-tube is removed. If the X-ray is clear, the T-tube can be taken out. Some surgeons prefer to clamp the tube intermittently before it is removed.
>
> The drain to the gall bladder bed can usually be removed at 48 h, although some surgeons prefer to leave it longer, particularly if they use catgut to tie off the cystic duct stump.

Biliary fistula

If the patient is not jaundiced, bile-stained drainage after a gall bladder operation is of ominous significance, and indicates a biliary fistula. If the patient is jaundiced, however, all serous collections in the peritoneum will be bile-stained and this may be nothing to worry about.

A biliary fistula can be demonstrated by doing a T-tube cholangiogram or a sinogram if there is no T-tube. An intravenous cholangiogram or HIDA scan may also be helpful. The drain should not be removed until the surgeon in charge has decided on the further course of action. Fistulae will often heal if there is adequate drainage of the biliary tree, but there is a danger of stricture formation later. The surgeon may arrange for an endoscopic retrograde cholangiopancreatograph (ERCP) and stent insertion in order to improve biliary drainage, or decide to re-explore the patient and repair the bile duct using a loop of jejunum.

After a cholecystectomy the patient is gradually returned to a normal diet and there is no need for him to keep off fatty foods in the convalescent period. He may need reassurance that his digestion should be normal after he has lost his gall bladder.

Surgical jaundice

Patients are referred to surgeons when their jaundice may be due to obstruction. The first task is to establish that the jaundice is indeed obstructive and then to determine the cause of the

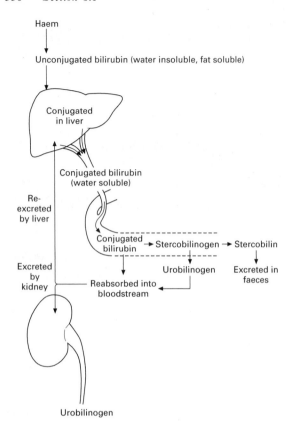

Fig. 64 Normal bilirubin metabolism: bilirubin is conjugated in the liver and excreted into the gut.

obstruction. An understanding of the physiology of bile metabolism is necessary.

Jaundice is due to excessive accumulation of bile pigment (bilirubin and its derivatives). The normal metabolism of bile is shown in Fig. 64. An excess of bilirubin may be due to any of the following:

1 Excessive production — prehepatic jaundice, e.g. haemolytic anaemia.

2 Defective processing of bilirubin in the liver — hepatic jaundice, e.g. hepatitis.

3 Blocked excretion of bile from the liver — posthepatic or obstructive jaundice, e.g. stone in the CBD or carcinoma of the pancreas.

The main features of these three types of jaundice are given below.

Prehepatic jaundice

This occurs in a younger age group and is common in children. There is an excessive production of bilirubin due to an increased red cell turnover. This may be due to a haemolytic disorder such as spherocytosis, drug-induced haemolysis or an incompatible blood transfusion. There is an increased unconjugated bilirubin in the peripheral blood and a low haemoglobin. The serum alkaline phosphatase, alanine transaminase (ALT) and the serum albumin are all normal. Blood clotting studies are also normal. The absence of liver damage makes this type of jaundice easy to separate from the other two. Because of the satisfactory liver function the jaundice is always mild and the patient is usually a lemon–yellow colour.

Hepatic jaundice

In this condition there is liver damage from one of a variety of causes including viral hepatitis, leptospirosis, alcoholic cirrhosis and drug- or chemical-induced liver damage. The patient is usually markedly jaundiced and ill from the effects of the liver disease. Laboratory tests show a raised serum ALT and a less marked rise in the serum alkaline phosphatase. Some bile is usually still being processed in the liver and the stools may remain a normal colour.

On examination the liver is enlarged and tender.

Posthepatic obstructive jaundice (Fig. 65)

In this condition the liver function is initially normal but the liver may become secondarily damaged due to back pressure or ascending infection. Characteristically the alkaline phosphatase is very high and the ALT less elevated. The serum albumin should be normal. The jaundice is usually deep but it may be intermittent if the obstruction is intermittent (e.g. gall stones).

Investigation of obstructive jaundice

1 Test the urine for urobilinogen and urobilin. Urobilinogen is raised in prehepatic jaundice and bilirubin is present in posthepatic jaundice. Urobilinogen is absent from the urine if the obstruction is complete.

2 Liver function tests. The pattern of results in various types of jaundice is shown in Table 19. In addition, the prothrombin time gives a useful indicator of liver function and may be important in the future management of the patient.

3 Ultrasound. If the intrahepatic bile ducts are dilated, the cause is obstructive. The investigation may also detect the presence of gall stones in the gall bladder or other masses within the liver parenchyma.

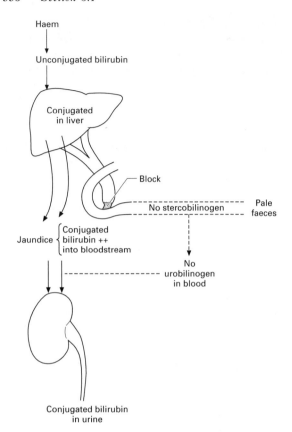

Fig. 65 Obstructive jaundice. When conjugated bilirubin cannot get into the gut it appears in the bloodstream and is excreted in the urine.

Table 19 Laboratory results in jaundice.

	Prehepatic (haemolytic)	Hepatic* (hepatitic)	Posthepatic (obstructive)
Bilirubin			
Unconjugated	Raised	Raised	May be raised
Conjugated	Normal	Raised	Raised
Alanine transaminase (ALT)	Normal	Raised	May be raised
Alkaline phosphatase	Normal	Slightly raised*	Raised
Plasma proteins	Normal	May be low	Normal

*There is often an element of obstruction in hepatic jaundice due to intrahepatic cholestasis.

4 Magnetic resonance scan: an excellent picture of the biliary tree can be obtained without the need for injections or endoscopy.

5 ERCP. The lower end of the CBD may also be cannulated using a fibroscope. The ampulla of Vater can be inspected during this procedure. This investigation should show the level of the obstruction and possibly its cause.

6 If the ducts in the liver are not dilated, a liver biopsy may be performed and may give a diagnosis of the cause of hepatic damage.

7 In cases where a carcinoma of the head of the pancreas is suspected a computed tomography (CT) scan may be helpful.

At any stage of this process the surgeon may decide that enough investigation has been done to warrant proceeding with a laparotomy or laparoscopy. This may also be indicated if the above work-up has failed to settle the question of whether the jaundice is obstructive or not. Such a laparotomy will be combined with intraoperative cholangiography and a liver biopsy.

Preoperative care

Patients with liver damage may have abnormal clotting factors and should be given vitamin K preoperatively. Where the jaundice is severe, there is a danger of induction of renal failure at the time of surgery (hepatorenal syndrome). This can be avoided by adequately hydrating the patient and by giving him a peroperative infusion of mannitol (dose 0.5 g/kg, e.g. 200 mL of 20%) intravenously. Before the operation is started, a urinary catheter should be inserted so that the urinary output can be monitored.

OPERATIONS: ERCP AND ENDOSCOPIC SPHINCTEROTOMY

Endoscopic sphincterotomy

The patient is heavily sedated or anaesthetized and an endoscope passed through the mouth into the duodenum. The ampulla is inspected and cannulated. The biliary and pancreatic ducts are visualized on an X-ray image intensifier. If a stone is seen a sphincterotomy can be performed using a diathermy wire stretched across an insulated cannula inserted into the ampulla. Stones can be pulled into the duodenum using a wire basket. They can also be crushed with a lithotrite, or a stent can be inserted. Suspicious lesions can be biopsied.

Continued on p. 340

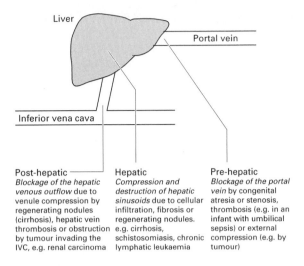

Post-hepatic
Blockage of the hepatic venous outflow due to venule compression by regenerating nodules (cirrhosis), hepatic vein thrombosis or obstruction by tumour invading the IVC, e.g. renal carcinoma

Hepatic
Compression and destruction of hepatic sinusoids due to cellular infiltration, fibrosis or regenerating nodules. e.g. cirrhosis, schistosomiasis, chronic lymphatic leukaemia

Pre-hepatic
Blockage of the portal vein by congenital atresia or stenosis, thrombosis (e.g. in an infant with umbilical sepsis) or external compression (e.g. by tumour)

Fig. 66 The causes of portal hypertension.

Codes

Blood	Group and save for ES
GA/LA	Sedation or GA
Opn time	0.5–2 h
Stay	0–24 h
Drains out	0
Sutures out	0
Off work	Depends on diagnosis

Continued.

> *Other operations*
> Other operations, to deal with obstructive jaundice are dealt with under the individual conditions.
> 1 Exploration of the CBD, p. 334
> 2 Whipple's operation, p. 358
> 3 Bypass operation for carcinoma of the pancreas, p. 359.

Portal hypertension

The portal venous pressure is raised when there is an obstruction in the portal system. This can be situated before, in or after the liver. The causes of such an obstruction are shown in Fig. 66. The commonest aetiology in Western countries is cirrhosis. Schistosomiasis is the main cause worldwide. The normal portal venous pressure is 5–10 mmHg and the pressure may reach 30–

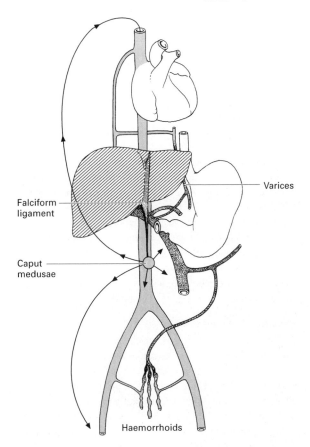

Fig. 67 Portal hypertension results in the enlargement of veins at the sites of portasystemic venous anastomoses.

40 mmHg in portal hypertension. Elevated portal pressure leads to the development of venous collaterals between the portal and systemic venous circulation. The most important of these are in the oesophagus, where varices may develop. Collaterals also develop at the umbilicus and in the rectum and anal canal (Fig. 67). The patient also develops ascites if there is coexistent liver failure with hypoproteinaemia and hyperaldosteronism. Splenomegaly is common and there may be a degree of hypersplenism with leucopenia and thrombocytopenia. Portal systemic encephalopathy may occur due to the fact that blood from the gut bypasses the liver and its filtering and detoxifying mechanisms.

Recognizing the pattern

The usual presentation of portal hypertension is haematemesis and melaena. This is described on p. 304. There may also be symptoms of anaemia. There is usually a past history suggestive of liver disease or alcoholism. The patient may have noticed easy bruising or a purpuric rash.

On examination the signs of portal hypertension include splenomegaly (80–90%), ascites and occasionally dilated veins around the umbilicus (caput medusae) over which there may be a venous hum on auscultation. Look for purpura and stigmata of chronic liver disease. These include jaundice, skin pigmentation, clubbing, spider naevi, palmar erythema, gynaecomastia, testicular atrophy and a female distribution of pubic hair.

The liver is a variable size in cirrhosis.

Hepatosplenomegaly and ascites with no history of alcohol abuse suggest hepatic vein obstruction.

Signs of encephalopathy include confusion, drowsiness and tremor, increased tendon reflexes, up-going plantar responses and constructional apraxia (e.g. inability to copy a star).

Proving the diagnosis

The presence of oesophageal varices can be demonstrated on barium swallow and fibroscopy. The latter is the investigation of choice, as the exact diagnosis is confirmed together with the source of bleeding. Ultrasound with Doppler study of the vessels allows visualization of the hepatic and portal veins and depicts directional flow. Ultrasound and CT scan also can be used to assess the liver texture. The precise anatomy of the portal system can be displayed by the venous phase of a coeliac or superior mesenteric arteriogram. Alternatively, splenoportography which involves percutaneous cannulation of a splenic venule followed by injection of contrast medium, may be used. ERCP may be useful if there is suspicion of cirrhosis secondary to extrahepatic biliary obstruction.

Evidence of liver disease may be found by measuring the serum bilirubin, serum albumin, hepatic enzymes and α-fetoprotein (to look for hepatoma). A liver biopsy may help to diagnose the nature of the disease. Serological assessment for evidence of hepatitis A, B and C, autoimmune disease and primary biliary cirrhosis is carried out. Finally the haemoglobin, platelets, clotting screen, urea and electrolytes, and calcium should also be measured.

Management

The long-term management of portal hypertension includes the elective management of ascites and the underlying liver disease associated with portal hypertension. This is dealt with in larger medical texts. Long-term β-blockers are at present under investigation.

Surgical management
1 Repeated injection sclerotherapy — this decreases recurrent bleeding, but does not change survival.
2 Repeated variceal ligation (banding).
3 Portosystemic shunts — these include the transjugular intrahepatic portosystemic shunt (TIPSS) procedure and there is a small role for open shunts in patients with extrahepatic portal hypertension (see below).
4 Oesophageal transection — although there is no complication with encephalopathy, 30% of patients will rebleed.
5 Gastric transection (see below).
6 Liver transplantation is the definitive treatment of portal hypertension and also deals with the underlying disease process and improves survival. While waiting for transplantation, sclerotherapy of oesophageal varices should be undertaken to prevent recurrent bleeding. If this fails to control bleeding then TIPSS is an alternative.

The emergency management of bleeding oesophageal varices is described on p. 347.

OPERATION: TIPSS
TIPSS involves the passage of a biopsy needle or stylet through the right internal jugular vein in order to create an intrahepatic track between the hepatic and portal vein under radiological guidance. This track is dilated with an angioplasty balloon catheter and a metallic stent inserted.

The main indication for TIPSS is to control and prevent variceal bleeding after failure of endoscopic methods.

Codes

Blood	2 units
GA/LA	LA
Opn time	2–3 h
Stay	About 48 h
Drains out	0
Sutures out	0
Off work	Variable

Postoperative care
There are usually no problems apart from those associated with the original disease process.

Continued on p. 344

Continued.

Complications
Early complications are rare. Check for a haematoma at the entry site. There is a possibility of the patient developing hepatic encephalopathy if liver function is marginal.

OPEN SHUNT PROCEDURES
These may be carried out in the following circumstances:
1 In patients with good liver function who are not suitable for TIPSS because they have no portal vein (extrahepatic portal vein obstruction), or where TIPSS has failed.
2 The serum albumin is more than 30 g/L.
3 The bilirubin is not significantly raised (< 35 mmol/L).
4 There is no medical history of encephalopathy.
5 Portal and systemic venography has shown that the planned anastomosis is possible. Venograms may be done during operation.

Preoperative management
Before an elective shunt the patient should be put on a low-protein high-carbohydrate diet if not on one already. The bowels should be cleared of all protein by careful bowel preparation (see p. 113). Neomycin (1 g 4–6-hourly) may also be given.

Additional preoperative measures include blood transfusion, platelet transfusion, correction of clotting defects, and a mannitol infusion to prevent the hepatorenal syndrome.

OPERATION: PORTACAVAL ANASTOMOSIS
A variety of shunt procedures have been performed in the past. These are rarely indicated now and are illustrated in Figs 68 and 69.

OPERATION: OESOPHAGEAL TRANSECTION
The oesophagus is exposed through a lower left thoracotomy, the vagal trunks are dissected clear and the oesophagus is transected. It is then resutured with continuous sutures to obliterate the vessel. Alternatively, the procedure can be performed through the abdomen with a stapling gun introduced through the stomach. This is technically easier and has the advantage that the chest is not opened.

Codes
Blood .... 6–10 units
GA/LA .... GA

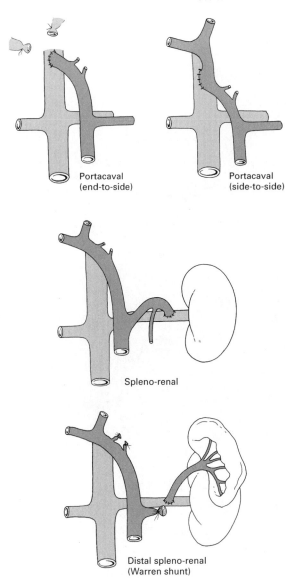

Fig. 68 Portacaval shunt operations.

Opn time .... 2–3 h
Stay .... Variable
Drains out .... Pleura 24 h; mediastinum 5–7 days
Sutures out .... 7–10 days
Off work .... Variable

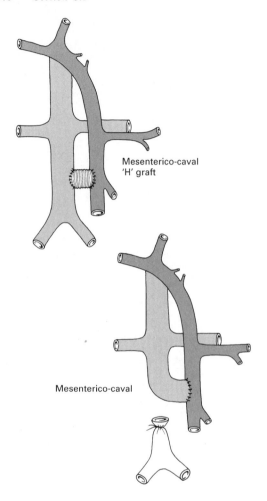

Mesenterico-caval
'H' graft

Mesenterico-caval

Fig. 69 Other portacaval shunts: mesentericocaval anastomoses.

Postoperative care
Fluids are reintroduced slowly as above.

OPERATION: GASTRIC TRANSECTION
The stomach is exposed through a left thoracoabdominal
incision and the stomach transected and resutured just below
the gastro-oesophageal junction.

Codes
Blood .... 10 units
GA/LA .... GA

Opn time .... 3–4 h
Stay .... Variable
Drains out .... Subphrenic space 7 days
Sutures out .... 7–10 days
Off work .... Variable

Postoperative care
This is similar to that described for gastrectomy on p. 294.

Bleeding oesophageal varices

These occur as part of the syndrome of portal hypertension and can bleed massively. Hospital mortality is high and 60% of those who recover rebleed within 1 year. Blood in the bowel may precipitate encephalopathy.

Patients with portal hypertension may bleed from other sites, usually a gastric or duodenal ulcer or haemorrhagic gastritis.

Recognizing the pattern

The haematemesis is usually profuse. There may be a history of similar episodes, and also of previous liver disease (e.g. cirrhosis, jaundice, hepatitis). The patient may be an alcoholic.

The patient is usually shocked. Stigmata of portal hypertension, liver disease and alcoholism are usually present to a varying degree. Look for the signs of encephalopathy (p. 342).

Proving the diagnosis

The bleeding site must be confirmed by a fibroscopy as soon as the patient is stabilized. Other emergency investigations include the following:

1 Haemoglobin, haematocrit and cross-match
2 Clotting screen
3 Platelet count
4 Urea, electrolytes and calcium
5 Liver function tests and serological assessment of hepatitis A, B and C, autoimmune disease and primary biliary cirrhosis.

Management

Resuscitation is carried out as on p. 305. A central venous pressure (CVP) line is usually needed. Use fresh blood if possible as this contains more clotting factors and platelets than stored blood. Fresh frozen plasma (FFP) and platelet transfusion may be required. Vitamin K (10 mg i.v.) is given. Neomycin (1 g 6-hourly) and lactulose (30–50 ml 8-hourly)

Continued on p. 348

Continued.

are given to decrease the urea-splitting organisms in the bowel and to clear the bowel of blood. This is done to prevent encephalopathy. Gastric and colonic washouts are also helpful.

If bleeding continues, a continuous infusion of octreotide (somatostatin analogue, 25–50 µg/h) can be given. This lowers portal venous pressure by reducing splanchnic blood flow, and is effective in controlling variceal bleeding in 65% of cases.

Injection sclerotherapy or variceal ligation is used to control the bleeding and is effective in the majority of patients. If, however, bleeding is too excessive and sclerotherapy is not possible then oesophageal tamponade using a Sengstaken tube is an effective method of achieving temporary control. This may allow further attempt at sclerotherapy or banding.

When sclerotherapy fails (less then 10% of patients) then one should consider performing TIPSS, oesophageal transection or gastric transection. The role of emergency open portosystemic shunts in this situation has virtually disappeared.

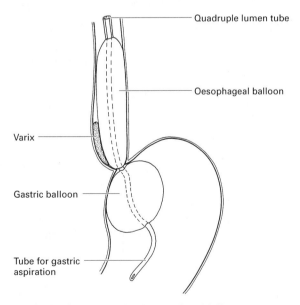

Fig. 70 The Sengstaken tube: the oesophageal balloon compresses the varices.

Sengstaken tube (Fig. 70)

This compresses the varices and fundal veins. The tube is passed into the stomach and the gastric balloon inflated. This balloon is impacted on the lower end of the gastro-oesophageal junction by traction on the tube. The upper oesophageal balloon is then inflated. Regular aspiration of the stomach is carried out through the tube to ensure that bleeding is not continuing. The oesophagus is aspirated to prevent inhalation of nasopharyngeal secretions. The tube is unpleasant for the patient and can be dangerous. Complications of its use include aspiration, pressure necrosis of the oesophageal and gastric mucosa, rupture of the oesophagus and respiratory obstruction.

If the bleeding is controlled after a few hours the tube is deflated and left *in situ* for up to 24 h before removal.

Surgical management

Preoperative management

Before operation the patient's haemoglobin, coagulation screen and platelet numbers must be as normal as possible. A mannitol infusion may be required to prevent the hepatorenal syndrome.

The operations described below are aimed at obliterating the bleeding varices. Operations for the general management of portal hypertension have already been described. In the emergency situation the varices may be either under-run or transected, or an emergency portacaval shunt may be performed. The choice depends on the rate of bleeding, the overall condition of the patient and the experience of the surgeon. Three other operations may be considered.

1 Oversewing of varices
2 Oesophageal transection (see p. 344)
3 Gastric transection (see p. 346).

Before operation the patient's haemoglobin, coagulation screen and platelet numbers must be as normal as possible. A mannitol infusion may be required to prevent the hepatorenal syndrome.

OPERATION: OVERSEWING OF OESOPHAGEAL VARICES

A left thoracotomy is performed and the oesophagus opened just above the diaphragm to expose the varices.

The varices (usually in three columns) are then oversewn using continuous chromic catgut sutures.

Codes

Blood .... 6–10 units
GA/LA .... GA
Opn time .... 90–120 min
Stay .... Variable
Drains out .... Pleura 24 h; mediastinum 5–7 days
Sutures out .... 7–10 days
Off work .... Variable

> *Postoperative care*
> A barium swallow can be performed on the fifth or sixth day
> and, if this is normal, fluids are reintroduced slowly.

Hepatic tumours
These may be benign or malignant.

Benign hepatic tumours
Benign hepatic tumours include the following:
1 Haemangioma
2 Focal nodular hyperplasia
3 Liver cell adenoma.

Benign tumours of the liver are uncommon and frequently asymptomatic, being found incidentally at laparotomy or laparoscopy. The cavernous haemangioma is the most common benign tumour of the liver. It presents in adults most commonly between 30 and 70 years of age and may grow to a very large size.

Focal nodular hyperplasia and liver cell adenoma are most commonly found in women of child-bearing age and are associated with the use of the oral contraceptive pill. Stopping this medication may result in regression of the tumour.

Recognizing the pattern
A cavernous haemangioma is usually asymptomatic but may present with vague abdominal symptoms (swelling, pain, nausea). The diagnosis is confirmed by ultrasound, CT scan and angiography. Biopsy is usually contraindicated in this condition.

Focal nodular hyperplasia tumours are usually small and found incidentally. Liver cell adenoma tumours are often larger and more likely to present with symptoms, particularly bleeding into the peritoneal cavity. The diagnosis is made by ultrasound, CT scan and biopsy. The latter may involve total excision depending on the location and size.

Management

The risk of spontaneous haemorrhage from a haemangioma is very small. However, resection may be indicated in the symptomatic case, the technique depending on the size and location of the lesion.

Patients with focal nodular hyperplasia or liver cell adenoma should be advised to stop the oral contraceptive pill. Distinguishing these tumours from malignant hepatoma may be difficult and justify excision. Having made the diagnosis, large tumours may require resection and small tumours may be managed conservatively.

There is no evidence that these lesions are premalignant.

Malignant hepatic tumours

Malignant hepatic tumours are of the following kinds:
1 Primary:
  (a) primary hepatocellular carcinoma (hepatoma)
  (b) cholangiocarcinoma
2 Secondary.

The incidence of primary hepatocellular carcinoma shows considerable geographical variation, being common in the Far East and Africa and relatively uncommon in Europe and North America. Its incidence is strongly associated both with chronic hepatitis B infection and with cirrhosis of other aetiologies. It is commoner in males (3 : 1). Other, less significant, aetiological agents include the groundnut fungal toxin (aflatoxin) and the oral contraceptive pill.

Cholangiocarcinoma (primary carcinoma of bile duct) most commonly occurs after 60 years of age and more frequently in males (2 : 1). It may develop at an earlier age, particularly in association with sclerosing cholangitis (10%) or (rarely) Caroli's disease (cystic disease of the biliary tract).

The majority of malignant tumours of the liver are secondary to primary tumours in the gastrointestinal tract (stomach, pancreas, colon) or elsewhere.

Proving the diagnosis

The diagnosis of a malignant neoplasm of the liver includes ultrasound and CT scan (this may also detect extrahepatic spread of disease, particularly to portal or para-aortic lymph nodes). Increased sensitivity for detecting small tumours has been achieved by using CT arterial portography (CTAP), spiral CT with prior injection of lipiodol (a radiodense substance taken up by all liver tumours) into the hepatic artery, and intraoperative ultrasound. The role of MRI has not yet been established. Coeliac arteriography may demonstrate an abnormal 'tumour' circulation. Histological confirmation is obtained by percutaneous CT-guided biopsy. Even after a needle biopsy, it is important to exclude the presence of a gastrointestinal primary tumour by endoscopy (stomach), CT scan (pancreas) and barium enema (colon). A cholangiocarcinoma may be very small and present with biliary obstruction; this may be difficult to biopsy and the diagnosis may be made by cholangiography (endoscopic or transhepatic).

Management

1 Resection.
2 Palliation.

If it appears that complete removal of the tumour is possible, the patient should undergo hepatic resection. Extensive hepatic resection carries high risks in patients with chronic liver disease, and must be carefully considered. In some cases where a primary liver tumour is small, patients should be considered for hepatic transplantation. Hepatic resection for secondary liver tumours should now be considered in all patients. The best results are obtained in fit patients with secondary colorectal metastasis with less than four deposits and no extrahepatic involvement.

In tumours unsuitable for resection and causing unacceptable symptoms, palliation is attempted. Most commonly this involves relief of jaundice either by transhepatic or endoscopic stenting of the biliary system or by surgical bypass.

OPERATION: HEPATIC RESECTION

1 Left hemi-hepatectomy (removal of the anatomical left lobe).
2 Right hemi-hepatectomy (removal of the anatomical right lobe).
3 Right trisegmentectomy (removal of the right lobe and medial segment of the left lobe).

The porta hepatis is explored and the appropriate branches of the portal vein, hepatic artery and hepatic duct ligated and divided. The liver parenchyma is then divided, carefully ligating or clipping all vessels which cross the line of section. The appropriate hepatic vein is identified, clamped and oversewn. A large silicone drain is placed in the region of the cut surface of the liver.

Codes

Blood .... 8 units

GA/LA .... GA

Opn time .... 2–6 h

Stay .... 10–21 days

Drains out .... Nasogastric tube 24 h; abdomen
7–10 days

Sutures out .... 10 days

Off work .... 2–3 months

Postoperative care

After hepatic resection, a patient requires monitoring on the intensive care unit or high-dependency unit for at least 24 h or until cardiovascular parameters are stable. The patient should be observed for postoperative haemorrhage, hepatocellular insufficiency, and particularly coagulopathy, hypoglycaemia, hypoalbuminaemia and later for signs of bile leak. (Full blood count, coagulation studies and liver function tests should be performed daily.)

Hepatic transplantation

Indications

The indications for liver transplantation include the following:

1 Chronic liver disease
2 Acute liver failure
3 Metabolic defects
4 Liver tumours.

Chronic liver disease

The common causes of chronic liver disease leading to transplantation are the following:

1 Primary biliary cirrhosis
2 Posthepatic cirrhosis (chronic active) hepatitis
3 Autoimmune chronic active hepatitis
4 Sclerosing cholangitis
5 Cryptogenic cirrhosis
6 Alcoholic cirrhosis (carefully selected cases).

Liver transplantation should be considered in patients with these diseases who develop life-threatening complications, particularly gastro-oesophageal variceal haemorrhage, encephalopathy, spontaneous bacterial peritonitis or intractable ascites and malnutrition. In some patients without such complications, symptoms of fatigue and itching may be so severe as to warrant transplantation.

Acute liver failure

Patients suffering from fulminant hepatic failure (liver failure within 8 weeks of the onset of symptoms) or subacute hepatic failure (liver failure between 8 and 26 weeks of the onset of symptoms) may require urgent liver transplantation. The most common aetiological agents are viral hepatitis (hepatitis B, non-A non-B), drug reactions and toxins.

Metabolic diseases

A number of life-threatening metabolic diseases are characterized by the deficiency of a hepatic enzyme. Examples of this include α_1-antitrypsin deficiency, primary hyperoxaluria and Wilson's disease. Successful replacement of the diseased liver results in permanent cure of the condition.

Liver tumours

Patients with primary liver tumours may be suitable candidates for liver transplantation if they have a small growth with no nodal involvement.

Preoperative care

The extent of liver disease is assessed by liver function tests, coagulation screen, and the presence or absence of complications of liver disease. The size of the portal vein can be assessed by Doppler ultrasound. The patients undergo a microbiological screen, including looking for cytomegalovirus. Blood grouping and antibody studies are undertaken. A full general medical and anaesthetic assessment is also carried out.

OPERATION: HEPATIC TRANSPLANTATION

The donor

Brain-dead, heart-beating donors are used. The liver is fully mobilized until it is attached only by its vascular connections (inferior vena cava (IVC), portal vein and hepatic artery). Cannulae are placed in the aorta and portal vein and, when the circulation stops (when the heart is excised for transplantation), *in situ* cooling is carried out. The liver, perfused and stored in suitable preservation solution, can remain ischaemic, at ice temperature, for up to 24 h.

The recipient

The recipient operation often has the following complications:

1 Portal hypertension
2 Coagulopathy
3 Adhesions due to previous upper abdominal surgery.

The liver is mobilized with careful attention to haemostasis. The bile duct is divided, the blood vessels clamped and the liver excised. The donor liver is then transplanted, anastomosing the suprahepatic IVC, infrahepatic IVC, portal vein, hepatic artery and bile duct. Some patients tolerate clamping of the IVC and portal vein poorly and require bypass from the infrahepatic IVC and portal vein, back to the right side of the heart.

Codes

Blood	12 units
GA/LA	GA
Opn time	5–6 h
Stay	2–3 weeks
Drains out	2–7 days
Sutures out	2 weeks
Off work	3 months

Postoperative management
Most liver transplant recipients require a period of ventilation and intensive monitoring of cardiopulmonary, renal and liver function. Immunosuppressive medication is started at the time of operation. Particular problems include bleeding, graft infarction, infection, rejection and biliary complications.

8.2 Pancreas and Spleen

For benign tumours of the pancreas, see section 4.3

Carcinoma of the pancreas

Carcinoma of the pancreas is an adenocarcinoma arising from the ductal epithelium. Histologically it is usually solid and fibrous (scirrhous) but may be medullary or rarely a cystadenocarcinoma. The incidence is increasing in the UK and the USA. Two-thirds of pancreatic carcinomas occur in the head of the gland and these tend to compress the CBD, causing jaundice. A carcinoma in the body and tail may remain undetected until it is quite large. Further spread occurs to the liver, lung and peritoneal cavity.

Recognizing the pattern

The patient with this disease is typically middle aged or elderly (aged 50–70 years).

The presentation is often non-specific with a gradual onset of ill health and weight loss. If pain is present, it is usually dull and situated deep in the epigastrium. It radiates through to the back. The pain is characteristically relieved by sitting forwards. The disease is sometimes associated with episodes of spontaneous venous thrombosis, 'thrombophlebitis migrans'.

The patient with a carcinoma of the head of the pancreas may be jaundiced and show signs of weight loss. In the presence of jaundice the gall bladder may be palpable as a smooth, rounded mass below the liver. Courvoisier's law states that if the gall bladder is palpable in a case of obstructive jaundice then the cause is unlikely to be gall stones. (Gall bladders containing stones are usually fibrotic and shrunken.)

Carcinomas of the tail of the pancreas present late and by then a mass is often palpable in the left upper quadrant.

Proving the diagnosis

This may be very difficult. A barium meal may show fixity and indentation of the posterior wall of the stomach, or indicate a mass enlarging and indenting the duodenal loop. Ultrasound or CT will show a mass in the pancreas gland and also whether there is any evidence of liver metastases. Ultrasound- and CT-guided biopsy of secondary deposits will confirm the diagnosis. The role of magnetic resonance imaging (MRI) is not yet established. An ERCP may show visible distortion of the duodenum and narrowing or kinking of the pancreatic duct. Cytology of pancreatic secretions, brushings or biopsy during ERCP may confirm the diagnosis. An ampullary carcinoma can be visualized directly and a biopsy taken. Arteriography and laparoscopic ultrasound are useful in assessing resectability. Liver function tests may confirm the obstructive nature of the jaundice (see Table 19). Faecal occult blood tests may be positive if the duodenum is involved. Carcinomas of the body and tail are often only diagnosed with certainty at exploratory laparotomy.

Management

Patients with evidence of secondary deposits of tumour or that are not resectable should be treated with tender loving care. If they are jaundiced then ERCP and stenting should be performed. Palliative gastric and biliary bypasses are also treatment options in young patients with irresectable tumours. Resectability can sometimes only be assessed at laparotomy. Periampullary tumours that are thought to be localized or resectable on diagnostic imaging in fit patients should be managed by a laparotomy and a Whipple's or pylorus-preserving pancreaticoduodenectomy. At operation if the tumour is not resectable then a bypass procedure is performed (triple bypass).

Preoperative management

A mannitol infusion may be required if the patient is jaundiced (see p. 339). We give prophylactic antibiotics (gentamicin and flucloxacillin). The patient's clotting factors should be checked and vitamin K_1 given if he is jaundiced.

OPERATION: DISTAL PANCREATECTOMY
(Fig. 71)
The splenic vessels are ligated and the spleen removed *en bloc* with the specimen. The cut end of the pancreas is closed and drained. This operation can be performed laparoscopically in advanced centres.

Codes

Blood	4 units
GA/LA	GA
Opn time	2–3 h
Stay	2–3 weeks
Drains out	7–10 days
Sutures out	7 days
Off work	About 2 months

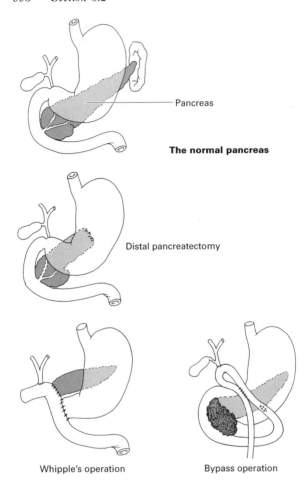

Pancreas

The normal pancreas

Distal pancreatectomy

Whipple's operation

Bypass operation

Fig. 71 Pancreatic operations.

OPERATION: WHIPPLE'S OPERATION
(see Fig. 71)
In this operation the neck of the pancreas is transected as it runs over the portal vein. The head of the pancreas is removed together with the distal part of the stomach, pylorus and complete duodenal loop up to the duodenojejunal flexure. The CBD is also divided. The gall bladder may or may not be removed. In the reconstructive phase of the operation the jejunal loop is brought up and anastomosed first to the CBD, then to the cut end of the body of the pancreas and finally to the stomach remnant. Drains are

inserted through this loop to splint the anastomoses to the CBD and pancreatic duct. These stents are usually brought out through the jejunal loop and thence to the surface. A larger drain is put up to the outer surface of the pancreatic anastomosis. A truncal vagotomy may be added in order to reduce gastric acidity and prevent stomal ulceration of the gastrojejunal anastomosis.

Codes

Blood	6 units
GA/LA	GA
Opn time	3–5 h
Stay	3 weeks
Drains out	7–10 days
Sutures out	7 days
Off work	2–3 months

Postoperative care

Individual surgeons vary widely in their postoperative management of this complex procedure. In the author's practice the patient is kept nil by mouth until flatus is passed. If there are no signs of anastomotic leakage (increased drainage or tenderness at the operation site), the various stents and drains are removed at about 7 days.

OPERATION: BYPASS OPERATION FOR CARCINOMA OF PANCREAS (see Fig. 71)

Three anastomoses are performed. In the first a loop of jejunum is anastomosed either to the CBD or to the distended gall bladder, thus relieving the biliary obstruction. Secondly, the stomach is anastomosed to the side of this loop forming a gastrojejunostomy. This relieves potential duodenal obstruction. Thirdly, an anastomosis is made between the two sides of the jejunal loop in order that food may bypass the loop going to the CBD.

Codes

Blood	2 units
GA/LA	GA
Opn time	90 min
Stay	7–10 days
Drains out	0
Sutures out	7 days
Off work	May be indefinite

Postoperative care
The objective is to produce good palliation and it is essential to keep the patient as comfortable as possible after the operation. Adequate pain relief is given. Care is taken to ensure that the urinary output remains adequate postoperatively and more mannitol may be required. Once the patient has recovered from the operation, a decision is made about whether he or she should also be given chemotherapy.

Pancreatitis

Pancreatitis is inflammation of the pancreas and may be acute, relapsing or chronic.

Acute pancreatitis

Acute pancreatitis is the term applied to a vicious circle of events, which follows damage to the pancreas from a variety of causes. Pancreatic enzyme precursors are released and activated by substances in the inflammatory exudate. The activated enzymes further damage the pancreas and subsequent inflammation and oedema tend to obstruct the pancreatic duct, aggravating the situation.

The disease progresses through well-recognized stages. Resolution may occur at any stage without progression to the next. It is important to understand these stages in order to monitor the patient's progress.

1 Oedema. In the first few days the pancreas is markedly oedematous and there is exudation of pancreatic enzymes into the peritoneal cavity resulting in autodigestion of fat and patchy fat necrosis throughout the peritoneum. During this stage the serum amylase will be high and if the process is severe there may be a fall in the serum calcium. The latter may be due to calcium being mopped up by the digested fats to form soaps.

2 Haemorrhage. In this next stage the digestion affects blood vessels and there is retroperitoneal bleeding. This phase also occurs early in severe disease, usually during the first week from onset.

3 Necrosis. Once blood vessels have become damaged, there may be infarction of large areas of the pancreatic gland, leading to slough formation.

4 Abscess and pseudocyst formation. This occurs in the second to third week. Pseudocyst formation probably occurs as the residual pancreas recovers. Secretions and transudate accumulate in a damaged pancreatic bed and in the lesser sac. If the

Table 20 Aetiological factors in acute pancreatitis.

Biliary disease (55–60% of cases in England)
Idiopathic (35–40%)
Alcoholic (1–5%)

Trauma
   crush injury
   abdominal surgery

Carcinoma of the pancreas
Mumps
Hypothermia
Drugs, e.g. steroids/thiazides
Polyarteritis nodosa
Hyperparathyroidism
Hyperlipidaemia

subsequent collection and residual slough become infected, a pancreatic abscess results.

Recognized causes of pancreatic damage are shown in Table 20.

Recognizing the pattern

The disease is more common in the middle aged and elderly. In the UK it is usually seen in the type of patient who suffers from gall stones (see p. 331).

The patient presents with a sudden onset of upper abdominal pain, which gradually becomes very severe. It tends to radiate through to the back and is usually associated with vomiting. Over the next 24 h the patient becomes gradually more and more ill.

On examination there is generalized abdominal tenderness, maximal in the upper abdomen. The patient also shows signs of dehydration and shock and is generally toxic with a fever. He may also be slightly jaundiced due to obstruction of the CBD by oedema or by the stone causing the pancreatitis.

Later careful examination may disclose bruising in the subcutaneous tissue of the flanks (Grey Turner's sign) or even around the umbilicus (Cullen's sign). These signs are due to bleeding from a severe haemorrhagic pancreatitis.

Both the history and signs are rather non-specific and the differential diagnosis includes perforated peptic ulcer, mesenteric infarction, intestinal obstruction and myocardial infarction.

Proving the diagnosis

The diagnosis is proved by measuring the serum amylase (normal range 80–150 Somogyi units). If this is above 1000–2000 units, acute pancreatitis is extremely likely. Other causes for a moderately raised amylase include a perforated duodenal ulcer, myocardial infarction and acute cholecystitis. The severity of the condition is not related to the amylase level. A falling haemoglobin or a falling calcium in the first few days after the onset or positive faecal occult blood are of grave prognostic significance and imply the onset of haemorrhagic pancreatitis. Methaemalbuminaemia is also ominous. It is these patients who are likely to progress to pseudocyst or abscess formation in the second and third weeks (see below).

Apart from the amylase, other baseline investigations should include the following:

1 Haemoglobin and white cell count.
2 Liver function tests and serum calcium.
3 Urine test for sugar and bilirubin.
4 A chest X-ray and an abdominal X-ray. These help to exclude a perforated ulcer or intestinal obstruction. They may show a solitary dilated loop of jejunum, which is suffering from localized ileus ('sentinel loop').
5 Electrocardiogram (ECG).
6 Blood gases.

After admission the daily progress of the disease is assessed by daily measurement of the following:

1 Urea and electrolytes
2 White cell count
3 Calcium
4 Urine for sugar content.

These detect any developing renal failure, hyperglycaemia (transient diabetes) or hypocalcaemia, which can then be treated accordingly.

Management

This condition is usually managed conservatively, though there are indications for surgical intervention.

Medical treatment

1 Bed rest.
2 Analgesia. The pain is often severe and the patient should be written up for pethidine (50–100 mg i.m. 4-hourly).
3 Blood and fluid replacement. The oedematous process is associated with a huge loss of fluid into the retroperitoneal

tissues, accompanied by a loss of protein and blood if the pancreatitis is severe. This results in oligaemia, which aggravates the tendency to renal failure. It is essential therefore to give the patient adequate fluid replacement early on. This should be sufficient to maintain a good urinary output. In the first 24 h this is mainly fluid and electrolyte replacement. Later plasma and blood should be given. In a severe case of pancreatitis a CVP line should be set up and a urinary catheter inserted to monitor the fluid replacement.

4 Resting the pancreas. Every effort is made to minimize the degree of pancreatic stimulation during the disease. The stomach is kept empty by aspiration through a nasogastric tube and no food is given.

5 Antibiotics. The use of antibiotics in acute pancreatitis is controversial. Some physicians believe it may delay or prevent the onset of late pancreatic sepsis but the evidence for this is not strong.

6 In severe gall stone pancreatitis, early ERCP and sphincterotomy and removal of CBD stones is advocated by some surgeons.

Surgical treatment

Although a few centres practice emergency total pancreatectomy for fulminant acute pancreatitis, operation is not generally required for the type of cases seen in the UK. There are, however, a few indications for operative intervention short of total pancreatectomy.

1 In the acute attack a laparotomy may be indicated to exclude other diseases and to prove the diagnosis of acute pancreatitis. This is, of course, best avoided as a laparotomy adds a further injury to the patient's problems. Where the diagnosis is in doubt, it can be justified. It is safe provided adequate fluid replacement is given preoperatively and postoperatively.

2 Late in the disease there may be a need to operate and remove necrotic and infected pancreatic tissue, or to drain a pancreatic pseudocyst or abscess. Occasionally patients also require operation because of persistent duodenal ileus (gastroenterostomy).

Management of complications

1 Renal failure. This occurs as a complication of the early stage of acute pancreatitis. Treatment is by peritoneal dialysis or in severe cases by haemodialysis.

Continued on p. 364

Continued.

2 Diabetes. A transient episode of hyperglycaemia is not uncommon in severe pancreatitis and insulin therapy may be needed. However, the diabetes usually recovers later.

3 Hypocalcaemia. Ten per cent calcium gluconate (10 ml) may be required once or twice a day.

4 Pseudocyst formation — see below.

5 Duodenal ileus. This is a rare complication. Although the patient's general health improves, he continues to show signs of duodenal obstruction with vomiting. The condition is due to persistent inflammation on the inner aspect of the duodenal loop. Occasionally a gastroenterostomy is required in order to start the patient feeding again (see p. 297).

6 Haematemesis and melaena. This is due to concurrent peptic ulceration.

After recovery

After recovery from the acute attack, identification and treatment of any underlying cause must be carried out so as to prevent recurrence. This may include cholecystectomy and exploration of the CBD, parathyroidectomy for hypercalcaemia or treatment of alcoholism. Whatever the cause of the pancreatitis, alcohol should be avoided for 3 months.

Pancreatic pseudocyst

Recognizing the pattern

The patient continues to run a swinging fever and a white count either remains elevated or begins to climb again. The abdomen should be examined regularly and a mass may become palpable in the epigastrium.

Proving the diagnosis

Performing an ultrasound scan proves the diagnosis. The mass may also be palpable and seen displacing the stomach anteriorly on a barium meal.

Most pseudocysts settle spontaneously and a policy of patient observation should be adopted. Indications for operation are failure to resolve after 2–3 weeks, the presence of unremitting distressing pain or a climbing fever. In the latter case the pseudocyst may have become infected and this is an indication for drainage. This may either be done percutaneously under ultrasound control by a radiologist, or by open operation.

OPERATION: DRAINAGE OF A PSEUDOCYST

The pseudocyst is either drained by a transgastric approach or into a loop of small bowel. A routine laparotomy is performed and the anterior wall of the stomach opened. The posterior wall of the stomach is then incised and the pseudocyst, which is adherent to it, is drained into the stomach. The walls of the cyst are sutured to the gastric mucosa. A tube drain is then placed in the pseudocyst and brought out across the lumen of the stomach through the anterior abdominal wall and skin to the exterior. This operation can be performed laparoscopically.

A pancreatic slough can also be removed endoscopically by passing a dilating cannula over a radiologically inserted drain in the left flank. A laparoscope is inserted together with secondary instruments through other ports. The necrotic tissue can then be aspirated under vision avoiding damage to the splenic vessels.

Codes

	Open drainage	Endoscopic drainage
Blood	4 units	4 units
GA/LA	GA	GA
Opn time	1–2 h	1–2 h
Stay	Variable, 1 week minimum	2–7 days
Drains out	14–21 days (see below)	2–7 days
Sutures out	7–10 days	Absorbable
Off work	Variable	Variable

Postoperative care

Oral fluids can be introduced once any ileus recovers. The transgastric tube is left in place until there is evidence that the cavity has shrunk down (usually about 2 weeks). The size of the cavity can be seen by injecting contrast down the drain and taking X-rays. The first of these is done on the tenth day. Once the tube has been removed, the gastrostomy is sealed with a pad of paraffin gauze and rapidly heals.

The recovery after the endoscopic procedure depends on how long drainage continues and whether the fever settles rapidly or not.

Chronic pancreatitis

In chronic pancreatitis there is gradual destruction and fibrosis of the gland. The pancreatic duct is narrowed and distorted and calculi or diffuse pancreatic calcification may occur.

This condition is associated with diabetes and malabsorption due to the failure of endocrine and exocrine function.

Recognizing the pattern

The patient is in poor health and may have chronic pain. Relapsing chronic pancreatitis is characterized by episodes of epigastric pain and vomiting with associated weakness. Obstructive jaundice may develop. Steatorrhoea, weight loss and diabetes indicate severe disease with failure of pancreatic function.

Proving the diagnosis

A plain abdominal X-ray may show calcification. The amylase is moderately elevated during a relapse. Stool analysis may show steatorrhoea (more than 6 g of fat lost per day). Pancreatic function can be measured by performing a glucose tolerance test and analysing pancreatic secretions (including bicarbonate and enzymes). These are obtained from a tube placed in the duodenum while the pancreas is stimulated with secretin/pancreozymin.

Management

Functional failure is treated medically with a high-protein, high-calorie diet, exogenous enzyme preparations and vitamin replacement. Insulin may be needed.

Surgery is required for a dilated pancreatic duct with strictures, and a bypass procedure may be needed for obstructive jaundice. In some cases of unremitting pain greater splanchnic nerve resection may be performed.

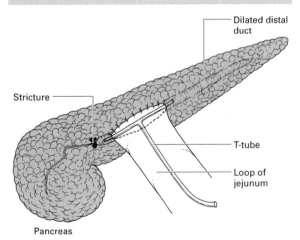

Fig. 72 Pancreaticojejunostomy for stricture. A loop of jejunum is anastomosed end-to-side to the dilated pancreatic duct.

OPERATION: FOR PANCREATIC DUCT
STRICTURE (Fig. 72)

If the stricture is in the head of the pancreas, a Whipple's operation may be performed. The distended distal duct is anastomosed to a Roux loop of jejunum. Where the stricture is in the neck or body of the gland, the distal distended pancreatic duct may be laid open and a loop of jejunum anastomosed to it side-by-side (pancreaticojejunostomy). Occasionally there are multiple strictures in the pancreatic duct and such a procedure is not then possible. In these circumstances the whole pancreatic duct may be laid open and anastomosed along the length of the gland to a loop of jejunum (Puestow's operation).

Codes

Blood .... 4 units
GA/LA .... GA
Opn time .... 2–3 h
Stay .... About 2 weeks
Drains out .... Pancreatic T-tube 10–14 days after pancreato-gram; main drainage tube about 7 days
Sutures out ...... 7 days
Off work .... 6–12 weeks

Surgical conditions of the spleen

The spleen is situated in the left upper quadrant of the abdomen protected by the ribcage. It receives blood from the splenic artery, which is a branch of the coeliac plexus. It also receives some blood from the short gastric and left gastroepiploic arteries. Blood returns to the portal system via the splenic vein. The spleen has important immunological functions, clearing antigens from the circulation and producing immunoglobulin M (IgM) and various factors that are important in the phagocytosis of encapsulated bacteria. It also produces lymphocytes and plays a role in red cell maturation.

The spleen can become enlarged as a result of a response to infection, connective tissue disorders, myelo- or lymphoproliferative disorders, infiltration by neoplastic cells from other sites and in various types of anaemia.

The indications for splenectomy can be grouped together as in Table 21. The operation can be performed laparoscopically in expert hands.

Table 21 Indications for splenectomy.

Hypersplenism

Myeloproliferative disorders, e.g. myelofibrosis, chronic myeloid leukaemia

Haemolytic anaemia: spherocytosis, elliptocytosis, pyruvate kinase deficiency, thalassaemia, immune haemolytic anaemia

Platelet disorders: thrombocytopenic purpura

Trauma (see p. 658)

Lymphoma (see p. 155)

Preoperative management
The patient should be immunized against *Pneumococcus* by giving 1 vial of Pneumovax II 2 weeks before an elective splenectomy. He or she should also be given pre- and post-operative penicillin (or erythromycin if allergic to penicillin).

OPERATION: OPEN SPLENECTOMY
A left subcostal or paramedian incision is performed. The short gastric vessels are divided. The peritoneum lateral to and above the spleen is opened and the spleen and tail of pancreas mobilized to the midline. The splenic flexure of the colon is freed, the splenic vessels divided between the pancreas and the spleen, and the spleen removed. Any splenunculi should also be removed.

Codes
Blood .... 2 units
GA/LA .... GA
Opn time .... 60–90 min
Stay .... 7–10 days
Drains out .... 3–7 days
Sutures out .... 7 days
Off work .... 4 weeks

OPERATION: LAPAROSCOPIC SPLENECTOMY
(Fig. 73)
The splenic vessels are usually approached through the lesser sac after dissecting the short gastric vessels. An ultrasonic scalpel is useful in this procedure. The artery and vein are

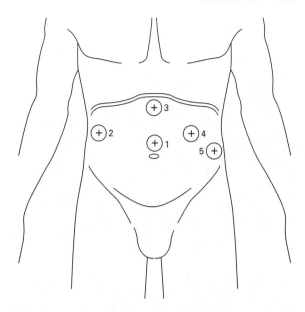

Fig. 73 Possible port sites for laparoscopic splenectomy.

ligated and the rest of the splenic pedicle divided with a linear stapler. The spleen is removed in a sialastic bag. It can either be broken up or removed intact through a short incision anywhere in the abdominal wall. (e.g. suprapubically for good cosmesis).

Codes

Blood	2 units
GA/LA	GA
Opn time	2–3 h
Stay	3–5 days
Drains out	24 h
Sutures out	Absorbable
Off work	2–3 weeks

Postoperative care
Following splenectomy a number of complications can arise.
1 Acute dilatation of the stomach. This is quite common after a splenectomy and can be avoided by adequate aspiration of the stomach until the gastric ileus has fully recovered.

Continued on p. 370

Continued.

2 Left basal pulmonary collapse and pneumonia. Movements of the left base are diminished and it is important to give adequate analgesia and physiotherapy to protect against this complication.

3 Subphrenic abscess. This may follow infection of a haematoma or damage to one of the organs in the neighbourhood of the spleen (see above). The abscess should drain spontaneously through the track provided.

4 Thrombotic complications. When the spleen is removed the platelet level rises and if the platelet count goes over $1000 \times 10^9/L$ there is a risk of thrombotic complications. Some surgeons use routine anticoagulant prophylaxis after this procedure or give dipyridamole (50–100 mg 8-hourly) or aspirin (75 mg daily or 150 mg on alternate days) to decrease platelet stickiness until the platelet count falls to less than $1000 \times 10^9/L$.

5 In the long term, patients, especially children, have an increased risk of dying from pneumococcal pneumonia and other infections, such as *Haemophilus influenzae*. They should be immunized after the operation if they have not been preoperatively. It is also reasonable to give penicillin V (250 mg b.d.) to patients for a year postoperatively or to children until the age of 21 years. Patients remain at a low risk of infection with penicillin-resistant organisms. Erythromycin can be substituted if the patient is allergic to penicillin.

9 Colorectal Surgery and Perianal Pain

9.1 Colorectal Surgery

Crohn's disease

Crohn's disease is a chronic inflammatory condition affecting the small or large bowel and rarely the oesophagus and stomach. It is of unknown aetiology. It produces characteristic granulomas through the full thickness of the bowel wall (unlike ulcerative colitis, which only involves the mucosa). These progress to fissure formation and sepsis around the bowel, and eventually to fistulae and strictures. There has been a modest increase in its incidence.

Recognizing the pattern

The patient will usually be between the ages of 15 and 55 years, and loss of weight is common in long-standing disease.

The history depends on the bowel involved:

1 Small bowel Crohn's disease presents either with chronic diarrhoea or with episodes of colicky abdominal pain due to obstruction. Severe inflammation in the terminal ileum may give a picture similar to appendicitis. In chronic disease there is often severe constitutional disturbance, e.g. lassitude, anaemia and weight loss. The patient may have fear of eating since this precipitates abdominal colic.

2 Large bowel Crohn's disease presents with diarrhoea or obstructive symptoms and can on occasion be difficult to distinguish from ulcerative colitis.

3 Perianal disease: fissures, skin tags, perianal abscesses and fistulae are characteristic of perianal Crohn's disease. These are difficult to treat and healing is slow. Lesions may be painless, but an undrained abscess can cause a great deal of distress.

On examination the patient may be pyrexial. In acute Crohn's disease a tubular mass may be palpable in the right iliac fossa. Otherwise there may be tenderness anywhere in the abdomen. Look carefully for signs of perianal sepsis.

Proving the diagnosis

Small bowel Crohn's disease can be diagnosed by a barium 'follow-through' or, more accurately, a small bowel enema. The affected gut is seen with a thick wall and a narrow lumen ('string sign'). There are ulcers and fissures in the bowel, which are seen as spicules of barium or cobblestoning. The affected areas of the bowel may be intermingled with normal intestine ('skip lesions'). Fistulae may be present. A barium enema will show discontinuous colonic disease. This can be assessed more accurately by colonoscopy. Biopsies will show the characteristic non-caseating granulomas. A computed tomography (CT) scan will show the intra-abdominal abscess or fistula and a magnetic resonance imaging (MRI) scan can be used to assess severe perianal and pelvic disease.

The patient may have abnormal liver function tests (hypoalbuminaemia), and anaemia and an elevated sedimentation rate. The affected area of the bowel shows up on an indium scan.

Management

The main treatment of Crohn's disease is medical. Drugs used are steroids and 5-aminosalicylic acid (5-ASA) compounds. Immunosuppression with azathioprine can also be effective.

The key to successful management is good medical therapy and timely surgery. The initial management of intestinal obstruction is medical but repeated episodes should be treated by surgical resection. If Crohn's disease is found at laparotomy for suspected appendicitis the appendix should be removed and if the ileocaecal disease is severe enough this should be resected at the same time.

Operative treatment is eventually required in 70–80% of cases. Surgical resection is kept to the absolute minimum to relieve symptoms. Where there are several areas of affected bowel, strictureplasty (widening of a strictured area) can be used to conserve gut length. In large bowel Crohn's disease the options are a segmental resection, a colectomy, anorectal anastomosis or, in severe cases, a panproctocolectomy.

Preoperative management

Check that the serum proteins are satisfactory. If they are not, a period of intravenous feeding may be indicated. With large bowel Crohn's disease a bowel preparation is undertaken (p. 113). The operation will usually be covered by antibiotics. If the patient is already on steroids, these must be increased preoperatively (p. 25).

OPERATION: ILEOCAECAL RESECTION FOR CROHN'S DISEASE

The affected bowel is resected with an adequate margin and an end-to-end anastomosis is performed.

Codes

Blood .... 2 units

GA/LA .... GA

Opn time .... 90–150 min

Stay .... 7–14 days

Drains out 0

Sutures out .... 7 days unless absorbable

Off work .... 6–8 weeks

Postoperative care

Nasogastric suction and intravenous fluids are continued until the patient has passed flatus. The care of patients on steroids postoperatively is dealt with on p. 25. The patient with severe Crohn's disease is often debilitated, and intravenous feeding may be continued postoperatively. Whenever an area of Crohn's disease has been resected, there is a danger of fistula formation. The patient should be kept in hospital long enough to make sure that this danger has passed (7–14 days).

Long-term follow-up will be needed, as there is a tendency for the disease to recur. Recurrent disease can be monitored by performing an indium scan and measuring acute phase proteins.

OPERATION: PANPROCTOCOLECTOMY
See p. 378.

Ulcerative colitis

Ulcerative colitis is a condition of unknown aetiology affecting the colon and rectum. It starts distally and may spread any distance proximally up the large bowel. Twenty per cent of cases involve the rectum only, 45% involve the rectum and part of the colon, while 35% involve the whole of the large bowel. The mucosa of the colon becomes ulcerated and tends to bleed. In severe acute disease the colonic wall may become very thin and perforate. This condition is called toxic megacolon and is an acute surgical emergency.

In long-standing disease there is a risk of carcinomatous change occurring in the large bowel. There are a number of extraintestinal manifestations including ankylosing spondylitis, iritis and sclerosing cholangitis.

Recognizing the pattern

The disease may affect patients of any age, although they are usually between the ages of 15 and 55 years. Patients with severe disease may be thin and malnourished. Ulcerative colitis patients may have an obsessive personality, but this is probably secondary to their chronic diarrhoea condition. The patient has a series of relapses and remissions. The bowel frequency may go up to 8–12 times a day during an attack. The stool is liquid and there is blood and mucus in the stool and there may be cramping, left-sided abdominal pain. Urgency and incontinence during these acute attacks will have a major impact on a patient's quality of life. On examination there may be tenderness over the colon in acute extensive disease, and the abdomen may be distended. On rectal examination there may be a velvety feel to the mucosa and blood and mucus are noted on the examining glove.

Proving the diagnosis

The diagnosis is proved on sigmoidoscopy when the inflamed, haemorrhagic mucosa can be clearly seen. During this examination it may be possible to determine the upper extent of the disease. A biopsy should always be taken, as this is diagnostic and may help to differentiate the disorder from Crohn's disease. Stool cultures are mandatory during a first attack and the possibility of amoebic dysentery should be considered. A barium enema or colonoscopy will also demonstrate the extent of the ulceration and in long-standing disease should be used to exclude secondary neoplastic change.

Management

An acute attack is treated with bed rest, intravenous infusion and replacement therapy, together with high doses of intravenous steroids (e.g. prednisolone 60 mg/day). Rectal steroids, 5-ASA compounds and antibiotics may also be used.

The management of a severe case of acute colitis is aimed at preventing the development of a toxic megacolon and either inducing a remission or removing the colon before it becomes so thin walled, dilated and irreversibly damaged that perforation occurs with peritonitis and a high mortality. A case of acute colitis should therefore be managed jointly by expert physicians and surgeons. Daily abdominal X-rays are performed and the colonic diameter measured. A trial of medical therapy over 5–7 days is standard practice. If a patient has not made a reasonable response by that stage then surgery should be considered.

Other investigations which help in assessing the severity

of the disease, and are usually monitored daily, include the following:

1 Haemoglobin and white cell count
2 Erythrocyte sedimentation rate (ESR)
3 Urea and electrolytes (especially the potassium)
4 Liver function tests (especially to monitor the serum albumin).

The indications for emergency surgery are as follows:

1 Toxic megacolon with a persistent colonic diameter of over 6 cm
2 Haemorrhage (though this is rare)
3 Perforation
4 Failed medical treatment: this can be said to occur if the patient, despite adequate therapy, has:
   (a) persistent diarrhoea
   (b) pyrexia more than 38°C
   (c) tachycardia or increasing abdominal tenderness, or
   (d) a falling haemoglobin or serum albumin.

The indications for elective surgery include the following:

1 Failed medical treatment, with chronic poor general health and interference with work and social activities
2 Frequent repeated attacks of acute colitis
3 Premalignant or malignant change.

Preoperative management

The patient must be made as fit as possible. Dehydration, anaemia and hypoproteinaemia are corrected. Bowel preparation is not usually indicated.

The possibility of surgery is explained to the patient early in the course of the episode of acute colitis. He must be told what the operation will entail and the dangers inherent in leaving the diseased colon *in situ*. Many patients will go on to have restorative surgery so that while they may have a temporary ileostomy, in many it is unlikely to be permanent. In the elective situation there is more time to discuss the various surgical alternatives. Patients should have the opportunity to meet others who have had an ileostomy or a restorative procedure. The involvement of the hospital's stoma therapy team is essential.

OPERATIONS

Four possible operations will be described here.

1 Total abdominal colectomy, ileostomy and preservation of the rectal stump.

Continued on p. 378

Continued.

2 Panproctocolectomy and terminal ileostomy.
3 Restorative proctocolectomy with a temporary loop ileostomy.
4 Closure of loop ileostomy.

OPERATION: TOTAL ABDOMINAL COLECTOMY, ILEOSTOMY WITH PRESERVATION OF THE RECTUM

The whole colon is removed from the caecum to the sacral promontory. If the omentum is adherent to the transverse colon this is also resected. A terminal ileostomy is brought out in the right iliac fossa. The rectum can either be closed at the sacral promontory, or brought out open at the lower end of the wound, or closed just beneath the skin.

Codes

Blood	2 units
GA/LA	GA
Opn time	2 h
Stay	10 days
Drains	0
Sutures out	Subcuticular or 7–10 days
Off work	2 months

Postoperative care

The new ileostomy may take time to adapt and high volumes of ileostomy effluent may cause dehydration.

OPERATION: PANPROCTOCOLECTOMY AND TERMINAL ILEOSTOMY

The whole colon is removed from the caecum to the anus using two incisions, one abdominal and the other perineal. The terminal ileostomy is brought out at the right iliac fossa. The anal canal is removed in the intersphincteric plane to make as small a perineal wound as possible. The empty pelvis is drained with suction drains via the abdominal wall.

Codes

Blood	2 units
GA/LA	GA
Opn time	3 h

Stay .... 10–14 days
Drains out .... 4–5 days; nasogastric tube
                                        until the ileostomy is working
Sutures out .... Subcuticular or 7–10 days
Off work .... 2–3 months

Postoperative care
This is the same as for an abdominoperineal resection of the
rectum and is described on p. 395.

OPERATION: RESTORATIVE
PROCTOCOLECTOMY
This is usually done as a second-stage procedure after a
previous total colectomy. The residual rectum is removed,
the ileostomy taken down and fashioned into an ileal reservoir. It is usually anastomosed to the top of the anal canal
using a stapling device and the operation is covered with a
temporary loop ileostomy.

Codes
Blood .... 2 units
GA/LA .... GA
Opn time .... 2–3 h
Stay .... 10 days
Drains out .... 3–4 days
Sutures out .... Subcuticular
Off work .... 2–3 months

OPERATION: CLOSURE OF LOOP ILEOSTOMY
This is usually a third-stage procedure after restorative
proctocolectomy. After checking with a pouchagram that the
pouch has healed and that there is no stenosis of the pouch–
anal anastomosis the loop ileostomy is mobilized,
reanastomosed and the abdomen closed.

Codes
Blood .... Group and save
GA/LA .... GA
Opn time .... 1 h
Stay .... 4–7 days
Drains out 0
Sutures out .... Subcuticular or 7–10 days
Off work .... Variable

Rectal bleeding in adults

Common causes of fresh rectal bleeding in adults include the following:

1 Haemorrhoids (p. 412)
2 Anal fissure (p. 411)
3 Inflammatory bowel disease (pp. 373–379)
4 Neoplasms — benign or malignant (pp. 382–397)
5 Diverticular disease (p. 397)
6 Meckel's diverticulum (p. 322).

Rectal bleeding in children is dealt with on p. 621.

If the blood is old and black, a bleeding lesion higher up in the bowel must obviously be considered. Blood from the upper colon and above will be mixed in with the motion. In lower rectal bleeding the blood is coated on the outside of the motion and is noted in the pan and on the toilet paper.

Investigation

A full history and examination should be taken and particular attention paid to the presence of abdominal masses and tenderness. On rectal examination, note whether the examination is painful or not and whether the anal sphincter is tight or not. A painful examination may indicate a fissure. A tight sphincter is often associated with other perianal pathology such as piles or fissures. Also on rectal examination, feel high up to note whether there is a palpable neoplasm in the rectum or even in the sigmoid colon. The latter is felt outside the rectum lying in the pelvis. An area of diverticulitis may be felt as a tender mass high up on the left side.

All adults presenting with rectal bleeding should have a proctoscopy and sigmoidoscopy.

On proctoscopy the surgeon can note the presence of piles and whether the surface is haemorrhagic or not. An anal fissure can be seen or excluded. If the examination is impossible due to pain, then a fissure is likely.

On sigmoidoscopy the presence of blood and mucus in the bowel can be seen and a tumour within the rectum looked for. The character of the rectal mucosa and any evidence of proctitis can be noted. Any tumour or suspicious area of mucosa can be biopsied.

Depending on local circumstances some patients will be investigated primarily with a flexible sigmoidoscopy. This gives a good view of the sigmoid and left colon up to the splenic flexure. It can be supplemented by a barium enema or a colonoscopy (which has the advantage of being able to demonstrate angiodysplasia). Polyps, carcinoma of the colon and the presence or absence of diverticular disease should all be noted.

The management of the condition found is dealt with under the appropriate sections.

Change in bowel habit

A change in bowel habit is a serious symptom and must always be investigated if it persists for more than 3 weeks, especially if the patient is over 30 years of age. It is most commonly due to colonic disease and possible causes include:

Inflammation: ulcerative colitis, Crohn's disease and diverticular disease.

Neoplasia: polyps, carcinoma of the colon.

Other less common causes of a change in bowel habit are pancreatic disease, chronic mesenteric ischaemia, and gastric and small bowel obstruction. These will not be considered further here.

Making a diagnosis

A full history is taken in order to determine the patient's normal bowel habit and the nature of the change. The changes in consistency and character of the motion and the presence of blood and mucus must be determined. With inflammatory large bowel disease (ulcerative colitis or Crohn's) there is a marked increase in frequency of defaecation and blood and mucus in the stool. This often lasts several weeks at a time with periods of normality between. The stools are watery.

With obstruction of the left side of the colon or rectum the patient suffers from continued alternating constipation and diarrhoea, usually occurring in cycles of a few days (see p. 386). This picture is seen in carcinoma of the left side of the colon or rectum or in diverticular disease with stricture formation.

With a sigmoid volvulus the patient has intermittent attacks of total constipation associated with abdominal pain and marked distension. In diverticular disease uncomplicated by stricture formation, there is an acute episode of severe, left-sided abdominal pain and diarrhoea which usually resolves completely. The motions are loose during the attack and may be pellet-like at other times.

A full examination is indicated and obviously a rectal examination must be included.

Sigmoidoscopy

This is done to look for a rectal lesion and the presence of blood and mucus coming down from a lesion higher up. Inflammatory disease of the mucosa is visible and can be biopsied. The nature of the stool in the rectum can provide valuable confirmatory evidence of the patient's history. Hard, rabbit pellet motions may be seen in the presence of diverticular disease.

Proctoscopy

This should be undertaken to look for the presence of piles. Patients sometimes complain of frequency of defaecation when they have piles as they believe they are not emptying their rectum fully due to the discomfort produced by the piles.

Barium enema

This is always indicated where there is a change in bowel habit in order to look for colonic polyps or a carcinoma.

The further management of a change in bowel habit is dealt with under the individual conditions as below.

1 Colonic polyps
2 Carcinoma of the colon (p. 384)
3 Carcinoma of the rectum (p. 391)
4 Diverticular disease (p. 397)
5 Sigmoid volvulus (p. 400)
6 Crohn's disease (p. 373)
7 Ulcerative colitis (p. 375).

Colonic polyps

There are a number of histological types of polyp in the colon, the most frequent and important of which is the adenoma. These may be either single or multiple. Familial adenomatous polyposis is a condition of extensive polyposis of the large bowel inherited as an autosomal dominant trait. There may be other associated growth disorders such as duodenal polyps, desmoid disease and exostoses.

Benign adenomas may be either sessile or pedunculated. Histologically they are described as tubular, tubulovillous or villous. Tubular adenomas have the appearance of a raspberry on a stalk. A villous adenoma is sessile with a frond-like surface. The larger the polyp the more likely is malignant change. Polyps may bleed or secrete mucus rich in potassium.

Rarer polyps include juvenile polyps, hamartomatous polyps of the Peutz–Jeghers syndrome, haemangiomas and lipomas. Metaplastic polyps are very common and probably a response to inflammation or injury and as far as is known have no potential for malignant change.

Recognizing the pattern

The patient is usually adult. Polyps of familial adenomatous polyposis appear around puberty. Solitary adenomas are rare before the age of 40 years. The patient may present with anaemia or increased bowel frequency with mucus diarrhoea. Polyps may cause intussusception and intestinal obstruction. Familial adenomatous polyposis may produce a picture resembling ulcerative colitis with episodes of abdominal pain, loss of weight, diarrhoea and the passage of blood and mucus. Symptoms suggesting malignant change include weight loss, anorexia and an increased change in bowel habit.

On examination there is often nothing abnormal to find. The polyp in the rectum may be palpable or seen on sigmoidoscopy and is usually a soft tumour protruding into the lumen. A hard area within it suggests malignant change.

Proving the diagnosis

The diagnosis is proved by sigmoidoscopy and barium enema or colonoscopy. The faeces may be positive for occult blood. Other relevant investigations include a full blood count to look for anaemia, and electrolytes to check the potassium level. Profuse haemorrhage from a haemangioma can sometimes be localized by arteriography.

Management

Adenomatous polyps over 5 mm in diameter are usually removed because of the risk of malignant change. Colonoscopic polypectomy using cold snaring for smaller polyps and diathermy for larger polyps is usually successful. Familial adenomatous polyposis is treated by prophylactic colectomy in patients in their late teens. If the rectum is not seriously involved an ileorectal anastomosis may be appropriate. Where there is extensive carpeting of the rectum by polyps a restorative proctocolectomy as for ulcerative colitis is the operation of choice. A minority of patients may prefer a proctocolectomy and ileostomy.

Postoperative care

Where there is a retained rectal stump in familial adenomatous polyposis coli, follow-up is by regular sigmoidoscopy and diathermy of any residual polyps. Other members of the family are offered genetic screening and/or flexible sigmoidoscopy until the age of 50 years. After colonoscopic polypectomy of a single adenoma further follow-up at 3–5-yearly intervals is sufficient.

Carcinoma of the colon

The clinical features of carcinoma of the colon depend on the site of the growth. They can be divided into those affecting the right side and those affecting the left. Because the contents of the right side of the colon are fluid and those of the left side semi-solid, right-sided lesions tend to obstruct late and left-sided lesions obstruct early. Both lesions tend to bleed quietly into the bowel and iron deficiency anaemia is therefore common. The importance of a family history is increasingly recognized.

Right-sided colonic carcinoma

Recognizing the pattern

The patient is usually over 40 years of age and the condition is common in 70–80 year olds. Women are more commonly affected than men. The patient may present with unexplained pain in the right iliac fossa or symptoms due to anaemia such as general malaise and weakness. He may notice a lump in the right iliac fossa and/or blood in the motions. Occasionally he presents with colicky abdominal pain when the lesion begins to obstruct the terminal ileum. On examination there may be a mass in the right iliac fossa and localized tenderness over the growth. Also look for hepatomegaly.

Proving the diagnosis

The stools may be positive for occult blood and the iron deficiency anaemia can be detected on a blood film. The ESR is often raised. The diagnosis is confirmed by performing a barium enema. The radiologist must be asked to give particular attention to the caecum. False-negative barium enemas are not uncommon and, if the condition is suspected and the barium enema negative, the investigation should be repeated after a few weeks. A colonoscopy may also help.

Management

In the general work-up of the patient, care is taken to look for metastases. Preoperative investigations include liver function tests, a liver scan and a chest X-ray. A barium enema is essential in order to exclude a second colonic lesion. Before operation is undertaken, the anaemia may have to be corrected by blood transfusion. Once the patient is prepared, surgical resection is performed to remove the tumour.

Preparation for surgery

The bowel must be adequately prepared so that hard faeces, which will cause obstruction below the anastomosis, are not present postoperatively (see p. 113). Prophylactic antibiotics are given for colonic surgery. Intravenous antibiotics are given on induction of anaesthesia and for 24 h. The antibiotic combination used is most frequently metronidazole and cefuroxime giving a broad spectrum of activity against mixed bowel organisms.

OPERATION: RIGHT HEMICOLECTOMY

The abdomen is opened and the terminal ileum, ascending colon and hepatic flexure of the colon are mobilized. The mesentery is divided and the growth and surrounding bowel removed. An anastomosis is made between the ileum and the transverse colon. It is not always possible to put an adequate drain to this anastomosis as it remains mobile within the peritoneal cavity.

Codes

Blood .... 2 units
GA/LA .... GA
Opn time .... 1–2 h
Stay .... 7–10 days
Drains out .... 5–7 days
Sutures out .... 7 days
Off work .... 6 weeks

Postoperative care

The patient will require analgesics but the dose of opiates should not be excessive as these cause colonic spasm and have been implicated in an increased anastomotic disruption rate. The patient usually has an ileus for 3–4 days and oral fluids can be increased once flatus has been passed. The patient commonly gets diarrhoea in the first few days after the bowel recovers and he should be reassured that this will gradually settle down. Antidiarrhoeal agents such as loperamide (Imodium) or diphenoxylate hydrochloride (Lomotil) may be helpful.

Left-sided colonic carcinoma

With left-sided lesions the main feature is the early onset of obstruction.

Recognizing the pattern

The patient is usually over the age of 40 years and the disease is common in the over-70s. Men are slightly more commonly affected. The patient presents with a change in bowel habit. There is constipation due to the hold-up of faeces at the site of the growth. The faeces then liquefy and after a few days the patient has spurious offensive diarrhoea. The cycle is then repeated. There is often associated left-sided colicky abdominal pain. In addition to the change in bowel habit the patient can present with rectal bleeding. This is always a serious symptom in the over-50s (see p. 380). As with right-sided lesions the patient may develop an iron deficiency anaemia. On examination the abdomen may be distended and the caecum may be palpable. There may be a mass in the left iliac fossa or localized tenderness over the growth. On rectal examination a mass may be noted anteriorly. Palpate for an enlarged liver due to metastases.

Proving the diagnosis

The diagnosis may sometimes be proved on sigmoidoscopy. A low growth may be visible and can be biopsied. Even when the growth is not visible, blood and mucus may be seen high up in the bowel together with semi-liquid faeces, indicating a lesion higher up. The proximal colon and caecum may be distended on straight abdominal X-rays. Where a carcinoma is suspected, a barium enema is mandatory. The radiologist should also be careful to exclude other lesions such as polyps or secondary carcinomas in the rest of the bowel. Colonoscopy may be helpful where the barium enema findings are equivocal, and is also a method of obtaining a biopsy from a lesion higher up in the bowel.

Preoperative management

A full bowel preparation is necessary (see p. 113). Antibiotic cover may also be given as for a right hemi-colectomy. The patient should be warned of the possibility of a colostomy. Colostomies are necessary either because the growth is unresectable (in which case the colostomy will be permanent), or in order to protect an anastomosis which was made under difficult conditions. In this case the colostomy will be of the loop type, usually in the transverse colon. Such a colostomy will be closed later (see below).

If a permanent colostomy is a possibility, then the site for this should be clearly marked on the patient when he is standing up. This should generally be done by a stoma therapist or by the surgeon.

OPERATION: LEFT HEMICOLECTOMY

The left side of the colon is mobilized and the growth resected. An end-to-end anastomosis is usually performed. If the operation is carried out as an emergency, however, the bowel ends may be brought out as a left iliac colostomy and this may be closed later.

Codes

Blood	2 units
GA/LA	GA
Opn time	1–2 h
Stay	7–10 days
Drains out	5–7 days
Sutures out	7 days
Off work	6 weeks

OPERATION: PAUL–MICKULICZ PROCEDURE

In this procedure the descending and sigmoid colon are mobilized and the growth brought out through a muscle-cutting incision in the left iliac fossa. It is then resected outside the abdomen. This operation is seldom performed now.

OPERATION: ANTERIOR RESECTION

This is a term applied to the operation required to resect growths in the upper rectum or rectosigmoid junction. This is described in the section dealing with carcinoma of the rectum (p. 394).

OPERATION: HARTMANN'S PROCEDURE

See Carcinoma of the rectum, p. 396.

Postoperative care

The patient has an ileus, but a nasogastric tube is not of much value and oral fluids should be kept to a minimum until flatus is passed.

The main postoperative danger is of anastomotic leakage and the best early warning of this is the temperature chart. The development of a swinging fever, a tachycardia and faecal discharge from the drain may make the diagnosis obvious. A colonic leak in the absence of a protective colos-

Continued on p. 388

Continued.

tomy can be a serious condition and it may be necessary to take the patient back to theatre to bring out the bowel ends as a colostomy.

If a temporary colostomy or loop ileostomy has been performed at the original operation, then arrangements will have to be made to close it at a suitable time.

Some surgeons perform an early limited barium enema at 10–14 days after the original resection. If this shows continuity of the anastomosis without leakage, the colostomy can be closed. Other surgeons prefer to wait longer than this and in that case a limited barium enema is usually undertaken 2–3 months after the original resection and the colostomy closed if all is well. Long-term follow-up of patients with cancer usually needs to be arranged.

OPERATION: TRANSVERSE LOOP COLOSTOMY

This operation is sometimes done on its own for acute colonic obstruction but it may also be part of a resection procedure as above. The transverse colon is mobilized through a laparotomy incision and the omentum separated from it. A transverse muscle-cutting incision is made in the right hypochondrium and a loop of colon brought out through it and maintained in position by passing it over a rubber tube or a glass rod. The abdominal wound is then closed and the colostomy opened by incising along the taenia. The edges of the colon are then sewn to the skin. Occasionally a loop colostomy is also formed from the sigmoid colon.

OPERATION: CLOSURE OF COLOSTOMY

The edges of the colostomy are freed from the skin and the piece of colon is either resected or the anterior wall is closed, restoring continuity. The operation is sometimes performed with the aid of a laparoscope.

Codes

Blood	0
GA/LA	GA
Opn time	1 h
Stay	7–10 days
Drains out	7 days
Sutures out	7 days
Off work	3–4 weeks

Postoperative care

The ileus is short-lived and free fluids can be given after 24–48 h. The wound commonly becomes infected and should be allowed to drain freely.

Other types of colostomy are shown in Fig. 74. A 'double-barrelled' colostomy is formed where part of the colon has been resected and the two ends are brought out next to each other. An 'end' colostomy is formed when the lower bowel is closed off or removed, as in an abdominoperineal resection (p. 395) or a Hartmann's procedure (p. 396).

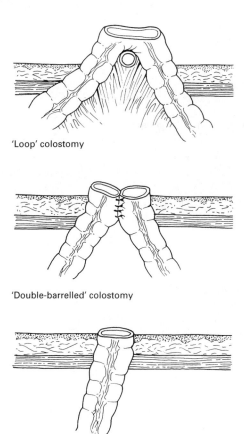

'Loop' colostomy

'Double-barrelled' colostomy

'End' colostomy

Fig. 74 Types of colostomy.

OPERATION: CLOSURE OF HARTMANN'S COLOSTOMY

The previous wound is reopened. There are usually a lot of adhesions to divide before the two ends of the bowel are ready for anastomosis. The latter may be performed with sutures or a stapling gun. This procedure can be performed laparoscopically.

Codes

Blood	2 units
GA/LA	GA
Opn time	3 h
Stay	3–7 days
Drains out	3 days
Sutures out	Subcutaneous
Off work	2–3 weeks

Carcinoma of the transverse colon

Recognizing the pattern

The patient presents with a picture intermediate between that of the right-sided lesion and the left-sided lesion, as might be expected. It is also not uncommon for the patient to notice a mass in his abdomen. On examination the mass may be palpable and is freely mobile in the early stages. If there is obstruction, the distended caecum may also be felt.

Management

This is identical to that described for other colonic lesions.

A colostomy will not usually be necessary, although, if the operation is particularly difficult, the surgeon may elect to bring out the bowel ends as a temporary colostomy rather than perform a primary anastomosis. The patient should be warned of this slight possibility.

OPERATION: TRANSVERSE COLECTOMY

The transverse colon is excised and an end-to-end anastomosis performed between the right colon and the left colon after full mobilization.

Codes

As for right hemi-colectomy.

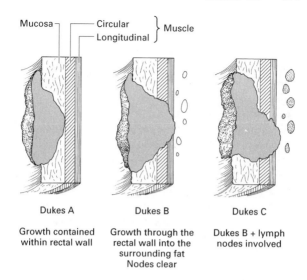

Mucosa — Circular ⎱ Muscle
— Longitudinal ⎰

Dukes A

Growth contained
within rectal wall

Dukes B

Growth through the
rectal wall into the
surrounding fat
Nodes clear

Dukes C

Dukes B + lymph
nodes involved

Fig. 75 Dukes' classification of carcinoma of the rectum.

Postoperative care
As for other colectomies.

Carcinoma of the rectum

An adenocarcinoma of the rectum usually forms a typical malignant ulcer with a necrotic base and raised everted edges. Growths are staged histologically according to Dukes' classification, which is based on histology and does not include distant metastases. The different stages are shown in Fig. 75. The TNM classification is being increasingly used for colorectal tumours.

T1: tumour confined to the submucosa

T2: tumour in the muscle coat but not through the bowel wall

T3: tumour through the bowel wall into perirectal or colonic fat

T4: tumour into an adjacent organ

N1: less than five local nodes involved

N2: more than five local nodes involved

N3: involved nodes at the high tie. (This is a ligature to mark the proximal end of the excised specimen and therefore the lymphatic drainage route from the tumour.)

M0: no metastases

M1: metastases.

The tumours are also classified as well differentiated (good prognosis) and average or poorly differentiated (poor prognosis).

The management of carcinoma of the rectum differs from that of other colonic carcinomas because much of the rectum is situated deep in the pelvis. Resection is not always possible through a laparotomy incision, and excision of the anus may be required.

Recognizing the pattern

The type of patient affected is similar to that for other colonic carcinomas. The presentation is usually in the form of bright rectal bleeding or of a change in bowel habit. The patient may experience a feeling of incomplete defaecation, which can be painful (tenesmus). On examination the diagnosis can often be made by rectal examination when the characteristic irregular everted edge is felt protruding into the bowel lumen.

Proving the diagnosis

On sigmoidoscopy the lesion may be visible and should be biopsied. A barium enema is performed to look for other lesions in the colon and may also be helpful in defining the extent of the local growth. A CT scan or rectal ultrasound can be used to stage the tumour and decide on possible preoperative radiotherapy.

Other investigations include the following:

1 Haemoglobin, white cell count and ESR
2 Liver function tests
3 Chest X-ray
4 Liver scan
5 Urea and electrolytes
6 Intravenous urogram. This should be performed if there is thought to be a possibility of ureteric involvement.

Management

The management is to excise the tumour and frequently this involves creating either a permanent or a temporary colostomy. In an anterior resection the growth is excised from above and continuity is restored. In an abdominoperineal resection the anus is also removed and a permanent colostomy made.

Preoperative management

Full bowel preparation is needed. If a permanent colostomy is a possibility, its site must be marked on the skin whilst the patient is standing. The possibility of a colostomy must be discussed with the patient and reassurance given about the implications of this procedure. It may be beneficial to introduce the patient to others who have had a colostomy performed. Prophylactic antibiotics are given and the patient is usually catheterized before the operation starts.

OPERATION: LOCAL EXCISION

When the patient is too old or frail to withstand a major operation, or where there is an accessible very early tumour of the rectum in younger patients, a local excision may be performed. There are a number of available techniques including perianal excision and transanal resection using a resectoscope. Malignant lesions recur quite quickly but palliation may be achieved for a while.

Codes

Blood	2 units
GA/LA	GA
Opn time	30 min to 1 h
Stay	3–5 days
Drains out	0
Sutures out	0
Off work	2–4 weeks

OPERATION: TEM PROCEDURE

Local excision may be acheived by transanal endoscopic microsurgery (TEM). This requires specialized expertise and expensive equipment. A large diameter operating proctoscope is placed in the rectum. A telescope attached to a video camera gives a good view of the rectal lumen and specialized instruments for manipulation, cutting and diathermy are inserted through ports in the proctoscope. Mucosal or full-thickness resections can be performed and the defect repaired by intraluminal suturing.

Codes

Blood	2 units
GA/LA	GA
Opn time	30 min to 3 h
Stay	3–5 days
Drains out	0
Sutures out	0
Off work	2–4 weeks

OPERATION: ANTERIOR RESECTION OF THE RECTUM

This is a widely used operation for cancer of the rectum. It implies restoration of continuity with an anastomosis and this can be achieved with tumours as low as 4 cm from the anal verge. Mobilization of the rectum within the pelvis is more difficult and time-consuming than operations within the abdomen. There is a risk of pelvic nerve damage and sexual dysfunction. The growth is resected with a satisfactory distal margin and an anastomosis performed between the rectal stump and the divided end of the mobilized left colon. The anastomosis is now easier with the introduction of mechanical stapling instruments. If these are used the stapling gun is inserted through the anus and the upper and lower ends of the rectum are snugged down on to it using purse-string sutures. When the gun is fired the anastomosis is completed with rings of metal staples. In a very low anastomosis a colon pouch is created by turning back the distal left colon into a J configuration, and creating a common lumen. This replaces the rectum's lost reservoir function. A protective loop ileostomy is frequently performed as part of the operation since anastomotic leakage is the most serious complication (see Codes for Hartmann's Procedure, p. 396).

OPERATION: LAPAROSCOPIC ANTERIOR RESECTION OF RECTUM

The operative principles are exactly the same as for the open procedure but the view is obtained laparoscopically. Four to five ports are used to introduce instruments. The bowel is divided using laparoscopic stapling guns and anastomosed with staples as in the open procedure, but using a detachable anvil in the proximal bowel which is 'leashed' to the staple gun in the rectal stump before firing. The specimen is subsequently removed in a watertight bag through a short incision in the iliac fossa. The operation may be converted to open at any stage if progress is not being made laparoscopically.

Codes

Blood	2 units
GA/LA	GA
Opn time	3–4 h
Stay	5–10 days
Drains out	3 days
Sutures out	Subcuticular
Off work	4–8 weeks

Postoperative care

Postoperatively the care of a patient with an anterior resection of the rectum is much the same as that for a left hemi-colectomy. A protective loop ileostomy is usually closed 2–3 months after the first operation. A limited barium enema may be performed at 10–14 days and the colostomy closed if the anastomosis has healed. Alternatively, this may be done 2–3 months after the operation.

OPERATION: ABDOMINOPERINEAL RESECTION OF THE RECTUM

This operation is used for tumours that are 5 cm or less from the anal verge. With such a low tumour, adequate clearance is not possible without removing the anus. A permanent colostomy is therefore unavoidable. The necessity for this must be explained to the patient preoperatively. The site of the colostomy is marked as mentioned above.

The rectum is mobilized from above as in the anterior resection operation. In addition to this, the lower rectum and anus are also excised through a perineal incision. At the start of this the anus is closed with a purse-string suture.

The rectum is then removed and the subcutaneous fat and skin are closed, leaving a drain to the space left in the pelvis. In women this drain may usefully be brought out through the vagina as this makes the postoperative recovery easier and more comfortable.

The abdominoperineal operation may be performed by one surgeon doing both the abdominal and the perineal resections, or by two surgeons. In the latter case it is known as a synchronous combined abdominoperineal excision of the rectum (SCAPER). The theatre staff will need to know whether one or two surgeons will be operating.

Codes

Blood	2 units
GA/LA	GA
Opn time	3 h
Stay	14 days
Drains out	3 days
Sutures out	Subcuticular or 7–10 days
Off work	2 months

Postoperative care

The postoperative care of an abdominoperineal resection is slightly more complicated than for an anterior resection.

Continued on p. 396

Continued.

There is a danger of haemorrhage in the first 24 h and a careful watch must be kept on the pelvic drain. Oral fluids can be increased when the colostomy starts to work. As far as the perineal wound is concerned, the best outcome is achieved when this heals by first intention. However, sepsis and breakdown of the perineal wound are not uncommon and in that case the sutures should be removed and free drainage established. The wound will then have to be regularly dressed until it heals from within. Long-term follow-up is required.

OPERATION: LAPAROSCOPIC ABDOMINOPERINEAL RESECTION OF THE RECTUM

The abdominal part of the operation can be performed laparoscopically and an excellent view obtained right down to the pelvic floor muscles. The perineal part of the procedure is completed as above and the specimen delivered through the perineal wound. This approach can be valuable in elderly or poor risk patients who benefit from less pain and therefore less of the depressant effects of postoperative analgesia.

Codes

Blood	2 units
GA/LA	GA
Opn time	3–4 h
Stay	7–14 days
Drains out	3 days
Sutures out	Subcuticular
Off work	4–8 weeks

OPERATION: HARTMANN'S PROCEDURE

This operation is used when a carcinoma of the rectum is found to be unresectable due to local invasion or when the patient is unfit for a more major resection. The term is also used in emergency surgery when an obstructing or perforated colonic mass is excised. The lower end of the rectum is closed and left *in situ*. The upper end of the bowel is brought out as a descending colostomy. In some cases continuity may be restored later.

Codes

Blood	2 units
GA/LA	GA

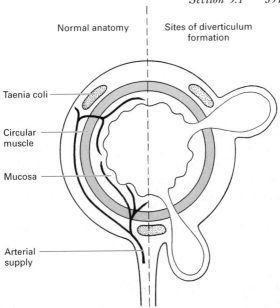

Normal anatomy | Sites of diverticulum formation

Taenia coli

Circular muscle

Mucosa

Arterial supply

Fig. 76 Diverticula are usually blown out at the entry points of vessels.

Opn time .... 2–3 h
Stay .... 10 days
Drains out .... 3 days
Sutures out .... Subcuticular or 7–10 days
Off work .... 6–8 weeks

Diverticular disease

Diverticular disease is a condition affecting the colon, which is more common in those who eat a Western diet low in roughage. The condition is associated with muscle hypertrophy and raised intraluminal pressure. Mucosa-lined pouches are pushed out through the colonic wall, usually at the entry points of vessels (Fig. 76). These pouches are the diverticula. The condition is thought to arise because of a lack of roughage in the bowel content. Roughage is present in raw foodstuffs such as whole wheat and raw cane sugar but is removed when these are purified to make white flour and white sugar. Roughage is not normally absorbed from the bowel lumen and acts like blotting paper. The moisture it retains makes the stool more bulky and soft, and more easily propelled along the colonic lumen. Without roughage and sufficient water the stool becomes dehydrated and harder and colonic pressures are raised.

Several conditions are thought to be associated with the lack of roughage, including diverticular disease, piles, anal fissure and fistula *in ano*.

Diverticular disease itself may present with acute inflammation in one or many pouches or as chronic disease with stricture formation due to recurrent inflammation.

Recognizing the pattern

The patient is usually over 40 years of age and frequently obese. The condition is more common in females, although it does occur in males quite regularly. In acute diverticulitis the patient experiences a rapid onset of pain, usually in the left iliac fossa. There may be associated diarrhoea and generalized abdominal colic. The pain in the left iliac fossa rapidly becomes worse and is exacerbated by coughing or moving. The patient develops a fever and feels generally unwell. On examination the patient is febrile with a tachycardia. He looks ill and is in obvious pain. The tongue may be furred and there is marked tenderness in the left iliac fossa with guarding and rebound tenderness. There may also be tenderness on rectal examination. In chronic diverticulosis the patient has often suffered from recurrent attacks of the type described above but then goes on to develop a more permanent change in bowel habit with alternating constipation and diarrhoea. There may be very little to find on general examination. He may also present with episodes of rectal bleeding.

Proving the diagnosis

A straight erect and supine abdominal X-ray may show some gas in the wall of the bowel in the left iliac fossa or fluid levels in loops of small bowel adherent to the area of inflammation. There may be distension of the colon proximal to the area of disease. In the acute situation a CT scan will demonstrate both the diverticula and any paracolic abscess. A water-soluble contrast examination will also demonstrate any possible perforations and the diverticular disease without aggravating the condition.

Once the acute episode has settled a barium enema is performed. Changes of diverticulosis are very common, however, and the presence of diverticula does not prove that these are causing the patient's symptoms. Other causes must be excluded.

When the disease becomes chronic, a narrowed area may develop in the descending or sigmoid colon and it can be difficult to decide whether this is benign or malignant. A repeat barium enema after a few weeks or a colonoscopy may decide the issue. Occasionally it is necessary to resort to laparotomy and resection in order to be sure that one is not dealing with a neoplasm.

Management

In the acute attack the patient is admitted and given a broad-spectrum combination of antibiotics such as metronidazole, gentamicin and penicillin or ampicillin. Analgesia may be needed. The condition usually settles rapidly unless there is abscess formation. If an abscess does form, it is best treated conservatively and will usually drain into the bowel. CT-guided drainage, however, may be helpful in difficult cases although there is a slight risk of development of a faecal fistula.

Chronic diverticular disease is treated by giving the patient adequate roughage in the diet, including wholemeal bread and bran. Bulk laxatives such as Isogel, Normacol or Fybogel may also be used. An adequate fluid intake must also be encouraged (see p. 414).

Surgery is indicated in diverticular disease where there are frequent recurrent inflammatory episodes; where complications such as perforation, stricture or fistula develop; or where there is doubt about the diagnosis.

Preoperative management

The patient should be advised to lose weight before surgery is undertaken. Patients with diverticular disease frequently have other problems, such as hiatus hernia, gall stones or late-onset diabetes. These should be considered in the general work-up. Preparation for the colectomy is described under Carcinoma of the descending colon (p. 384).

OPERATION: LAPAROTOMY FOR ACUTE DIVERTICULITIS

Operation should be avoided in the acute stage if possible. Where it is necessary, because of perforation or generalized peritonitis, the abdomen is opened and the acute diverticular disease confirmed. In experienced hands the most suitable operation is a Hartmann's procedure (p. 396) or occasionally an on-table lavage and primary anastomosis. If the abdomen is opened and acute diverticular disease is found, then it is best left alone unless perforation has occurred.

Postoperative care

This is as for left hemi-colectomy if the bowel has been resected. If a perforation has been closed and drained,

Continued on p. 400

Continued.

antibiotics should be continued postoperatively and the drain removed after 5–7 days when an adequate track has formed. A decision will have to be made later about closing the colostomy and before this is done the affected piece of bowel must be resected. This may be undertaken in either one or two stages.

Sigmoid volvulus

A sigmoid volvulus occurs in patients who have redundant sigmoid colon on a long mesentery with a narrow base. The sigmoid loop tends to twist, causing intestinal obstruction with massive dilatation of the bowel. The loop may become ischaemic. Constipation and excessive use of laxatives are common precipitating factors. This disease is more common in patients on tranquillizers and particularly occurs in mental hospitals.

Recognizing the pattern

The patient is usually elderly and may have suffered from constipation and taken laxatives for many years. The history is one of an acute onset of marked abdominal distension and colicky pain. There is complete constipation and no flatus is passed per rectum. There may be a history of repeated attacks as the colonic loop twists and spontaneously untwists. On examination the abdomen is grossly distended and tympanitic. There is tenderness, particularly in the left iliac fossa. Rectal examination shows an empty bowel, which may be ballooned. There is tenderness high up.

Proving the diagnosis

The diagnosis is proved by straight erect and supine abdominal X-rays, which show the grossly distended sigmoid colon stretching across to the right upper quadrant. The erect film shows large fluid levels within this loop.

Management

The management in the acute stage is to perform a sigmoidoscopy and pass a large-bore flatus tube up into the volvulus. This procedure releases the flatus and faeces in the obstructed loop and gives the patient instant relief. The tube should be well lubricated before it is passed up and a bucket should be available. A more sophisticated version of this technique is to use colonoscopy to decompress the twisted loop.

The patient is then put on a high-roughage diet and if possible tranquillizers are withdrawn. The condition frequently recurs but the loop can be deflated many times if the patient is frail and not suitable for a definitive operation.

Occasionally the loop cannot be deflated and emergency laparotomy and resection may be required.

If the patient is fit and the condition becomes recurrent, then resection is also indicated. This may be done as a one-stage procedure with an end-to-end anastomosis or two ends of the bowel may be brought out as a left iliac colostomy (see p. 387). The codes for this operation and the postoperative care are the same as for a left hemi-colectomy.

Rectal prolapse

Rectal prolapse occurs in two age groups.
1 In very young children (under the age of 2 years, see p. 621).
2 In elderly females (over the age of 60 years).

There are two anatomical types of prolapse, mucosal and complete. In mucosal prolapse the bowel musculature remains in position but redundant mucosa prolapses out of the anal canal. This is the type that occurs in children and also in adults with third-degree piles (see p. 413).

In complete rectal prolapse there is effectively an intussusception of the upper rectum into the lower anal canal. It is associated with weakness of the pelvic musculature, often following multiple childbirth. In this case the whole bowel wall is inverted and passed out through the anus. There may be associated prolapse of the uterus. The difference between these two types of prolapse is illustrated in Fig. 77.

Complete rectal prolapse in adults

Recognizing the pattern

This usually occurs in elderly multiparous women. The rectal prolapse is of variable length and causes a profuse mucous discharge which soils the patient's underclothes. There may be associated bleeding. In advanced cases the prolapse may come down very readily and it may become impossible for the patient to get out of the house.

Proving the diagnosis

Asking the patient to strain and seeing the complete prolapse appear can prove the diagnosis. It will be noted that the head of the prolapse is separate from the anal margins.

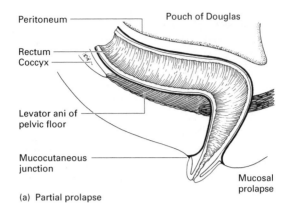

Peritoneum

Pouch of Douglas

Rectum
Coccyx

Levator ani of
pelvic floor

Mucocutaneous
junction

Mucosal
prolapse

(a) Partial prolapse

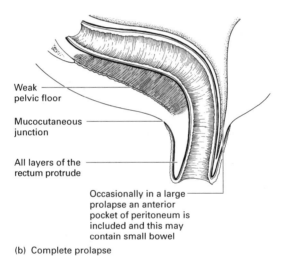

Weak
pelvic floor

Mucocutaneous
junction

All layers of the
rectum protrude

Occasionally in a large
prolapse an anterior
pocket of peritoneum is
included and this may
contain small bowel

(b) Complete prolapse

Fig. 77 Two types of rectal prolapse. (a) Partial prolapse and (b)
complete prolapse.

Management

In the early stages conservative management may be helpful
but is not usually of much value once the prolapse has
become well established. It consists of using stool softeners
and perineal exercises. Operative measures include the following:

1 Delorme's operation.

2 A rectopexy fixing the mobilized rectum to the sacral
promontory with or without the use of a mesh.

3 Resection rectopexy excising the redundant sigmoid colon at the same time.

Preoperative management

A bowel preparation is given. Antibiotics are not required.

OPERATION: DELORME'S PROCEDURE

With the prolapse everted through the anus, a solution of 1/400 000 adrenaline is injected subcutaneously. The mucosa over the prolapse is then excised to within a centimetre of the dentate line. The upper mucosal margin is then sutured to the distal mucosa, bunching up the underlying rectal muscle within the pelvis.

Codes

Blood	Group and save serum
GA/LA	GA
Opn time	45–60 min
Stay	3–4 days
Drains out	0
Sutures out	Absorbable only
Off work	Not applicable

Postoperative care

Faecal softeners are given from the time of operation. The procedure is relatively non-invasive and recovery is usually rapid and uncomplicated. Recurrence is rare but if it occurs the procedure can be repeated. Patients who were incontinent before the operation may continue to be so afterwards and should be warned of this.

OPERATION: RECTOPEXY OR RESECTION RECTOPEXY

Preoperative management

A full bowel preparation is necessary. Antibiotics should be given with the premedication.

OPERATION: OPEN RECTOPEXY

The rectum is mobilized as for anterior resection. An implant or mesh (Ivalon, Teflon or Marlex) may be sewn into the presacral space and attached to the rectum laterally. The implanted mesh gives rise to considerable fibrosis glueing the rectum to the sacrum. In some patients the implant can cause a functional constipation and for this reason resection rectopexy may be more effective. Here the rectopexy is performed and the sigmoid resected with a primary anastomosis.

Codes

Blood .... 2 units
GA/LA .... GA
Opn time .... 60–90 min
Stay .... 5–7 days
Drains out 0
Sutures out.. 7 days
Off work .... Not applicable

OPERATION: LAPAROSCOPIC MESH RECTOPEXY
This operation lends itself well to the laparoscopic approach. The mesh is usually stapled to the sacrum and sutured to the rectum anteriorly. The redundant rectum is 'hitched up' to the presacral fascia using two sutures. Very little analgesia is required postoperatively, a factor which may be critical in the survival of these frail patients.

Codes

Blood .... 2 units
GA/LA .... GA
Opn time .... 1–2 h
Stay .... 2–3 days
Drains out 0
Sutures out.. Subcuticular
Off work .... Not applicable

Postoperative care
It is not uncommon for one episode of prolapse to occur in the early postoperative stages before the fibrosis has become established. It should be replaced and the patient reassured. Faecal softeners should be given as soon as the patient has recovered from ileus. A close watch should be kept for signs of developing sepsis and prolonged antibiotic treatment should be given if there is any suspicion of this.

9.2 Perianal Pain

This section deals with a number of related perianal conditions which present with pain or discomfort in the perineum. In order to understand their aetiology, it is necessary to be familiar with the anatomy of the perianal structures and these are depicted in Figs. 78 and 79. The conditions include perianal abscesses, fistulae and fissures, haemorrhoids and perianal haematomas.

Perianal abscess

The most common cause of perianal abscess formation is infection arising in a perianal gland. These glands lie between the internal and external sphincters and open into the anal canal via the anal crypts at the pectinate line. The pectinate line is made up of flaps of mucosa (anal valves) above which are small recesses (anal sinuses). If the opening of the gland becomes blocked or damaged, stasis can result and lead to infection. The resulting abscess lies between the anal sphincters and tends to point towards the skin at the anal margin (Fig. 80). It may spread laterally into the ischiorectal fossa, or more rarely, superiorly above the levator ani into the pararectal fossa.

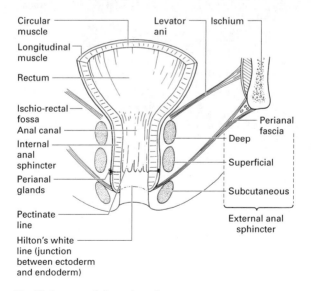

Fig. 78 Anatomy of the anal canal.

Sagittal section

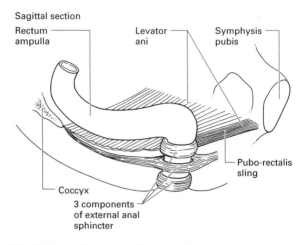

Fig. 79 Anal sphincters seen from the side.

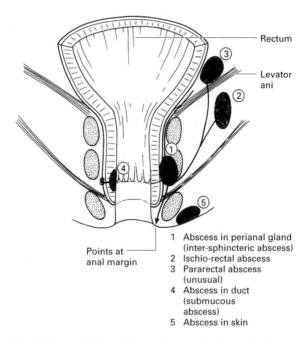

1 Abscess in perianal gland (inter-sphincteric abscess)
2 Ischio-rectal abscess
3 Pararectal abscess (unusual)
4 Abscess in duct (submucous abscess)
5 Abscess in skin

Fig. 80 Anatomical sites of abscess formation in the perianal region.

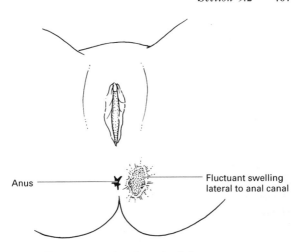

Anus

Fluctuant swelling
lateral to anal canal

Fig. 81 Clinical presentation of a perianal abscess.

Recognizing the pattern

Patients of any age including children may be affected. The characteristic sitting posture with one buttock raised may make the diagnosis obvious. This is due to gradual onset of pain around the anus, which becomes throbbing and severe. Defaecation and sitting are painful. On examination the abscess may be seen deep in the skin next to the anus (Fig. 81). There is much surrounding oedema. On proctoscopy the damaged opening to the affected gland may be seen and there may even be pus discharging from the opening.

Proving the diagnosis

The diagnosis is obvious on examination and no other tests are indicated.

Management

The abscess should be drained unless it is secondary to pelvic abscesses above the levator ani. Such abscesses should not, if possible, be drained into the perineum as this may give rise to a high rectal fistula. The management of pelvic abscesses is described on p. 73.

OPERATION: DRAINAGE OF PERIANAL ABSCESS
A cruciate incision is made over the abscess next to the anus. The contents are evacuated. Loculi within the abscess are gently broken down but care must be taken not to extend the abscess upward through the levator ani.

A proctoscopy and rectal examination are carried out and if an internal opening can be seen within the anal canal then the whole tract must be laid open as for a perianal fistula (see below).

Codes
Blood 0
GA/LA .... GA
Opn time .... 15 min
Stay .... 3–7 days, depending on size of abscess cavity
Drains out .... 48 h
Sutures out 0
Off work .... 1–4 weeks

Postoperative care
The abscess is dressed daily, leaving paraffin gauze in the cavity so that the wound heals without bridging over. A gauze wick should not be used, as pushing this in tends to deepen the cavity and also obstructs normal drainage. Antibiotics may be indicated if the organism is a group A *Streptococcus*.

Perianal fistula

A perianal fistula is an abnormal connection between the lumen of the anus (or rectum) and the skin. It usually develops from a perianal abscess that bursts onto the skin or is drained surgically. If the internal opening of the original infected perianal gland remains patent, a fistula results.

Various types of fistula are described according to the level at which they transgress the anal sphincters. The important distinction is between those that open into the bowel below the deep external anal sphincter ('low') and those that open above this ('high', Fig. 82). The latter are fortunately rare and are often due to other disease such as Crohn's, ulcerative colitis, carcinoma, trauma or a foreign body. A low fistula can be laid open and allowed to heal without endangering continence. A high fistula requires more complicated management.

Recognizing the pattern

The patient complains of persistent perianal discharge and recurrent abscesses. On examination the external opening is usually seen lateral to the anus and the internal opening may

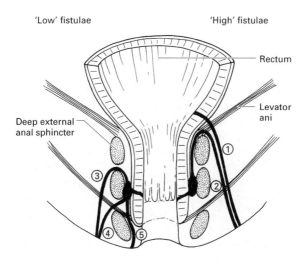

'Low' fistulae   'High' fistulae

Fig. 82 The types of perianal fistula. High: 1, extrasphincteric; 2, suprasphincteric. Low: 3, high transphincteric; 4, low transphincteric; 5, intersphincteric.

be palpable on rectal examination. Proctoscopy should be undertaken to try and visualize the opening. This is sometimes difficult to detect especially if it is not exuding pus at the time.

Goodsall's rule states that a fistula lying in the anterior half of the anal area opens directly into the anal canal, while a fistula lying in the posterior half tracks around the anus and opens in the mid-line posteriorly (Fig. 83).

During rectal examination assess the tone of the anal sphincter. It may be weaker in the elderly, meaning that less muscle can be cut at operation.

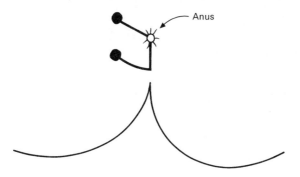

Fig. 83 Goodsall's rule.

Management

The treatment of a perianal fistula is to lay it open. Faecal continence is lost when major parts of the external anal sphincter, the puborectalis sling and the internal sphincter are divided. Therefore, low fistulae can be laid open, with only slight danger of minor incontinence due to damage to the internal anal sphincter. When in doubt fistulae should be managed with the use of seton. This is a silk, nylon or plastic thread placed around the tract to act as a chronic drain. Setons can be tightened and used as a cutting seton but this can also cause problems with continence. The internal opening of a high fistula may need to be closed operatively with an advancement flap repair. Occasionally a covering colostomy may be required. Any predisposing cause such as Crohn's disease must also be treated.

Preoperative management
The patient should be given a laxative on the night before the operation and the bowel emptied with enemas if necessary.

OPERATION: LAYING OPEN OF LOW PERIANAL
FISTULA
A probe is passed into the external opening and carefully passed along the fistulous tract until it goes through the internal opening into the anal canal. A knife is used to cut down on the probe and the tract thus laid open completely. Any lateral extensions of the tract must also be laid open.

Codes
Blood 0
GA/LA .... GA
Opn time .... 15 min
Stay .... 3–10 days, depending on size
                                                       of cavity laid open
Drains out 0
Sutures out 0
Off work .... 2–4 weeks

Postoperative care
The wound is dressed daily and the patient can have regular twice-daily saline baths. The wound often takes 6–8 weeks

to heal. In the final stages it is very little trouble to the patient and normal life can usually be resumed. The patient is put on a regime of bulk laxatives (e.g. Normacol or bran).

OPERATION: HIGH PERIANAL FISTULA

The whole tract cannot be laid open because of the danger of incontinence. The lower part is opened and drained but care is taken to cut the least amount of external and internal sphincter necessary. A seton is passed through the tract to allow fibrosis and healing and a possible subsequent anal advancement flap.

Codes

Blood 0
GA/LA .... GA
Opn time .... 1 h
Stay .... 3–10 days
Drains out 0
Sutures out 0
Off work .... 4–6 weeks

Anal fissure

In this condition the anal mucosa is torn so that the circular muscle layer is exposed. Intense muscle spasm results which is worse after each bowel movement. The tear usually starts at the pectinate line when an anal valve is torn downwards by the passage of a hard stool.

The fissure is usually on the posterior aspect of the anal canal as most of the pressure during defaecation occurs at this point.

Recognizing the pattern

The patient can be of any age. The condition is not uncommon in babies. There is a history of pain on defaecation, often occurring first during a period of constipation. The pain then recurs each time the bowels are opened and there is often fresh rectal bleeding ('bright red blood on the paper'). On examination a 'sentinel' pile may be visible if the anus is inspected with the buttocks gently parted. This 'sentinel' pile represents the bunched up, torn strip of mucosa at the base of the fissure. A rectal examination may be exquisitely tender or impossible because of severe pain and muscle spasm. This finding alone is enough to confirm the diagnosis.

Management

In the early stages the introduction of bran into the diet together with analgesic suppositories may give relief. Glyceryl trinitrate 0.2% ointment has recently been used successfully in the treatment of anal fissures since this causes a reduction in anal canal pressure and improves healing. An anal stretch was the treatment of choice at one time but concerns over continence mean that this has been largely replaced by lateral anal sphincterotomy. This too can cause incontinence unless carried out very carefully.

OPERATION: SPHINCTEROTOMY

Where the fissure has become chronic, a sphincterotomy may be performed. The lowermost fibres of the internal anal sphincter are divided in the 3 or 9 o'clock position up to the height of the topmost level of the fissure itself. The base of the fissure is not divided, especially if this is in the mid-line posteriorly, since it causes guttering and continence problems. The fissure itself is simply scraped and the edges freshened up.

Codes

Blood	0
GA/LA	GA
Opn time	15–30 min
Stay	48 h
Drains out	0
Sutures out	0
Off work	1–2 weeks

Postoperative care

The patient should be put on a high-fibre diet and perhaps some lactulose for a week or so.

Haemorrhoids

The condition haemorrhoids (or 'piles') is extremely common in Western civilization. The normal anal canal, just above the anal sphincter, is closed by soft 'cushions' of mucosa containing a submucosal plexus of veins. If excessive pressure is generated during defaecation, the mucosal cushions are stretched and can prolapse through the anal canal as 'piles'. The excessive pressure may be due to any of the following:

1 Hard dry stools (due to lack of roughage in the diet or inadequate water intake).

2 Failure to allow the sphincter to relax before the stool is pushed through the canal. Piles are usually worse at times of stress.

3 Excessive straining during defaecation.

4 Decreased relaxation of the anal canal due to the presence of pecten bands (fibrous bands in the upper anal canal).

Once formed, piles may gradually increase in size due to congestion and hypertrophy. Three degrees of piles are described and the recognition of these degrees is important as the method of treatment is related to them.

First degree

These piles remain within the anal canal. They present with discomfort or rectal bleeding.

Second degree

These prolapse out of the anal verge but are easily replaced. They present with perianal discharge or irritation, together with discomfort and rectal bleeding. The patient may also complain of the presence of the prolapsed piles themselves.

Third degree

These are permanently prolapsed. Third-degree piles may become strangulated. The piles prolapse and the circulation is obstructed by the anal sphincter, which goes into intense spasm as the inflammation develops. The haemorrhoids thrombose.

Recognizing the pattern

The characteristic patient is a tense young executive but piles can affect people of any age and either sex. In the older age groups the patient is frequently obese. The history is of perianal discomfort or discharge with or without rectal bleeding. The bleeding is fresh and is noted on the paper or in the pan after defaecation. The blood is on the outside of the stool. The patient may also experience a feeling of incomplete emptying of the rectum, which occurs after defaecation and is due to the bulk of the piles in the anal canal.

With first-degree piles there is nothing visible externally or on rectal examination. Proctoscopy shows the haemorrhoids bulging over the end of the proctoscope placed just within the anal canal. Piles are never palpable on rectal examination unless they are actually thrombosed.

Second-degree haemorrhoids may be seen to prolapse out of the anal verge on straining. They are also clearly visible on proctoscopy.

Third-degree piles are visible as soon as the anus is inspected and if they can be replaced within the anal canal they rapidly prolapse again.

Strangulated third-degree piles present as inflamed bunches of tissue surrounding the anal canal. They are exquisitely painful and tender.

Management

First-degree piles may be treated conservatively or by injections.

Second-degree piles can be treated either by injections, 'banding' or, in recurrent cases, haemorrhoidectomy.

Third-degree piles require haemorrhoidectomy.

Conservative treatment

This is important, whatever other measures are indicated. The patient must be educated to modify his diet and to avoid excessive straining. Stools become bulky, soft and easy to pass if they contain enough fibre (e.g. bran). Fibre is not absorbed during digestion and acts like blotting paper keeping water in the stool. It must therefore be combined with an adequate water intake. Excessive straining may be due to nervous tension or due to a feeling of incomplete emptying associated with the bulk of the piles.

PROCEDURE: INJECTION OF PILES

The injection of piles is an outpatient procedure. The object is to cause scarring between the stretched anal cushions within the anal canal and the underlying muscle. A proctoscope is inserted in the anal canal and the piles bulge over the rim of the instrument. Injections of 5% phenol in *Arachis* oil are put into the submucosal layer above the pectinate line. The injections should be painless. Injections should not be put in too superficially (when blanching of the mucosa will be seen) as this will cause sloughing of the mucosa.

The patient may experience some discomfort in the first 2–3 days after injection of piles but this settles rapidly. The beneficial effect is noted after 6–10 days. It may be necessary to repeat the treatment.

Some centres use cryotherapy or photocoagulation as alternative methods of mucosal fixation. Both are relatively pain-free but the equipment is expensive and the results are not significantly better than injection therapy.

PROCEDURE: BANDING OF PILES

The pile is grasped through a proctoscope and a tight rubber band positioned around its neck. Thrombosis and separation of the pile then follow.

OPERATION: HAEMORRHOIDECTOMY

Preoperative management

The bowels should be emptied using laxatives on the day before the operation.

Operation

The patient is placed in the lithotomy position and the prolapsing piles are grasped with clamps. They are excised together with the surrounding anal skin tags and the dissection is advanced to the neck of the pile in the submucosal layer. The piles are ligated within the anal canal. It is important to leave mucosal skin bridges between each group of piles excised, otherwise an anal stricture may result.

Codes

Blood	2 units
GA/LA	GA
Opn time	30 min
Stay	3–7 days
Drains out	0
Sutures out	0
Off work	3–4 weeks

Postoperative care

Reactionary haemorrhage may occur in the first few hours after the operation. Patients should always be nursed with the foot of the bed elevated. This elevation can be increased if haemorrhage does occur. Blood transfusion is then given if necessary. If the bleeding does not settle, the patient should be taken back to theatre and the individual bleeding point found, using a suitable proctoscope. It is then ligated.

The patient is given Normacol and Milpar postoperatively and encouraged to have his bowels open as soon as possible.

Continued on p. 416

Continued.

The first defaecation is often painful but if he becomes constipated it is worse. Daily baths postoperatively are helpful in keeping the anal area clean and increasing the patient's comfort.

There is often a slight secondary haemorrhage at 7–10 days after the operation and the patient should be warned about this. It is usually minimal.

The patient may be incontinent of flatus for 2–3 weeks after the operation until the mucosal cushions have healed. He should be warned of this and reassured it will settle down.

The patient should be put on bran after any perianal operation and should remain on it indefinitely thereafter.

Management of strangulated piles

The conservative management consists of the following:

1 Bed rest
2 Elevation of the foot of the bed
3 Analgesia
4 Topical icepacks.

If this produces relief, a haemorrhoidectomy is performed later. If not, an early anal stretch or haemorrhoidectomy is carried out.

Perianal haematoma (thrombosed external pile)

This is due to a ruptured superficial perianal vein, which gives rise to a subcutaneous haematoma.

Recognizing the pattern

The patient may be of any age. There is frequently a history of straining at stool. The condition presents with a sudden onset of severe perianal pain. Left untreated the pain gradually settles over a week or so and the haematoma resolves. On examination there is a cherry-like, rounded, blue haematoma in the subcutaneous tissue next to the anal verge. It is exquisitely tender.

Management

In the first 2–3 days the treatment is to evacuate the haematoma after infiltrating with local anaesthetic. This gives immediate relief. If the haematoma has been present for longer than a week, it is probably best left to resolve naturally.

10 Hernias

10.1 Hernias and Other Groin Lumps

Anatomy of the groin

A wide variety of interesting conditions can present as a lump in the groin and for this reason such lumps are popular as examination cases. Students are often confused about the anatomy of this area and hence uncertain of the interpretation of physical signs and the surgical approach to a hernia. The femoral sheath is usefully conceived as a gap between the anterior abdominal wall and the posterior abdominal wall as these two structures meet in the groin. Through this gap pass the main vessels to the leg and medial to them is the femoral canal. This part of the anterior abdominal wall consists of the external oblique, internal oblique and transversus abdominus muscles. These are all attached to the inguinal ligament. The ligament is attached to the pubic tubercle medially and the anterosuperior iliac spine laterally. Behind the inguinal ligament are the muscles of the posterior abdominal wall running into the anterior thigh (psoas and iliacus) and also the pectineus. The femoral vessels lie on top of these muscles and behind the inguinal ligament (Fig. 84).

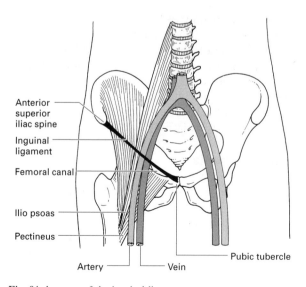

Fig. 84 Anatomy of the inguinal ligament.

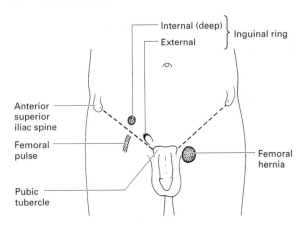

Fig. 85 Landmarks in the groin.

Inguinal hernias occur through the inguinal canal in the lower part of the anterior abdominal wall and are therefore above the inguinal ligament. Femoral hernias occur down the femoral canal and are therefore posterior to the inguinal ligament and appear in the thigh below and lateral to the pubic tubercle. Obturator hernias occur from within the true pelvis and they can be palpated within the adductor compartment of the thigh.

General assessment

In approaching a groin lump it is first necessary to define the anatomical landmarks and thus to decide which anatomical structure is involved. It is particularly important to define the line of the inguinal ligament by palpating the bony points from which it arises (Fig. 85).

A list of possible groin lumps and their relationship to the inguinal canal is given in Table 22.

Inguinal hernia

Inguinal hernias are protuberances of the peritoneal contents through the abdominal wall where it is weakened by the presence of the inguinal canal.

Indirect hernias follow the path of the spermatic cord or round ligament down the inguinal canal. Their origin is therefore lateral to the inferior epigastric artery, which defines the medial edge of the internal ring.

Direct inguinal hernias arise from a different cause, the weakness being in the posterior wall of the inguinal canal rather

Table 22 Lumps in the groin.

Anatomical structure	Pathology	Above or below the inguinal ligament
In the skin	Lipoma, fibroma, haemangioma, etc.	Either
Deep to the skin		
Femoral vein	Saphena varix (see Varicose veins, p. 552)	Below
Femoral artery	Aneurysm (see p. 539, Vascular disorders)	Below
Lymph nodes, inguinal or femoral	Primary or secondary neoplasia or infection	Either
Hernias	Inguinal, direct or indirect	Above
	Femoral	Below

than down the canal itself. They therefore arise medial to the inferior epigastric vessels.

Strangulated hernias are described on p. 428.

Recognizing the pattern

Indirect hernias can occur at any age and are common in children. They are more common in males than females as the inguinal canal is wider in the male. Direct hernias are rare in children and more common in the elderly.

The patient presents with a swelling in the groin that may cause some discomfort or restrict activity. In both types of hernia there may be a family history of the condition and there may also be an immediate precipitating cause such as an episode of heavy lifting or severe coughing due to chronic bronchitis.

On examination there is a bulge in the groin above the line of the inguinal ligament. In the early stages the hernia is lateral to the pubic tubercle and as it enlarges it may protrude over the pubic tubercle and down into the scrotum or vulva. The lump has a cough impulse over it unless it is incarcerated. After reduction an indirect hernia is controlled during coughing by pressure over the deep inguinal ring (see Fig. 85). On relieving the pressure the hernia runs obliquely down the canal. A direct hernia is not so controlled and bulges straight forward.

Management

Conservative

If the hernia is indirect a truss can be considered. This works by compressing the inguinal canal from front to back and thus preventing an indirect hernia protruding. A truss is not suitable for treatment of a direct inguinal hernia unless the defect is very small. Direct inguinal hernias will tend to bulge round the sides of the truss before long.

Most patients find a truss rather uncomfortable and irksome to wear but it has its place in elderly and frail patients who would prefer to avoid an operation.

Surgical

Most inguinal hernias will be repaired operatively.

Preoperative management

The patient should be advised to stop smoking and to lose any excess weight. Patients who continue smoking up to the time of a hernia repair tend to have a severe bronchitis after the operation and this puts added strain on the repair in the early stages. Obesity makes the operation more difficult and also puts more strain on the repair postoperatively.

If the patient is bronchitic, he should have a few days of physiotherapy to the chest before the operation is undertaken.

Patients with recurrent inguinal hernias may have to be warned that a satisfactory repair of the abdominal wall may only be possible if the testicle and spermatic cord are removed. Their consent must be obtained if this is being considered. This is not necessary if a recurrent hernia is being repaired laparoscopically.

OPERATION: OPEN REPAIR OF INGUINAL HERNIA

The indirect hernial sac is ligated at its neck and excised after the contents have been reduced back into the abdomen. A direct hernial sac is not usually excised. It is inverted and the defect in the posterior wall of the inguinal canal is repaired. The posterior wall of the inguinal canal can then be strengthened by sewing the conjoint tendon to the inguinal ligament (Bassini repair). Some surgeons also use a nylon darn which criss-crosses backwards and forwards between the inguinal ligament and the conjoint tendon.

In the Shouldice operation a Bassini repair is performed with division of the transversalis fascia transversely and then repaired by overlapping the proximal and distal flaps.

In a Lichtenstein repair the posterior wall of the canal is strengthened with a piece of Prolene mesh sited under the spermatic cord and the external oblique aponeurosis. This repair is less painful than previous repairs and can be done under a local anaesthetic.*

In the Stoppa repair a large piece of Prolene mesh is placed inside the abdominal wall between the peritoneum and the muscle. This is done through a lower abdominal incision.

In children and young adults it is only necessary to excise the sac (herniotomy) and no attention is needed to the posterior inguinal canal wall (herniorrhaphy).

All of these repairs can be made more comfortable for a few hours by local infiltration of bupivacaine.

Codes

Blood	0
GA/LA	GA or LA
Opn time	15–30 min
Stay	2–5 days
Drains out	0
Sutures out	5 days
Off work	4 weeks

Postoperative care

The patient is mobilized early and can leave hospital as soon as he can walk independently. Hernias are increasingly repaired as day-case procedures.

Pain may increase when the local anaesthetic wears off. Warn the patient to expect this. Strong analgesia is usually required for the first 48 h but mild analgesics such as aspirin or paracetamol will suffice thereafter. The patient is usually advised to take things gently for 2 weeks from the operation date. Thereafter he should undertake gradually increasing exercise in order to regain muscular fitness. There is no evidence that early return to work increases the recurrence rate.

*For more detailed descriptions of these hernia repairs see Dunn, DC and Menzies D, *Inguinal Hernia Repair, the Laparoscopic Approach*, Blackwell Science 1996.

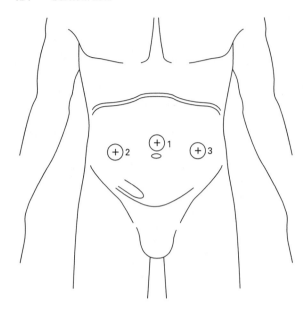

Fig. 86 Possible port sites for transperitioneal repair of right inguinal hernia.

OPERATION: LAPAROSCOPIC REPAIR OF INGUINAL HERNIAS (see Fig. 86)

The approach may either be across the peritoneum (transperitoneal repair), or through the retroperitoneal tissues (retroperitoneal aproach). A large piece of Prolene mesh is placed on the inner aspect of the groin between the muscle and the peritoneum. Only stab wounds 5–10 mm in diameter are required and the operation is remarkably painless. Fifty per cent of patients require no analgesia after leaving hospital. This method is the operation of choice for recurrent and bilateral hernia repairs where the recovery, unlike that of the open counterpart procedures, is the same as after a unilateral primary repair. The surgeon must be thoroughly skilled in laparoscopic techniques.

Codes

Blood	0
GA/LA	GA
Opn time	30–90 min
Stay	1 day
Drains out	0
Sutures out	Absorbable
Off work	3–7 days

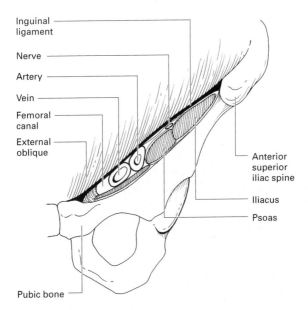

Fig. 87 Femoral canal lies behind the inguinal ligament medial to the femoral vein.

Femoral hernia

Femoral hernias protrude down the femoral canal, which is medial to the femoral vessels and lateral to the pubic tubercle. From an understanding of the anatomy of the femoral canal, it can be seen that femoral hernias will always have a narrow neck. This is because it is constricted by the inguinal ligament anteriorly; the pubic bone and reflected part of the inguinal ligament (lacunar ligament) medially; the pectineal part of the pubic bone posteriorly; and the femoral vein laterally (Fig. 87). Consequently, the risk of strangulation is high. As the angle between the inguinal ligament and the pectineal part of the pubic bone is greater in females than males, the femoral canal is wider in females and femoral hernias are more common.

Recognizing the pattern

The patient is usually female and middle aged or elderly, although femoral hernias can occur in either sex and at any age.

The history is of a lump appearing in the groin, which is frequently painful. Femoral hernias often present with an episode of strangulation and small bowel obstruction is not uncommon. A strangulated hernia will be missed if the groin is not adequately exposed during the general examination.

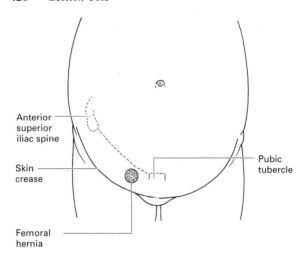

Fig. 88 Groin crease is not a guide to the position of the inguinal ligament. Always define the bony landmarks, especially in obese patients and children.

Strangulated femoral hernias are frequently missed in obese patients (Fig. 88).

On examination there is a rounded swelling tucked in medially in the groin. It is below and lateral to the pubic tubercle. It may be of any size but is frequently 2–3 cm in diameter. Even when the main bulk of the hernia has been reduced, a soft palpable lump can usually be found. If the hernia enlarges sufficiently, it tends to spread upwards over the inguinal ligament and pubic tubercle and this can be confusing. If the groin is carefully palpated, however, its origin can be determined. Definition of a femoral hernia from an inguinal one is important as the former are much more likely to strangulate and should therefore be repaired without undue delay.

Management
The management of a femoral hernia is surgical repair. A truss should never be prescribed.

OPERATION: REPAIR OF FEMORAL HERNIA
Two main approaches are possible.
1 Below the inguinal ligament.
2 Above the inguinal ligament.
    A strangulated hernia will usually have to be approached from above in order to deal with possible bowel infarction.

APPROACH FROM BELOW (LOCKWOOD'S OPERATION)

An incision is made in the groin below the inguinal ligament and the hernia found in the subcutaneous tissue. Its neck is isolated, the contents reduced back into the abdomen and the sac excised. The femoral canal is closed at its lower end by suturing the inguinal ligament to the pectineal fascia posteriorly. This operation is very minor and can be done under a local anaesthetic.

Codes

Blood	0
GA/LA	GA or LA
Opn time	15 min
Stay	2–3 days
Drains out	0
Sutures out	5–7 days
Off work	2–3 weeks

APPROACH FROM ABOVE

In this approach the abdominal muscles of the inguinal region are opened and the upper end of the femoral canal visualized within the abdominal cavity. The approach may be via either a vertical incision in the conjoint tendon (McEvedy's operation) or a transverse incision through the posterior wall of the inguinal canal (Lotheissen's operation). If the hernia is strangulated, the peritoneum is opened and the contents of the sac inspected. Non-viable bowel may then be resected. The femoral canal is then exposed in the retroperitoneal layer and closed with sutures between the inguinal ligament and the pectineal fascia.

Codes

Blood	0
GA/LA	GA
Opn time	30 min
Stay	5–7 days
Drains out	0
Sutures out	5–7 days
Off work	4 weeks

Postoperative care

This is much the same as for an open inguinal hernia repair. Where a femoral hernia has been approached from below the inguinal ligament, the recovery is rapid.

Strangulated hernia

Most types of hernia may become irreducible. Various stages are recognized.

1 In a simple irreducible hernia, the contents cannot be reduced but the blood supply is intact and there are no symptoms of intestinal obstruction. The usual cause is adhesions between the sac and its contents — almost certainly omentum.

2 In an obstructed hernia, the sac contains bowel which has become obstructed.

3 In a strangulated hernia, the blood supply of the contents is compromised and there is a danger of, or actual, necrosis of the tissues enclosed in the hernia. Both the preceding types of irreducible hernia predispose to strangulation.

Other terms used for irreducible hernias are as follows:

1 Richter's hernia. A knuckle of the sidewall of the bowel is caught in the sac but the continuity of the bowel is maintained (Fig. 89a). In this case the bowel wall is strangulated but there is no intestinal obstruction.

2 Reduction *en masse*. If a strangulated hernia is reduced the strangulation is normally relieved. Occasionally, however, it is possible to reduce the visible mass of the hernia but for the sac and its neck to be reduced as well. In this case the contents remain strangulated even though the external hernia has disappeared (Fig. 89b). Any clinician attempting to reduce a strangulated hernia must be aware of this possibility. If the patient's symptoms (e.g. of bowel obstruction and abdominal pain) persist after reduction of the hernia, it must be considered and early operation may be indicated.

Recognizing the pattern

The hernia suddenly becomes irreducible, painful and tender. There may be accompanying symptoms of intestinal obstruction. Occasionally patients present only with general abdominal symptoms and have not themselves noticed the hernia.

On examination the hernia is irreducible and tender. A distended abdomen and obstructive bowel sounds may confirm suspicions of intestinal obstruction. Similarly, an erect and supine abdominal X-ray may be helpful.

Management

A strangulated hernia must be explored surgically, the hernia reduced and the contents examined and removed if non-viable.

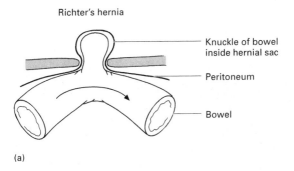

Richter's hernia

— Knuckle of bowel inside hernial sac

— Peritoneum

— Bowel

(a)

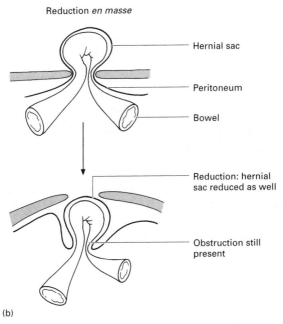

Reduction *en masse*

— Hernial sac

— Peritoneum

— Bowel

— Reduction: hernial sac reduced as well

— Obstruction still present

(b)

Fig. 89 (a,b) Some terms used for special types of strangulation.

Preoperative management
If the hernia cannot be reduced, urgent operation is required. The patient may need rapid rehydration first. The serum electrolytes should be within the normal range before the anaesthetic is given. Make sure the patient is shaved before the operation starts. A strangulated hernia is often infected and antibiotics (gentamicin, metronidazole and either penicillin or ampicillin) should be given with the premedication.

OPERATION: FOR STRANGULATED HERNIAS

The details are given under individual hernias and small bowel resection. In general, the sac is opened and the contents inspected and then the strangulation released. The affected bowel is wrapped in a warm saline swab. It may be necessary to wait several minutes in order to be sure that it is viable. If it is not, it is resected. If there is gross contamination, the wound will need to be drained. Such a drain can be removed after 3–4 days.

Codes

Blood 0
GA/LA .... GA
Opn time .... 60–90 min
Stay .... About 7 days
Drains out .... 3–5 days
Sutures out .... 5–7 days
Off work .... 4 weeks

Postoperative care

The patient may have an ileus for 1–2 days. Apart from this the postoperative course is as for any other hernia.

Incisional hernia

An incisional hernia occurs where there has been breakdown of the muscle closure in a previous abdominal wound. There is often a history of postoperative wound haematoma or sepsis but the hernia itself may not appear for several weeks or months after the operation.

Recognizing the pattern

The patient is nearly always obese.

The patient notices a bulge at the side of the previous operation scar associated with discomfort. He may also suffer from more general abdominal pain associated with obstruction of loops of bowel within the hernia.

On examination the incisional hernia is easily visible when the patient stands up or strains but it may be invisible as he lies flat. It can usually be demonstrated by asking the patient either to cough or to tense his abdominal muscles by straight leg raising. The margins of the muscular defect are palpable beneath the skin and the size of the defect should be determined. Note whether the contents of the incisional hernia are fully reducible or not.

Management

Once the muscle layers of a laparotomy wound have separated, it is difficult to be certain of obtaining a sound repair at a second closure. Frequently the tissues are poor anyway, and the patient's obesity is against obtaining a good result. A conservative approach may therefore be advocated. If an operation is advised, the patient should be told that it carries a high failure rate.

Conservative management
The patient is strongly advised to lose weight and a surgical belt is provided.

Preoperative management
The patient should stop smoking and lose weight before an operative repair is considered. The theatre staff frequently regard an incisional hernia as a minor operation and do not realize that its repair will entail a full laparotomy. The hernia cannot be repaired until the adherent loops of bowel have been freed and the edges of the muscle clearly defined. Deep instruments may therefore be necessary.

OPERATION: REPAIR OF INCISIONAL HERNIA
The stretched scar in the skin is excised. The muscle edges are defined and adhesions divided. Several different types of repair are possible and deep tension sutures will usually be used for the muscle layer.
1 Mesh repair. A large incisional hernia is best closed using a piece of mesh which is placed on the inner aspect of the abdominal wall and considerably 'underlaps' the previous defect.
2 Simple closure with deep-tension nylon. In this type of closure continuous nylon suture is inserted taking wide bites of tissue. Only the superficial layers of skin are not included. This repair is suitable for small hernias.
3 Deep-tension figure-of-eight nylon sutures. These can be placed through all layers including the skin. This method of closure is also used for dehisced abdominal wounds in the postoperative period (see pp. 68–69).

Codes

Blood	0–2 units
GA/LA	GA
Opn time	1 h
Stay	3–7 days
Drains out	1–2 days
Sutures out	Skin 7–10 days; deep-tension sutures 10–14 days
Off work	4–6 weeks

Postoperative care
If the closure is very tight the patient may develop chest problems postoperatively and chest physiotherapy will be important. An external binder can sometimes be used to take the tension off the wound. Any sign of a wound infection must be treated early and most surgeons cover these operations with antibiotics prophylactically.

Umbilical hernia

Umbilical hernias in infants are dealt with on p. 619.

Paraumbilical hernias in adults

A hernia in this site in adults does not occur at the umbilicus, but rather just above it or below it, due to a weakness in the linea alba. It is commoner in women, and obesity, multiparity and weak abdominal muscles are predisposing causes. The sac may contain both omentum and bowel and in this age group gastrointestinal symptoms of subacute obstruction are more common. The hernia may become quite large and irreducible. Strangulation may occur.

Management
The patient should lose weight. Operation is usually advised because of the risk of strangulation.

OPERATION: PARAUMBILICAL HERNIA REPAIR
The sac is dissected clear and then opened. The adhesions holding the bowel and omentum are freed and the bowel returned to the abdomen. The defect is then closed.

Codes

Blood 0
GA/LA .... GA
Opn time .... 30–45 min
Stay .... 1–3 days
Drains out .... Subcutaneous 24 h
Sutures out .... 5–7 days
Off work .... 1 month

Postoperative care
This is similar to that for an incisional hernia.

Epigastric hernia

This is a midline hernia through a defect in the linea alba above
the umbilicus. The initial weakness may be at the site of penetrating vessels. It usually contains extraperitoneal fat
(epiplocoele), although if it enlarges a true peritoneal sac may
protrude. In this case it may contain omentum. However, it
never contains bowel.

Recognizing the pattern

The hernia may be symptomless or present as a small pattern
swelling in the epigastrium, which may be painful, particularly
on exercise. Occasionally it causes episodes of severe epigastric
pain and vomiting. These may have been extensively investigated but no cause found.

On examination the small epigastric mass is palpable and
more prominent when the patient coughs or tenses the abdominal muscles.

Management
These hernias usually require operative repair.

OPERATION: REPAIR OF EPIGASTRIC HERNIA
The hernia is excised and the defect in the linea alba closed
with non-absorbable sutures. There may be other epigastric
hernias present which should also be removed.

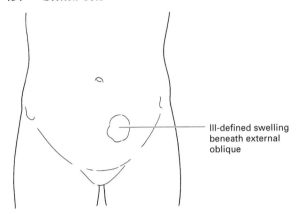

Ill-defined swelling beneath external oblique

Fig. 90 Spigelian hernia.

Codes

Blood 0
GA/LA .... GA
Opn time .... 15–30 min
Stay .... Day case
Drains out 0
Sutures out .... 5–7 days or absorbable
Off work .... 2–3 weeks

Spigelian hernia

The hernial sac protrudes through the linea semilunaris (the lateral edge of the rectus sheath), at the level of the semi-circular fold of Douglas (Fig. 90). It usually lies underneath the external oblique. It has a narrow neck and strangulation may occur.

Recognizing the pattern

It is usually seen in obese people over the age of 50 years and presents as a swelling below and lateral to the umbilicus. It may cause some discomfort, which is worse on exertion, and occasionally it causes nausea and vomiting.

Management

The management is by surgical repair.

OPERATION: REPAIR OF SPIGELIAN HERNIA
The sac is isolated, emptied and ligated, and the defect closed in layers. The operation can be performed laparoscopically when a piece of mesh could be placed internal to the defect in the preperitoneal space.

Codes

Blood 0
GA/LA .... GA
Opn time .... 30 min
Stay .... 0–3 days
Drains out 0
Sutures out .... Absorbable
Off work .... 2–3 weeks

Obturator hernia

This is a hernia that protrudes from the pelvis out through the obturator canal. It lies beneath the adductor muscles of the floor of the femoral triangle in the upper thigh.

Recognizing the pattern

It is commoner in women. The swelling is usually hidden, although it may be more obvious if the leg is laterally rotated, abducted and flexed. Strangulation is common and this usually causes intestinal obstruction. A Richter's hernia is quite common in this site (see p. 429). Pain is often referred along the obturator nerve to the knee.

Management

The management is by surgical repair.

OPERATION: REPAIR OF OBTURATOR HERNIA
The hernia is repaired from above, usually through a lower paramedian laparotomy incision.

Codes

Blood 0
GA/LA .... GA
Opn time .... 30 min
Stay .... 1–2 days
Drains out 0
Sutures out .... 7 days
Off work .... 1 month

Umbilical discharge in adults

Umbilical discharge in children is dealt with on p. 620. In adults a vitellointestinal or urachal cyst or fistula may also be considered.

Other causes in adults include an umbilical stone or a simple skin abscess.

An umbilical stone consists of inspissated secretions and exfoliated squamous cells that collect at the base of a deep uncleaned umbilicus. Eventually infection may occur and a persistent discharge, either through the umbilicus or through an adjoining sinus, may result.

Management
The managemement is by surgical exploration.

Preoperative care
The patient should lose weight. A swab is taken from the discharge and relevant antibiotic cover started with the pre-medication. An ultrasound examination may demonstrate a urachal cyst. A sinogram may also be useful.

OPERATION: EXPLORATION OF THE UMBILICUS
The umbilical scar is detached from the linea alba and the umbilical pit everted. Any deep connections can be isolated and divided. The umbilicus is cleared of all debris and its deeper part may be excised, resulting in a shallower depression. If a urachal abnormality or vitellointestinal abnormality is present, it is excised.

Codes
Blood 0
GA/LA .... GA
Opn time .... 30–60 min (depending on extent)
Stay .... 2–3 days
Drains out .... 48 h
Sutures out .... 5–7 days
Off work .... 1 week

10.2 Skeletal Pain

Skeletal pain (referred pain)

'Skeletal pain' felt in the abdomen is probably due to pressure on thoracic or lumbar nerve roots as they leave the spinal column. Alternatively, the pain may radiate from one of the many joints or ligaments in the spinal column. The stimulus to the nerve root is interpreted as pain anywhere in the distribution of that nerve. Thus T8 nerve root pressure may give rise to epigastric pain and T12 root pressure to loin or suprapubic pain.

Skeletal pain is the great mimic of all abdominal conditions. Because of this there is a tendency to label any undiagnosed abdominal pain as skeletal and thus avoid trying to reach an accurate diagnosis. This tendency must be resisted.

Recognizing the pattern

The patient is of any age. There is often a history of associated anxiety or tension. With anxiety muscle tone is raised and hence the danger of nerve root pressure is increased. There may be a previous history of other skeletal pains such as sciatica or cervical spondylosis.

The pain is related to posture or movement. It is usually worse in certain postures (but beware, this is also true of acute appendicitis). The patient may relate the pain to being in a fixed position such as when driving or watching television or even lying in bed. The pain is eased by certain movements and exacerbated by others. It is frequently better during the night and gets worse towards the end of the day. It may radiate to other areas supplied by the same spinal nerve.

On examination there may be no physical signs. Tenderness over the spine or pain on femoral nerve or sciatic nerve stretching are helpful positive signs when present. The patient often feels tenderness over the area where the pain is felt even though there is no localized lesion at that site. Localized tenderness is not therefore very helpful in defining whether a pain is skeletal or not.

Proving the diagnosis

There is no clinical test which will prove that a pain is skeletal.

An X-ray of the spine may show spondylosis in the area of the root supplying the painful area but since such changes are very common they do not prove that the lesion found is the cause of the pain.

Management

Spinal exercises may be helpful and analgesics and reassurance should be given as necessary. Relaxants such as Valium can be very useful to relieve both the painful muscle spasms and the overlying anxiety.

11 Urinary Tract Surgery

11.1 Disorders of the upper urinary tract
Renal tract stones
Pyelonephritis
Renal tumours
Renal cysts
Haematuria
Renal transplantation

11.2 Conditions of the lower urinary tract
Bladder stones
Bladder tumours
Bladder diverticulum
Cystitis
Incontinence
Acute retention of urine
Bladder outflow obstruction
Benign prostatic hyperplasia (BPH)
Prostatic carcinoma
Acute prostatitis
Chronic prostatitis
Urethral stricture

11.3 Male genitalia
Conditions of the foreskin
Carcinoma of the penis
Scrotal conditions
Absent testis (cryptorchidism)
Lumps in the scrotum
Painful testis

11.1 Disorders of the Upper Urinary Tract

Renal pain is felt in the loin between the twelfth rib and the iliac crest. The pain is usually more or less constant. Ureteric pain radiates down and forwards from the loin to the groin and on to the vulva or scrotum. Ureteric pain is usually a true colic.

Common surgical causes of renal pain are stones, pyelonephritis and renal tumours.

Renal tract stones

Stones form in the renal tract due to increased concentration of solutes in the urine such as calcium (e.g. in hyperparathyroidism), uric acid (gout) or oxalic acid, or due to a general increased concentration of the urine during dehydration. Roughened areas within the renal pelvis and calyces may act as focal points for the formation of stones (Randall's plaques). Other predisposing factors include stasis and pooling of urine due to obstruction and urinary infection.

The commonest type of stone is composed of calcium and magnesium phosphates and carbonates. These precipitate in alkaline urine such as occurs in a *Proteus* urinary infection. The stone is soft and friable. The commonest pure stones are calcium oxalate. They are hard and rough and may cause haematuria. The formation of both calcium oxalate and uric acid stones is favoured by acid urine. Oxalate stones are radio-opaque and cystine and uric acid calculi are radiolucent.

The stones are usually formed in the renal calyces or pelvis. They may continue growing to fill the whole of the renal pelvis (staghorn calculus). Alternatively, they may remain small and pass down the ureter into the bladder causing ureteric colic. The stone may become stuck at any point in this passage, but particularly at the pelviureteric junction, where the ureter crosses the iliac artery, and at the entrance of the ureter into the bladder. Infection may develop proximal to an impacted stone, and if the upper tract is obstructed, a pyonephrosis may develop. This condition, in which the renal pelvis and proximal ureter are filled with pus, constitutes a grave surgical emergency, since it requires urgent decompression and drainage to prevent septicaemia and shock.

Recognizing the pattern

The patient may be of any age, although stones are unusual before adolescence. Males are more commonly affected than females in a ratio of 2 : 1.

Stones within the kidney give rise to pain in the loin and often present with episodes of urinary infection. If a stone passes down the ureter, the patient experiences excruciating bouts of severe colic starting in the loin and radiating round into the flank and groin. The pain is so severe that the sufferer tends to roll around in agony unable to find a comfortable position. He may vomit. Haematuria may discolour the urine after an attack of pain. These symptoms may be mimicked by individuals seeking opiate analgesia, in an attempt to convince the doctor that that they are suffering from renal colic.

On examination there may be tenderness in the renal angle or along the line of the ureter but the physical signs are minimal compared with the severity of the pain. Constitutional upset with fever and malaise indicate secondary infection.

Proving the diagnosis

The presence of red cells in the urine on microscopy is the most helpful finding. In the early stages these may be absent and in that case the examination should be repeated after 24–48 h. Evidence of infection should also be sought.

A straight abdominal X-ray may show the stone lying in the kidney substance or along the line of the ureter (Fig. 91). Ninety per cent of urinary stones are radio-opaque (compared with 10% of gall stones). If a stone is seen, its diameter should be measured, since this will indicate whether it is likely to pass spontaneously.

An emergency intravenous urogram (IVU) will confirm the diagnosis and show the position of the stone. Ultrasound may also demonstrate hydro- or pyonephrosis.

Screening tests for raised serum calcium and uric acid should always be performed.

Management principles

This is either conservative or operative, the choice depending on the size of the stone. Try to decide whether the stone will pass spontaneously. The critical size is 0.5 cm.

If it is clearly too large to travel down the ureter, then it must be removed. If, however, natural passage is possible, then the initial management is always conservative. If there is infection in an obstructed upper tract, drainage must be established. This is usually achieved by means of a

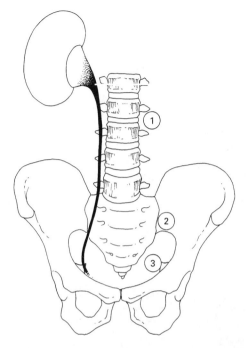

Fig. 91 The landmarks for the ureter on an abdominal X-ray.
1, Lumbar transverse processes. 2, Sacroiliac joint. 3, Ischial spine.

nephrostomy tube, inserted by a radiologist under ultrasound guidance.

Conservative management
The patient is put on a regular non-steroidal analgesic, although pethidine may be required in severe colic. The patient should be encouraged to drink plenty of fluid and the urine sieved to see if a stone has passed. If found it should be analysed.

Surgical management
The treatment of urinary calculi has advanced rapidly in the last decade. Using percutaneous renal surgery a track can be created between the skin and the intrarenal collecting system. A nephroscope can then be passed and the stone removed with forceps. If the stone is too large, it can be disintegrated by ultrasound or shattered by an electrohydraulic discharge. The fragments are then removed.

Continued on p. 444

Continued.

Extracorporeal shock–wave lithotripsy (ESWL) was first developed in Germany. In the early lithotriptors, a shock wave was created by an underwater spark generator and the energy was focused onto the stone by positioning the patient in a bath, using X-ray screening to locate the stone. A general anaesthetic was often necessary. More modern lithotriptors use electromagnetic or piezoelectric generated shock waves and are preferable because they require minimal analgesia.

Surgical intervention is indicated for renal stones if lithotripsy is not available or fails, or if the stone is too large (e.g. some staghorn calculi). The surgical management of the stone depends on whether it lies in the kidney or in the ureter and, if in the ureter, at what level. Surgical intervention for ureteric stones is indicated if there is increasing renal impairment or if there is infection above the site of obstruction.

Management of stones in the ureter

Previously stones were removed from the ureter endoscopically by passing a Dormia basket. Rigid and flexible ureteroscopes are now available and allow the stones to be removed under direct vision. They may first be disintegrated by ultrasound or electrohydraulic shock waves. Alternatively, a self-retaining ureteric stent, which has curled proximal and distal ends (called a 'double J stent'), may be passed from the bladder to the renal pelvis. This will permit drainage of urine and cause the ureter to dilate, so that spontaneous passage of the stone may occur. This technique is often used in the acute management of a ureteric stone, since it provides immediate pain relief for the patient. The stent should be removed within a month, as encrustation may occur. Ureteric stents can also cause distress to the patient, who may complain of back pain or urinary frequency.

Stones in the upper ureter may also be treated by ESWL, or they may be pushed into the renal pelvis and treated as a renal stone by percutaneous renal surgery or by ESWL. Rarely, if non-invasive methods fail, open surgery is performed.

OPERATION: ENDOSCOPIC TREATMENT OF URETERIC STONE

Stones in the lower third of the ureter may be removed by passing a cystoscope into the bladder through which a Dormia basket is passed beyond the stone. The basket is opened and pulled back, hopefully engaging the stone. Several passes of the basket may be required. It is best to perform this with X-ray guidance.

If the above procedure fails, or the stone is above the lower third of the ureter, the ureteric orifice is dilated and a ureteroscope is passed into it. The instrument is carefully advanced until the stone is encountered and extracted. A ureteric stent may alternatively be passed, via the cystoscope, leaving the stone in the ureter.

Codes

Blood	0
GA/LA	GA
Opn time	Variable
Stay	1–3 days
Drains out	0
Sutures out	0
Off work	Variable

Postoperative care

If the stone has been extracted, send it for biochemical analysis after the patient has seen it. If a stent has been inserted, obtain a plain X-ray, to ensure that it is correctly positioned with the proximal end in the renal pelvis and the distal end in the bladder.

OPERATION: URETEROLITHOTOMY

The incision depends on the site of the stone. The retroperitoneal area is exposed and the peritoneum and its contents retracted medially. The ureter is found and slings passed above and below the stone to prevent it displacing upwards or down-wards. The ureter is incised and the stone removed. The ureterostomy is closed with absorbable sutures and the wound drained.

Codes

Blood	2 units
GA/LA	GA
Opn time	30–60 min
Stay	7–10 days
Drains out	3–5 days
Sutures out	7 days
Off work	4–6 weeks

Postoperative care

There is usually very little ileus and no nasogastric tube is required. The patient is encouraged to drink 2–3 L a day after the first 24 h. The drain is removed once it is clear that there is no ureteric fistula. If a urinary leak does occur, the drain is left *in situ* and the leak will usually close. If leakage continues longer than a week, the passage of a ureteric catheter will usually solve the problem.

Management of stones in the kidney

Ninety per cent of renal stones can be treated by percutaneous renal surgery and/or ESWL. For the rest, open surgery is required. It may be necessary to perform a partial or total nephrectomy. The latter is especially indicated for a staghorn calculus, if a preoperative radionuclide (diethylenetriaminepentacetic acid or DTPA) scan has demonstrated that the kidney contributes less than 15% of the overall renal function.

Preoperative management

If the urine is infected, antibiotics are commenced preoperatively. The stone or stones must be adequately demonstrated radiologically. The timing of the surgery should be coordinated with the radiologist if percutaneous surgery is planned. The radiographers should also be warned that they may be required during the operation.

OPERATION: PERCUTANEOUS
NEPHROLITHOTOMY

A cystoscope is passed and a ureteric catheter inserted into the ureteric orifice on the appropriate side. Radio-opaque contrast solution is introduced. Under X-ray screening a trocar needle is inserted into the renal pelvis via a percutaneous puncture in the flank. The tract is then dilated over a guide wire, so that it will admit a larger sheath, through which a rigid nephroscope is inserted. Calculi in the renal pelvis are extracted. It may be necessary to fragment larger stones using a lithoclast or other technique. The renal pelvis is irrigated and an X-ray obtained to confirm that all the stones have been removed. A nephrostomy drain is inserted, via the tract, into the renal pelvis. Staghorn calculi may require more than one percutaneous puncture for removal.

Codes

Blood .... Group and save
GA/LA .... GA
Opn time .... 1–3 h
Stay .... 3–5 days
Drains out .... Nephrostomy removed when the
urine is clear, usually after about 48 h
Sutures out .... 7–10 days
Off work .... 2 weeks

Postoperative care

When the urine draining through the nephrostomy tube is clear, a nephrostogram is performed to ensure that there is free passage of urine down the ureter, before the nephrostomy is removed.

OPERATION: OPEN REMOVAL OF RENAL STONES

The kidney is exposed via a posterolateral incision over the twelfth rib. The stone may be removed from the renal pelvis (pyelolithotomy), the renal substance (nephrolithotomy) or both (pyelonephrolithotomy). An intraoperative X-ray may be taken to ensure that all the stones have been removed. Occasionally, if the stones are numerous or there is associated renal damage, a partial or even total nephrectomy is required. A drain is put down to the kidney bed and occasionally, if the operation has been difficult, a nephrostomy tube is inserted to remove any blood clot that may form in the renal pelvis.

Codes

Blood .... 2 units
GA/LA .... GA
Opn time .... 60–120 min
Stay .... 7–10 days
Drains out .... 3–5 days, nephrostomy 48 h
Sutures out .... 7–10 days
Off work .... 4–6 weeks

Postoperative care

This is similar to that after ureterolithotomy.

Prevention of recurrence

The patient should be encouraged to drink as much fluid as possible. Any cause of renal stones found on screening must be treated.

Pyelonephritis

This is due to parenchymal infection of the kidney secondary either to ascending infection from the bladder or problems in the kidney itself such as renal stones or pelviureteric obstruction. Occasionally the kidney may become infected as a complication of septicaemia. The organism is usually a Gram-negative bacillus. Pyelonephritis with urinary tract obstruction is an emergency and should be diagnosed without delay. Rapid progression to septicaemia and shock can occur.

Recognizing the pattern

The patient is of any age but more frequently female and of child-bearing age.

There is a sudden onset of illness with a high fever and vomiting. The systemic symptoms are often dominant and the patient may not complain of any symptoms referable to the urinary tract in the early stages. On questioning, however, there may be pain in the loin and this can be severe. The patient may describe symptoms of a urinary tract infection, such as frequency and dysuria, and may give a past history of similar episodes.

On examination there may be a tachycardia and a high fever (up to 39.5°C) often with rigors. There is localized tenderness over the affected kidney.

Proving the diagnosis

The diagnosis is confirmed by finding bacteria and pus cells in the urine. Pus cells may be absent in the early stages if the affected kidney shuts down and fails to excrete infected urine into the bladder. One negative midstream urine specimen (MSU) should not therefore be taken as excluding the diagnosis but must be repeated.

An ultrasound is performed to exclude pyonephrosis. A plain abdominal X-ray may show an associated calculus in the position of the kidney or ureter, which should subsequently be confirmed on an IVU.

Management

It is important to set up urinary and blood cultures before treatment is commenced. If the kidney is obstructed it is urgently decompressed by inserting a percutaneous nephrostomy tube. Antibiotics are given in high dosage, intravenously if necessary. Analgesia with opiates or non-steroidals may be needed, and the patient is encouraged to drink at least 3 L of fluid daily. If a perinephric abscess forms, it is drained through a loin incision.

Renal tumours

Renal tumours may be either benign or malignant. Benign tumours include cysts and true benign neoplasms. Malignant tumours may be primary or secondary. Primary renal tumours arise either from the urothelium of the calyces and pelvis (pelviureteric tumour) or from the kidney substance itself (hypernephroma).

Pelviureteric tumours

Urothelial tumours can arise anywhere where there is transitional cell epithelium. They are associated with the ingestion of carcinogens (transitional cell carcinomas or TCCs) or the presence of chronic renal calculi (squamous cell carcinoma) (see p. 441).

Recognizing the pattern

The patient is usually over the age of 40 years. He presents with a history of painless haematuria or occasionally ureteric colic associated with the passage of a clot. There are usually no physical signs.

Proving the diagnosis

An IVU will show either a filling defect in the renal tract, evidence of obstruction, with hydronephrosis, or a non-functioning kidney. If the filling defect is not demonstrated, a retrograde ureteropyelogram, via a ureteric catheter inserted at cystoscopy, is indicated. Urinary cytology may show carcinoma cells.

Management

As a urothelial tumour represents instability in the epithelium of the renal tract, it is usually considered necessary to remove the whole of the renal tract on the affected side. The need for this must be explained to the patient. Occasionally two incisions are necessary, one in the loin to remove the kidney and a second in the lower abdomen to remove the pelvic part of the ureter.

OPERATION: NEPHROURETERECTOMY

The kidney is explored and its vessels isolated and ligated. The kidney is removed and the ureter is followed down into the pelvis and excised together with a patch of the bladder mucosa. The bladder muscle is repaired. A urinary catheter is left *in situ* and the renal bed drained.

Codes

Blood	2 units
GA/LA	GA
Opn time	1–2 h
Stay	7–10 days
Drains out	48 h
Sutures out	7–10 days
Off work	4–6 weeks

Postoperative care

In the early stages there is a danger of haemorrhage in the renal bed and the vital signs must be carefully monitored. The urinary catheter should not be removed until it is clear that the bladder repair has healed. This usually occurs within 7 days. If there is any doubt, a cystogram is helpful.

The patient should be followed up by cystoscopy and with regular review of the other kidney by IVU. This is in order to detect the development of further tumours.

Hypernephroma

Hypernephroma is an adenocarcinoma arising from the substance of the kidney. The tumour may grow very large. It tends to spread up the renal vein and grow into the inferior vena cava. It may even extend into the right atrium of the heart. Metastasis occurs via the lymphatics to para-aortic lymph nodes and via the blood stream to the lungs, brain and bone. It may be clinically silent until it has grown to a large size, and systemic symptoms often divert attention away from the local disease.

Recognizing the pattern

The patient is usually over 50 years old and more commonly male. However, the disease can also affect young people and can present with a wide variety of symptoms. The typical triad is a palpable mass, loin pain and haematuria.

It may present in less typical ways such as with a pyrexia of unknown origin associated with night sweats. The tumour may bleed into the renal tract, producing 'clot colic' or anaemia. Patients may also present with symptoms from metastases (e.g. pathological fracture). A hypernephroma spreading along the renal vein sometimes obstructs the testicular vein on the left, causing a varicocoele. Finally, hormonal secretion from the growth may cause hypertension (renin), polycythaemia (erythropoietin) or hypercalcaemia (parathormone). Not infrequently a hypernephroma presents as an incidental 'cannon ball' metastasis found on a chest X-ray.

On examination the lump in the loin may be easily palpable. It is usually only possible to feel the lower pole, which may be ballotted and moves down on respiration. It is resonant to percussion due to the overlying colon.

Proving the diagnosis

Investigation of the urine will often show microscopic haematuria. An ultrasound of the renal area shows a solid mass arising from the kidney. The ultrasound may also be used to investigate whether or not there is growth in the renal vein and vena cava. An IVU will show a renal mass distorting the calyces and will also demonstrate contralateral renal function. This investigation is not required if an abdominal computed tomography (CT) scan, with intravenous contrast, is performed to assess the degree of local spread and the presence of para-aortic lymph node metastases. This will also demonstrate a normal functioning contralateral kidney, which is crucial if a total nephrectomy is contemplated. Bilateral hypernephromas are occasionally demonstrated on a CT scan and may be associated with a familial condition called von Hippel–Lindau disease. If spread into the renal vein is considered, then vena cavography should be performed.

Management

During the preoperative work-up, a careful search should be made for the presence of metastases. A chest X-ray should be performed. A biochemical profile and full blood count are helpful in detecting metabolic or haematological complications of the tumour.

The standard treatment for patients with hypernephroma is radical nephrectomy. Even if metastases are present, this operation will control symptoms related to the primary tumour, such as haematuria and pain.

OPERATION: RADICAL NEPHRECTOMY

The tumour may be very bulky and this can make the operation difficult and increase the blood loss. Occasionally it is necessary to open the chest and divide the diaphragm in order to get adequate exposure.

The kidney is usually exposed via an anterior, transperitoneal approach. A loin incision may be employed, though exposure is not so good. You should determine which approach the surgeon intends and inform the theatre staff

Continued on p. 452

Continued.

and anaesthetist. When the approach is through the bed of a rib, a pneumothorax is not uncommon. A chest drain may be needed postoperatively (p. 253).

If the tumour is invading the inferior vena cava, then the surgeon will have to control that vessel in order to effect an adequate removal. He may open the chest to achieve this. The renal vessels are ligated and the kidney, together with the adrenal, the surrounding fat and fascia and the upper ureter are removed. A drain is left in the renal bed.

Codes

Blood .... 4–6 units
GA/LA .... GA
Opn time .... 2–3 h
Stay .... 5–10 days
Drains out .... 48 h; chest 24–48 h
Sutures out .... 7–10 days
Off work .... 4–6 weeks

Postoperative care

Where a pneumothorax has occurred, a postoperative chest X-ray should be carried out in the erect position in the first few hours after the operation to check that the lung has fully re-expanded.

There is a danger of haemorrhage in the first 24 h and careful monitoring of pulse, blood pressure and fluid balance is necessary during this period. There may be an ileus but this is not usually prolonged beyond 48 h. Very occasionally surrounding organs are damaged during the removal of a large tumour. Examples of this are damage to the tail of the pancreas on the left side (pancreatic fistula) and damage to the stomach, colon or spleen.

Radiotherapy may be given to skeletal metastases for symptomatic control of pain. Local radiotherapy and systemic chemotherapy do not appear helpful. Recently use of immunotherapy (interferon and interleukin-2) has appeared to give some survival advantage, with response rates of up to 30%.

Renal cysts

Renal cysts may be single or present as part of polycystic disease of the kidney. The latter is a familial condition and may affect both kidneys and be associated with cysts in other organs. A single cyst is quite common and usually produces no symptoms. It may be found during investigations for other renal conditions.

Management

Polycystic kidneys may give rise to hypertension and may progress to renal failure. There is little that can be done to prevent this. Eventually renal transplantation may be needed.

Most single renal cysts have a characteristic appearance on ultrasound or CT and reassurance of the patient is usually the only treatment that is required. Occasionally a cyst and a carcinoma may coexist, however, and ultrasound-guided aspiration of the cyst, with cytological examination of the aspirate, is performed on patients who are under 65 years of age, or in whom pain or haematuria is present.

Haematuria

Haematuria is a common presenting complaint and a routine series of investigations is undertaken.

Making the diagnosis

There are three important points to establish in the history.

Is it true haematuria?

Other causes of red urine include the following:

1 Drugs, i.e. rifampicin, para-aminosalicylic acid (PAS), nitrofurantoin and phenindione
2 Foodstuffs such as beetroot
3 Porphyria
4 Haemoglobinuria
5 Factitious haematuria.

The differentiation can be made on the history and on urine microscopy. Ward testing 'stix' for blood are also helpful, though they may also be positive in porphyria and haemoglobinuria.

It is also important to make certain that the blood is not coming from the vagina or rectum. This can be discovered by a careful history and examination.

The causes of true haematuria are listed in Table 23.

Timing of the bleeding in the urinary stream

Blood at the start of the urinary stream suggests a urethral lesion. Blood at the end of the urinary stream suggests a localized bladder lesion. Blood showing throughout micturition

Table 23 Causes of haematuria.

General
Bleeding disorders
Anticoagulants
Haemoglobinopathy

Local
Kidney
Glomerulonephritis
Carcinoma
Trauma
Infarction
Papillary necrosis

Ureter
Tumours
Stones

Bladder
Cystitis
Trauma
Foreign body
Stones
Tumours

Urethra
Benign prostatic hyperplasia
Prostatic carcinoma
Urothelial tumours

suggests a renal, ureteric or diffuse bladder disorder. If there are clots, the shape of these clots may indicate their source. For example, long, thin, worm-like clots come from the kidneys or ureters, and represent casts of the ureters.

Is the haematuria painful or not?

Painful haematuria
The bleeding is usually secondary to a cystitis, which may itself be secondary to other problems such as bladder neck obstruction or stones. You have to remember, however, that infection is a common complication of urothelial tumours.

A diagnosis of cystitis can be confirmed by examining the urine, when an excess of red and white cells will be found and there may be a positive growth on culture.

Painless haematuria
Further investigation is mandatory in order to exclude a carcinoma.

Routine investigations

1 Microscopy and culture of MSU. Red cell casts or protein indicates glomerular disease. Pus cells are present in an acute infection. If they are present and the urine is sterile, the possibility of tuberculosis, tumour or calculi must be considered.

2 Exfoliative cytology of a fresh specimen of urine may show tumour cells.

3 An IVU is mandatory in all cases of painless haematuria and in most cases of painful haematuria. Ultrasound may also be needed.

4 Cystoscopy is nearly always necessary in adults.

5 Full blood count, looking for anaemia.

Management

The treatment of cystitis is with antibiotics, and, if it is the first episode in a young woman, no further investigation may be needed providing the haematuria settles. If it persists, if the infection recurs or if the patient is male, further investigation of the urinary tract by cystoscopy and IVU is required. This is in order to exclude causes such as urothelial tumours, calculi or prostatic hypertrophy.

The management of hypernephroma is dealt with on p. 450, pelviureteric tumours on p. 449 and bladder tumours on p. 460.

Recurrent bleeding due to enlarged veins on a benign prostate may necessitate prostatectomy (p. 476).

Renal transplantation

This operation is indicated for the treatment of terminal renal failure, commonly as an end result of chronic glomerulonephritis, chronic pyelonephritis, polycystic kidneys, obstructive uropathy, hypertensive or diabetic renal failure, or rare metabolic diseases affecting the kidney such as oxalosis. Such patients are usually maintained on a chronic dialysis regimen and after full counselling their name may be placed on a transplant waiting list.

Preoperative management

The patient is grouped, tissue typed and screened for antibodies. The donor may be a living relative or a cadaver. Cadaveric donors may be heart beating donors, when there must be a diagnosis of 'brainstem death', or they may be

Continued on p. 456

Continued.

non-heart beating donors. Once a donor becomes available and the potential recipient is known to have a negative cross-match, arrangements are made to admit him to hospital.

Donor operation

Removal of a kidney from a living donor is similar to a nephrectomy for other reasons (see p. 449). Great care is taken not to damage the renal vessels and the kidney is then perfused as below. This procedure carries the disadvantage of the risk to the health of the donor. It is preferable that a separate team of surgeons looks after the donor.

When a living donor kidney is not available, a cadaveric kidney is used. Once permission has been gained from the relatives, the kidneys are removed through a cruciate or subcostal incision. This operation is often combined with the removal of other organs, including the heart and liver. The renal artery, vein and ureter are all carefully dissected out. The aorta is then cannulated and the kidney perfused with a preserving solution. The kidney is removed, together with the ureter, renal vein and renal artery, which includes a patch of aorta. It is stored in a preservation solution in a sterile plastic bag surrounded by ice.

Recipient operation

The recipient may be dialysed immediately preoperatively. The kidney is transplanted into the retroperitoneal tissues of the iliac fossa. The renal vein is usually anastomosed to the external iliac vein and the renal artery to the external iliac artery. The ureter is implanted into the bladder.

Codes

Blood	2 units
GA/LA	GA
Opn time	2 h
Stay	Variable
Drains out	48 h
Sutures out	10 days
Off work	Variable

Postoperative care

Fluid management in the immediate postoperative period must be meticulous, since there may be a dramatic diuresis of up to 20 L of urine per day for the first 2–3 days. The patient should have a central line and intravenous fluids should be administered to replace measured losses and to maintain a normal central venous pressure (CVP). Not all kidneys function immediately, however, and dialysis may be necessary until the renal function is satisfactory. Standard triple therapy immuno-suppression with cyclosporin, aza-thioprine and prednisolone are started immediately. A full blood count, electrolytes, urea and creatinine should be measured daily. Cyclosporin levels should initially be moni-tored weekly until stable.

The pulse, blood pressure and temperature must be care-fully monitored. Fever in the first 3–4 days, with deteriorating urine output, may indicate early (accelerated) graft rejec-tion. Common complications of renal transplantation, apart from rejection, include infection, ureteric obstruction and fluid collections around the kidney. In the long term, these patients are at increased risk of certain malignancies, par-ticularly skin cancers. Long-term immunosuppression, to prevent acute rejection and follow-up are mandatory.

11.2 Conditions of the Lower Urinary Tract

Bladder stones

Bladder calculi have the same aetiology as renal calculi. A stone in the bladder may have originated in the renal pelvis, although if a stone can pass down the ureter it usually manages to pass out through the urethra. In most cases bladder stones form primarily in the bladder. Stone formation is favoured by urinary stasis (e.g. bladder diverticulum, bladder outflow obstruction), infection or the presence of a foreign body.

Recognizing the pattern

Bladder stones can occur in any age group. Males are more commonly affected than females.

The typical pattern of symptoms is pain, frequency and haematuria. The pain is felt in the suprapubic area, perineum and tip of the penis or labium majus. It is worse when the patient is upright and the stone is lying on the trigone. The pain increases with any jolting movements or at the end of micturition. Urinary frequency is also more troublesome during the day and there may be a feeling of incomplete emptying after micturition. Haematuria commonly occurs at the end of the stream. Occasionally there may be intermittent obstruction to urinary flow.

On examination the prostate may be enlarged. In women it may be possible to feel a bladder stone on bimanual vaginal examination.

Proving the diagnosis

1 Test the urine for blood, pus cells and evidence of infection.
2 Request a plain abdominal X-ray. Ninety per cent of bladder stones are radio-opaque.
3 Cystoscopy. This enables one to see the bladder stone and also to look for any predisposing pathology (e.g. prostatic hypertrophy or bladder diverticulum).

Management

A very small stone may be managed conservatively in the hope that it may pass. Larger stones are removed. This may be done either endoscopically or at open operation.

OPERATION: ENDOSCOPIC REMOVAL OF BLADDER STONE (LITHOLAPAXY)

The stone is visualized, using a rigid cystoscope. It must be fragmented prior to removal by using an electrohydraulic lithotriptor, or alternatively by crushing it with a lithotrite. The smaller pieces of the stone are then washed out from the bladder. If there is a urethral stricture or enlarged prostate, this is usually treated at the same time, e.g. by dilatation or transurethral resection of the prostate (TURP) (see pp. 484 and 476).

Codes

Blood	0
GA/LA	GA
Opn time	30–60 min
Stay	2–5 days
Drains out	0
Sutures out	0
Off work	1–2 weeks

Litholapaxy is not suitable for larger or particularly hard stones, or for stones that have formed around a foreign body. In these cases, or if there is another lesion which will require open operation (e.g. a very large prostate or a bladder diverticulum) the stone is removed via an open cystostomy.

OPERATION: CYSTOSTOMY

The bladder is approached by either a transverse suprapubic (Pfannenstiel) incision or a vertical midline incision. The rectus muscles are retracted and the bladder opened. The stone is removed and any predisposing cause also treated. A supra-pubic catheter is left in the bladder, and a urethral catheter if a prostatectomy has been performed. A drain is left in the wound.

Codes

Blood	2 units
GA/LA	GA
Opn time	1–2 h
Stay	10 days
Drains out	Wound 3–5 days; suprapubic catheter 7 days; urethral catheter 5–10 days
Sutures out	5–7 days
Off work	4–6 weeks

Postoperative care
The bladder wound heals in 5–7 days and the catheter is then removed. It is important to avoid urinary infection and prophylactic antibiotics are given over the early postoperative course.

Bladder tumours

Virtually all bladder tumours are malignant and of these, 95% are TCCs. The remainder are rare and are either squamous cell carcinomas (associated with chronic irritation and squamous metaplasia due to bilharzia, bladder stones or indwelling urinary catheters) or adenocarcinomas (associated with ectopia vesicae or persistent urachal remnants).

The majority of TCCs have no known aetiology. However, there is an increased incidence in those who have worked in the dye, rubber and printing industries. β-naphthylamine and benzidine have been implicated as the carcinogens. Smokers have an increased risk of developing TCCs, as have those who have had pelvic irradiation or who have been treated with cyclophosphamide.

Staging (Fig. 92)

TCCs are staged according to the TNM classification (T = tumour, N = nodes, M = metastases). The tumour staging is as follows:

Tis: *in situ* carcinoma affects multiple areas in the bladder and has a tendency to progress to anaplastic and invasive disease

Ta: papillary, no invasion of lamina propria

T_1: invades lamina propria

T_2: invades superficial muscle

T_{3a}: invades deep muscle

T_{3b}: invades perivesical fat

T_4: invades adjoining organs.

If the tumour is staged by the pathologist, then the stage is prefixed by 'p' (i.e. Ta becomes pTa).

Tumours are also graded on histological appearance:

G1: well differentiated

G2: moderately differentiated

G3: poorly differentiated.

The patient is usually elderly and the disease is four times more common in men.

Ninety per cent of patients present with painless haematuria, occasionally passing clots which may lead to clot retention. Fifteen per cent have frequency and dysuria due to carcinoma

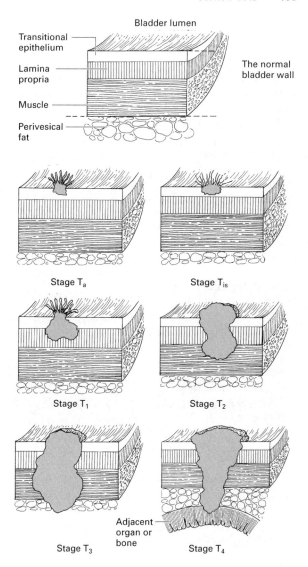

Bladder lumen

Transitional epithelium

Lamina propria

Muscle

Perivesical fat

The normal bladder wall

Stage T_a

Stage T_{is}

Stage T_1

Stage T_2

Stage T_3

Adjacent organ or bone

Stage T_4

Fig. 92 The staging of bladder tumours.

in situ or to associated infection. Obstruction of the bladder neck may cause the symptoms of retention of urine. Involvement of the ureteric orifices can cause hydronephrosis and loin pain. Nerve involvement causes continuous suprapubic pain radiating to the groin and perineum.

Usually there are no signs. The patient may be anaemic secondary to prolonged or severe blood loss. In advanced cases abdominal examination may reveal a palpable mass in the pelvis, enlarged lymph nodes in the groin or a palpable liver.

Proving the diagnosis

1 Urine microscopy and culture. This will demonstrate the presence of red cells due to bleeding and white cells due to infection, or occasionally sterile pyuria due to the tumour.

2 Urine cytology. This may show the presence of malignant cells, particularly if there is carcinoma *in situ*.

3 IVU. The tumour may appear as a filling defect in the bladder and the function of both kidneys can be assessed.

4 Flexible cystoscopy. This is the gold standard investigation, since it allows the tumour to be visualized.

Assessment and staging

This is performed under general (or spinal) anaesthetic. The tumour is viewed through a rigid cystoscope, biopsied and a bimanual examination is performed to assess the degree of invasion. For invasive tumours (T2 and above) a CT scan is performed.

A chest X-ray is performed and blood is taken for a full blood count and urea, creatinine and electrolytes to assess renal function.

OPERATION: CYSTOSCOPY AND EXAMINATION UNDER ANAESTHESIA

Typical well-differentiated non-invasive tumours look like a sea anemone and may be multiple. An invasive tumour appears solid and may be ulcerated. The lesion is biopsied, taking normal surrounding tissue and muscle if possible. If the tumour appears superficial, a full transurethral resection may be performed (see below). Biopsies should also be taken of 'normal' mucosa away from the tumour, to check for carcinoma *in situ*.

Bimanual examination is performed both before and after biopsy/resection of the tumour.

Codes

Blood	Group and save
GA/LA	GA
Opn time	20–30 min
Stay	1–2 days
Drains out	Catheter out 24 h
Sutures out	0
Off work	Variable, depending on need for further treatment

Management

Carcinoma *in situ* may be treated with a course of intravesical immunotherapy (bacille Calmette–Guérin or BCG), following which a further cystoscopy is performed and biopsies taken. If there is evidence of residual disease, then cystectomy should be considered.

Superficial TCCs (stages T_a and T_1) are treated initially by transurethral resection. For multiple tumours, a course of intravesical chemotherapy (mitomycin C or epirubicin) or immunotherapy (BCG) is appropriate. All patients with superficial bladder tumours need to be followed up with regular check cystoscopies, initially after 3 months, as recurrence is likely. Recurrences are treated by cystodiathermy. Five per cent of superficial tumours become invasive.

Invasive TCCs (stages T_2, T_3 and T_4) are treated by radiotherapy and a salvage cystectomy is performed if tumour recurrence occurs or severe radiation cystitis ensues. Alternatively, some surgeons prefer to perform a primary cystectomy.

Radiotherapy may also be used for palliation of advanced carcinoma, to relieve symptoms of haematuria, local pain, frequency of micturition and incontinence. It must be remembered, however, that radiotherapy may also cause these symptoms.

OPERATION: TRANSURETHRAL RESECTION OF BLADDER TUMOUR (TURBT)

The tumour is excised completely, including the superficial layer of bladder wall muscle in its base, using the resectoscope. The specimens are sent for histological staging. The main danger of this procedure is bladder wall perforation.

Codes

Blood	Group and save
GA/LA	GA
Opn time	30–60 min
Stay	3–4 days
Drains out	Catheter out 2–5 days, when bleeding stopped
Sutures out	0
Off work	1–2 weeks

OPERATION: CYSTECTOMY

If the patient is to have an ileal conduit, the site of this should be established preoperatively and the skin marked.

A lower midline incision is made and a full laparotomy performed. The bladder is removed *en bloc* with the iliac and obturator lymph nodes. In males, the prostate is also removed and in females, the uterus, fallopian tubes and ovaries. The urethra is only excised if there is evidence of urethral disease.

Following the cystectomy, one of several procedures is performed in order to provide a means of draining the urine.

1 Ileal conduit. The ureters are sutured to a segment of isolated ileum, which drains the urine continuously via an ileostomy, into a bag on the patient's abdomen.

2 Continent ileal pouch. The principle is the same as above, except that the urine is stored in a pouch fashioned from a segment of ileum and/or caecum. This is catheterized intermittently by the patient through a small abdominal stoma.

3 Neobladder. A 'new bladder' is fashioned from a segment of ileum or colon, sutured to the internal urethral meatus and the ureters are implanted into this.

Codes

Blood	4–6 units
GA/LA	GA
Opn time	3–4 h
Stay	3 weeks
Drains out	5 days
Sutures out	10 days
Off work	2 months

Postoperative care

There may be much blood loss during this procedure, so the patient must be monitored carefully postoperatively, for signs of haemodynamic instability or evidence of further bleeding. Often these patients are kept in the intensive care or high-dependency unit for the first 24 h. The urine output must be watched closely, as must the patient's renal function. Breakdown of the urinary anastomosis may result in a urinary fistula (see p. 64). If there is an ileostomy, it should be checked regularly for signs of ischaemia (oedema, dusky blue colour). The long-term sequelae of diverting the ureters into a segment of bowel include chronic urinary infections and, in the long term, pyelonephritis.

Bladder diverticulum

This is an extrusion of bladder mucosa through the hypertro-phied muscle of the bladder wall. It is most often acquired as a pulsion diverticulum secondary to outflow obstruction and is usually close to the ureteric orifice. Very occasionally it is con-genital, arising from remnants of the urachus in the midline.

Symptoms are due to urinary stasis and secondary infection, with calculus formation. A diverticulum may cause a hydrone-phrosis by compressing the ureter. Occasionally a carcinoma develops in a diverticulum and, because of the lack of a muscle coat, extravesical spread occurs early.

Recognizing the pattern

The patient is usually male and over the age of 50 years.

Haematuria or recurrent cystitis may occur. Sometimes there is a history of double voiding of urine (pis-en-deux), the first batch being clear and the second batch being cloudy as the diverticulum drains its contents into the bladder. Diverticula are not infrequently found inadvertently on an IVU and may be symptomless.

Usually no signs are found on examination. Rectal examina-tion may reveal a large prostate.

Proving the diagnosis

1 An IVU or retrograde cystogram will demonstrate the diver-ticulum by filling it with contrast.

2 Cystoscopy with the bladder distended demonstrates the opening of the diverticulum.

Management

Provided any outflow obstruction of the bladder is treated, and provided the diverticulum itself is asymptomatic and uninfected, it can be left alone. However, if symptoms or the complications listed above ensue, then the diverticulum should be removed.

Preoperative management

The patient should be given a course of antibiotics and, if necessary, bladder washouts for 4 days before operation, if there is evidence of infection.

OPERATION: RESECTION OF DIVERTICULUM

A cystoscopy is performed initially and the ureteric orifice catheterized for identification. The bladder is approached

Continued on p. 466

Continued.

extraperitoneally. The diverticulum is dissected out, separated from the ureter and then excised and the hole in the bladder closed.

Codes

Blood .... Group and save
GA/LA .... GA
Opn time .... 90 min
Stay .... 7–10 days
Drains out .... Catheter 10 days; extravesical drain
                                          3 days
Sutures out .... 7–10 days
Off work .... 4–6 weeks

Postoperative care
A short course of antibiotics may be given to cover the operation and the first few days afterwards. The only major complications to watch for are urinary tract infection and urinary fistula (see p. 64).

Cystitis

Cystitis is the term used to describe inflammation of the bladder. There are several causes (see Table 24) although infection is the commonest and is dealt with in section 1.8.

Recognizing the pattern

The typical symptoms of cystitis are frequency of micturition and burning dysuria. The patient may also complain of suprapubic pain, haematuria, urgency, urge incontinence and nocturia.

Table 24 Causes of cystitis

Infective	Idiopathic
	Secondary to
	diabetes mellitus
	pregnancy
	residual urine
	stone
	foreign body (e.g. catheter)
	enterovesical fistula
Interstitial cystitis	
Radiation cystitis	
Drugs	e.g. Surgam, cyclophosphamide

On examination there are often no physical signs, although there may be suprapubic tenderness. There is often an associated pyrexia.

Proving the diagnosis

1 MSU. White cells are characteristically found. There may also be red cells in the urine. If there is infection, the organisms may be seen on direct microscopy or may be grown in culture. This is often the only investigation that is required.

2 Cystoscopy. This investigation is required for recurrent infective cystitis as well as for persistent symptoms without evidence of infection. The appearance of radiation cystitis is typical, showing multiple areas of friable mucosa and telangiectasia. The bladder capacity is often very small. In interstitial cystitis the bladder capacity is often very small also, and on filling, an ulcer (Hunner's ulcer) may appear.

3 Bladder biopsy. This is indicated if interstitial cystitis is suspected, and also to exclude carcinoma *in situ* which may present is a similar way.

4 IVU and ultrasound of the urinary tract are indicated if there is recurrent infective cystitis in a female, or a single episode in males and children, or persistent infection despite adequate antibiotic treatment.

Management

Infective cystitis is treated with the appropriate antibiotic. Prophylactic antibiotics (e.g. trimethoprim 200 mg *nocte*) may help prevent infections.

Radiation cystitis may require repeated cystoscopies and diathermy of bleeding vessels. If the bleeding is persistent or excessive, a cystectomy is sometimes performed.

Interstitial cystitis (cause unknown, but may be related to an autoimmune aetiology) is also difficult to treat. Various treatments have been tried, including bladder distension to increase capacity, oral steroids or antihistamines and intravesical dimethyl sulphoxide or heparin. As with radiation cystitis, cystectomy may be the final solution for these patients.

Incontinence

This is the involuntary loss of urine. It occurs when the pressure in the bladder exceeds the resistance in the outflow tract. It may be classified as follows:

1 *Overflow incontinence.* This is due to overdistension of the bladder as a result of outflow obstruction or neurological disease.

2 *Urge incontinence.* The patient experiences a strong urge to micturate and is unable to inhibit the passage of urine. It is a result of overactivity of the detrusor muscle of the bladder and may be due to neurological disease, outflow obstruction or there may be no apparent cause.

3 *Stress incontinence.* The patient passes urine following rises in intra-abdominal pressure (e.g. on standing or coughing). It is due to reduced competence of the urethral sphincter mechanism. This occurs most commonly in women following childbirth. It may also occur in neurological diseases or following menopause in females.

4 *Passive incontinence.* There is continuous loss of urine. This may be via a vesicovaginal fistula or may occur if the urethral sphincter mechanism is totally incompetent.

Recognizing the pattern

The patient is usually elderly. As well as the history of incontinence, factors relating to the aetiology of the incontinence may be elicited. In both overflow and urge incontinence the patient may have associated neurological symptoms or a history of poor urinary flow. In stress incontinence female patients often describe difficult or multiple births.

On examination patients with overflow incontinence may have a palpable bladder. A neurological examination should be performed. In females, a vaginal speculum examination may show the impression of the bladder (cystocoele) or rectum (rectocoele) in the vagina.

Proving the diagnosis

An MSU should be examined since urinary tract infection often causes bladder irritability and urge incontinence, especially in the elderly. An ultrasound of the bladder may reveal chronic retention of urine in patients with overflow incontinence. Urodynamic studies are the definitive examination. Fluid is instilled into the bladder, while the intravesical pressure is monitored. In urge incontinence, characteristic rises in intravesical pressure are found as a result of abnormal detrusor muscle contractions. Any loss of urine associated with stress incontinence can also be noted.

Management

Infection is treated with the appropriate antibiotic. If there is neurological disease causing overflow incontinence, the bladder may be emptied by intermittent self-catheterization or an indwelling catheter. Incontinence due to outflow obstruction is treated by relieving the obstruction. Urge incontinence due to bladder instability may be helped by the use of anticholinergic medication (e.g. oxybutynin).

Stress incontinence should be treated initially by weight loss and physiotherapy, aiming to strengthen the pelvic floor musculature. More severe stress incontinence, which is not helped by these techniques, may be treated by an operation such as colposuspension. Other methods of increasing urethral resistance include topical application of oestrogen in postmenopausal women and injection of plastics around the urethra. In some men with incompetent sphincters, it may be possible to insert an artificial sphincter.

OPERATION: COLPOSUSPENSION
This is performed via a suprapubic transverse (Pfannenstiel) incision. The vagina is lifted out of the pelvis and sutured to the pubic bone, thus increasing the urethrovesical angle. A catheter is usually left in the bladder.

Codes

Blood	Group and save
GA/LA	GA
Opn time	40 min
Stay	4–5 days
Drains out	Catheter out 3 days
Sutures out	7–10 days
Off work	4 weeks

It is often not possible to render incontinent patients totally dry. It is important to provide continence aids such as pads (for men and women) and urine collecting devices (for men).

Acute retention of urine

This is painful complete inability to pass urine of sudden onset. It is most commonly due to an enlarged prostate in an elderly man. Other less common causes include urethral stricture, prostatic carcinoma, stones or blood clot in the urethra, urinary tract infection, constipation, neurological disease (e.g. cauda equina compression and multiple sclerosis), pregnancy, pelvic tumour and drugs (e.g. alcohol and anticholinergics). Trauma causing acute retention is considered on p. 664. Postoperative retention of urine is considered on p. 60.

Recognizing the pattern

The patient presents complaining of an inability to pass urine, and suprapubic pain, which characteristically comes in spasms. There may be a history of chronic symptoms secondary to bladder outflow obstruction.

On examination the bladder is enlarged and tender. The urethra should be palpated for stones or stricture and a rectal examination should be done to assess the size of the prostate and to exclude constipation (particularly in the elderly).

Proving the diagnosis

The diagnosis is proved by catheterization (see below).

Further investigations should be arranged to try and discover the cause.

1 Test the urine for blood or signs of infection
2 Perform a white cell count and haemoglobin
3 Measure the urea and electrolytes to assess renal function
4 Perform an abdominal X-ray to look for bladder calculi. This may also show constipation or bony secondaries from carcinoma.

Management

The patient should be admitted. If he is not in too much distress, conservative measures may be attempted first. These include strong opiate analgesia, privacy, the sound of running water and standing the patient up. A hot bath also helps.

If conservative methods fail or if he is very distressed or uncomfortable, then the patient must be catheterized. This is a technique that every medical student must learn properly. Although it appears easy, if it is done badly or carelessly, urinary tract infection and urethral damage may result.

PROCEDURE: URETHRAL CATHETERIZATION

A 12- or 14-gauge Foley catheter is usually large enough and is inserted with strict, aseptic technique. An assistant should be available. Firstly, prepare the trolley and make sure that everything you require is there. After cleansing the penis or vulva, squeeze plenty of local anaesthetic lubricant gel into the urethra. Poor lubrication is a frequent cause of failure to catheterize. After allowing time for the anaesthesia to work, pass the catheter gently but firmly. If resistance occurs, maintain this gentle firm pressure. Do not force the catheter as this may cause further spasm and oedema, and could create a false tract. As the bladder is entered, urine flows. This may take a few seconds as the lubricant is cleared from the inside of the catheter.

Pass most of the catheter up into the bladder and then inflate the balloon (if present). Connect the catheter to a bag. If you encounter difficulty passing the catheter, call someone with more experience before you damage the urethra. After catheterizing a male, pull the foreskin over the glans again or a paraphimosis may result. After catheterization the urine is drained into a bag. Failure to pass a catheter may be evidence of a urethral stricture.

PROCEDURE: SUPRAPUBIC CATHETERIZATION

If urethral catheterization is not successful, suprapubic catheterization is required. Local anaesthetic is infiltrated above the symphysis pubis and a catheter is inserted through a small incision via a trocar. It is important to keep in the midline. Make sure that you can feel the bladder and that you can aspirate urine with the needle used for infiltrating the local anaesthetic. Once the catheter is in the bladder, inflate the balloon (if present) to secure it. The catheter is then secured with a stitch. Remember to push enough catheter into the bladder to allow it to remain inside once the bladder has emptied. If the catheter does come out, it must not be reintroduced when the bladder is empty as the trocar may enter the peritoneum and damage the bowel.

Further management

Postoperative or bed-ridden patients who have gone into acute retention can have the catheter removed once they are mobile. If acute retention recurs, the catheter is reinserted for 24–48 h. Once the patient is up and in less pain, the problem usually resolves. Similarly, following acute retention secondary to constipation or urinary tract infection, the catheter may be removed once the condition has been treated.

Patients with acute retention due to prostatic enlargement and who are fit can be treated by early prostatectomy. With 'acute on chronic' retention time must be allowed for a general assessment and the detection and treatment of any chronic renal failure before a prostatectomy can be undertaken.

In a very elderly patient who is quite clearly unfit for operation, the only solution may be long-term catheter drainage. Small, soft, silastic catheters are available for this and the patient may either change this himself or have it done by a district nurse at home.

Continued on p. 472

Continued.

Antibiotics and catheter management

1 When antibiotic prophylaxis is required on a patient with chronic obstruction and probable infection, either ampicillin with intravenous gentamicin or cefotaxime can be used. If the organism is known to be resistant to these, try ciprofloxacin which may be given either intravenously or orally.

2 If the patient is asymptomatic or has local symptoms only, even in the presence of urinary growth, do not treat until the catheter is removed. Gram-positive organisms (e.g. faecal streptococci and coagulase-negative staphylococci) are then likely to clear spontaneously whereas Gram-negative bacilli (e.g. *Escherichia coli*) often require 3 days of oral antibiotic to clear (prescribe according to susceptibility).

3 If the catheter has to be removed and then replaced because of blockage, then use a chlorhexidine washout (inject 100 ml of 0.02% aqueous chlorhexidine solution, hold for 30 min, then release and change catheter).

4 If the patient's catheter is functioning and should not be removed, but there are systemic symptoms including pyrexia, then the drug of choice is probably oral ciprofloxacin 100–250 mg b.d. Also check the organism's susceptibility.

Bladder outflow obstruction

This is usually due to disease of the prostate (particularly benign prostatic hyperplasia, BPH) and urethra.

Recognizing the pattern

It usually affects men, who may present with either obstructive symptoms (hesitancy, poor flow and terminal dribbling) or irritative symptoms (frequency of micturition, urgency and nocturia) or a combination of both. Eventually, acute or chronic retention of urine may occur.

Proving the diagnosis

As with the investigation of incontinence, bladder outflow obstruction can be investigated by carrying out urodynamic studies, which should include measurement of the urinary flow rate. In some centres, a videocystometrogram is performed using contrast material and the bladder and urethra observed under X-ray screening during filling and voiding.

Certain patients require further investigation by urethrocystoscopy. This may be performed as an outpatient procedure using the flexible cystoscope. Alternatively, a rigid cystoscope may be used, when the procedure should be performed under general anaesthesia.

Management

Preoperative management
It is common practice, on completion of this examination, to proceed to definitive treatment under the same anaesthetic. If this is intended, make sure that theatres know and that the appropriate instruments are ready (e.g. a resectoscope or urethrotome).

OPERATION: URETHROCYSTOSCOPY
The urethra is examined on the way into the bladder. A forward-viewing cystoscope is used. This is later changed to a side-viewing cystoscope to examine the bladder.

Codes

Blood	0/group and save
GA/LA	GA
Opn time	10–20 min
Stay	Day case/24 h
Drains out	0
Sutures out	0
Off work	Variable

Benign prostatic hyperplasia (BPH)

This is a benign nodular or diffuse proliferation of both the musculofibrous and glandular elements in the prostate gland. It involves the inner zone of the gland, unlike carcinoma. The rest of the gland is compressed to form a capsule. It occurs to a varying degree in all men over the age of 50 years. The cause is uncertain but possible factors are an imbalance between androgens and oestrogens in later life or a benign neoplastic process. The enlargement causes elongation, narrowing and kinking of the prostatic urethra.

There is no relation between the size of the prostate on examination and the degree of obstruction. The obstruction results in hypertrophy of the detrusor muscle, producing a trabeculated appearance of the bladder wall. The mucosa may protrude between bands of muscle, forming saccules or diverticula. Eventually the muscle may become atonic, leading to chronic urinary retention, infection and stone formation. Alternatively, the muscle may become unstable, leading to abnormal contractions. Engorged veins at the base of the bladder may burst and cause haematuria. Back pressure may eventually cause obstruction of the upper tracts with hydronephrosis and eventually renal failure.

Recognizing the pattern

The patient is usually aged between 55 and 75 years.

The history is of a poor urinary stream with hesitancy and terminal dribbling. Micturition is incomplete, resulting in a gradually increasing volume of residual urine. As the bladder hypertrophies, the detrusor becomes unstable, resulting in urinary frequency and nocturia. There may be associated urgency of micturition and urge incontinence. The patient may present with an episode of acute retention, commonly precipitated by drinking, bed rest or being trapped in a situation where he has to hold on too long due to lack of toilet facilities.

Excess residual urine may cause overflow incontinence. Haematuria may occur. Finally, there are symptoms such as loin pain, thirst, malaise or mental impairment due to chronic renal failure.

The prostate is examined through the rectum. Make sure the patient's bladder is empty. Assess the following:

1 Shape
2 Symmetry
3 Surface
4 Size
5 Sulcus of the prostate.

The sulcus is the median groove on its posterior surface. It is preserved in BPH but may disappear in malignant disease. In a normal prostate it is possible to slide the finger forward round each side of the convex surface of the gland. It is 2–3 cm across. In BPH the gland is smooth but symmetrical, the surface is flattened and it is difficult or impossible to get the examining finger forward round each side.

There may be general evidence of chronic renal failure and uraemia, e.g. dehydration, anaemia, skin pallor or hypotension. Abdominal examination may reveal loin tenderness and a palpable bladder.

Proving the diagnosis

Investigations performed to confirm the diagnosis of BPH are as follows:

1 An ultrasound of the urinary tract. This looks for hydronephrosis secondary to back pressure, postmicturition

residual urine in the bladder and the size of the prostate gland.

2 Test MSU for blood, protein and glucose and to exclude infection.

3 Send blood for urea, creatinine and electrolytes to assess renal function, prostate-specific antigen (PSA) to screen for prostate cancer and full blood count in case of anaemia secondary to blood loss or renal failure.

4 Urodynamic studies.

5 Urethrocystoscopy.

Management

If the symptoms are mild and renal function is normal, a policy of 'watchful waiting' may be undertaken. Otherwise, medical or surgical treatment should be considered.

Medical

Antiandrogens (e.g. finasteride) are used to reduce the volume of the prostate gland, and α-adrenoceptor antagonists (e.g. terazosin) to relax the smooth muscle of the prostate and the proximal urethra. These may be used to improve urinary flow, particularly in men with minor to moderate symptoms or those awaiting prostatectomy.

Surgical

The usual treatment of this condition is surgical removal of the prostate gland via the following procedures:

1 Transurethral resection of the prostate (TURP)

2 Retropubic prostatectomy

3 Laser prostatectomy — this is available in some centres and is gaining popularity since it may offer the prospect of day-case prostatic surgery.

The indications for prostatectomy for proven BPH include the following:

1 Severe symptoms secondary to BPH

2 Complications of BPH (acute retention, renal failure, bladder stone formation, recurrent infection, heavy haematuria, detrusor instability).

Preoperative management

If the urine is infected, this must be sterilized with antibiotics before operation. Any uraemia is improved by a few days of catheter drainage. Dehydration and anaemia must also be corrected.

Continued on p. 476

Continued.

The patient should be told that one result of prostatectomy is retrograde ejaculation, resulting in a reduction in the quantity of ejaculate on sexual intercourse. In younger patients this may mean a reduction in fertility and this should be discussed with them preoperatively.

OPERATION: TRANSURETHRAL RESECTION OF THE PROSTATE (TURP)

The operation is a specialist procedure requiring experience with a resectoscope. The whole of the lateral and middle lobes of the prostate are resected. On completion a urethral catheter is inserted. The prostatic chippings must be sent for histology to exclude a prostatic carcinoma.

Codes

Blood .... 2 units
GA/LA .... GA
Opn time .... 30–90 min
Stay .... 3–5 days
Drains out .... Urethral catheter 2–3 days
Sutures out 0
Off work .... 4 weeks

Postoperative care
See below.

OPERATION: RETROPUBIC PROSTATECTOMY (MILLIN'S)

A preliminary cystoscopy is performed. The bladder and prostate are approached via a suprapubic extraperitoneal abdominal incision. The anterior prostatic capsule is opened transversely and the adenoma identified and enucleated. The veru montanum and external sphincter are carefully preserved. A wide-bore three-way irrigating urethral catheter is inserted and the prostatic capsule closed.

Codes

Blood .... 2 units
GA/LA .... GA
Opn time .... 60–90 min
Stay .... 10–14 days
Drains out .... Irrigating urethral catheter
                                            3–5 days; retropubic drain 24 h
Sutures out .... 7–10 days
Off work .... 4–6 weeks

Postoperative care

Ensure that the catheter drains satisfactorily. A bladder irrigation system is usually set up, using either a triple-lumen urethral catheter or a separate suprapubic catheter. Normal saline or sterile water are instilled daily (3–4 L). This is left running for 24 h or until the urine is sufficiently clear of clots to drain freely.

Should clot retention occur, it is relieved by syringing the bladder with 50–100 cm³ of normal saline (do not withdraw the syringe too forcefully as this causes the catheter to collapse). Occasionally it may be necessary to take the patient back to theatre to control severe bleeding.

The catheter is removed once the urine is clear of blood. Do not remove it too soon as it may be difficult to reintroduce in the early postoperative period.

Early postoperative complications include primary and secondary haemorrhage, urinary tract infection, septicaemia, the 'TUR syndrome' (which is due to absorption of irrigant fluid and may cause hyponatraemia or hypotension if extreme), failed trial without catheter and deep vein thrombosis. Long-term complications include urinary incontinence, retrograde ejaculation and urethral stricture.

Prostatic carcinoma

This is an adenocarcinoma. There is no known aetiological factor, although it often coexists with BPH. The tumour is usually androgen dependent.

It arises in the outer zone of the gland (unlike BPH). It can still occur therefore after a transurethral prostatectomy for BPH. Local direct spread may involve the bladder, the ureters or the urethra. Direct invasion posteriorly is hindered by the fascia of Denonvilliers and involvement of the rectum is unusual.

Blood-borne spread occurs to bone, particularly the pelvis, lumbar vertebrae or greater trochanter of the femur via the communications of the prostatic venous plexus. Bony secondaries are characteristically osteosclerotic and appear on X-ray film as areas of increased density.

The stages of the tumour's development are shown in Fig. 93.

Recognizing the pattern

The patient is usually over the age of 65 years, though the condition is being diagnosed more frequently in younger men.

Prostatic carcinoma usually presents with a disturbance of flow similar to BPH. The history of flow disturbance is usually

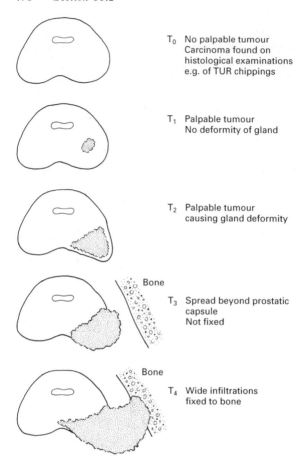

T_0 No palpable tumour
Carcinoma found on
histological examinations
e.g. of TUR chippings

T_1 Palpable tumour
No deformity of gland

T_2 Palpable tumour
causing gland deformity

Bone

T_3 Spread beyond prostatic
capsule
Not fixed

Bone

T_4 Wide infiltrations
fixed to bone

Fig. 93 The stages of prostatic carcinoma.

shorter. Other presentations are with back pain or bilateral
sciatica (due to vertebral secondaries), neurological lesions due
to compression of the spinal cord or the general symptoms of
carcinomatosis.

Rectal examination characteristically shows asymmetrical,
nodular enlargement of the prostate, which feels hard and irregular with obliteration of the posterior median sulcus.
Metastases in bone may cause areas of tenderness, particularly
in the pelvis, femur and lumbar region of the back.

Proving the diagnosis

The diagnosis is proved by the following investigations:
1 Prostatic specific antigen (PSA) is the most specific tumour

marker for prostatic carcinoma. It may also be raised in some patients with BPH, prostatitis and following TURP. In prostatic carcinoma, its level correlates to a degree with the stage and grade of the tumour. In metastatic disease it may be elevated to a level more than 10 times normal. It is also used as a follow-up investigation in patients with prostatic carcinoma, since an increase in levels may herald the development of metastases. In centres where this test is not available, prostatic acid phosphatase may be measured instead.

2 Histology. Tissue may be obtained for histological diagnosis and grading by either biopsy or, more often, at prostatectomy. Biopsy is done with a Trucut needle by the transrectal or transperineal route, under antibiotic cover. Transrectal ultrasound may help in guiding the needle toward suspicious lesions for transrectal biopsy.

Other investigations to assess and stage the disease are as follows:

1 Test the urine for signs of infection
2 Full blood count
3 Urea and electrolytes to assess renal function
4 Alkaline phosphatase (raised if there are bony secondaries)
5 Chest X-ray to look for metastases
6 Technetium bone scan. This will demonstrate the presence of bony metastases. It is sometimes necessary to supplement this with plain X-rays of suspicious areas.

IVU and CT scan may also be helpful. An IVU will demonstrate any upper tract dilatation secondary to obstruction by infiltration of tumour around the ureteric orifices. A CT scan will demonstrate pelvic lymph node metastases and can help in showing whether there is extracapsular spread of the tumour.

Management

Disease which is localized to the prostate may be treated by observation alone, since many prostatic cancers do not progress within the patient's life span, particularly in older men. For younger men, however, localized disease should be treated by external beam radiotherapy or radical prostatectomy.

The mainstay of treatment of metastatic disease is to decrease androgen activity. This may be done either by bilateral orchidectomy (subcapsular orchidectomy is usually performed) or using hormonal therapy. The available hormonal treatments include antiandrogens such as flutamide

Continued on p. 480

Continued.

or luteinizing hormone-releasing hormone (LHRH) agonists such as goserelin (Zoladex). Oestrogens are rarely used, despite their efficacy, because of the high incidence of thromboses (coronary thrombosis, strokes and deep venous thrombosis) associated with these drugs. Pain from bony metastases may be alleviated by external beam radiotherapy.

If there is bladder outflow obstruction then this is usually treated by TURP.

OPERATION: SUBCAPSULAR ORCHIDECTOMY

The scrotum is incised and the testes exposed. The capsule of each testicle (tunica albuginea) is incised vertically and the testicular tissue inside removed. The tunica is then resutured after careful haemostasis, and the testicle replaced in the scrotum. Occasionally a silastic prosthesis is placed inside the tunica albuginea.

Codes

Blood	Group and save
GA/LA	GA
Opn time	30–60 min
Stay	2 days
Drains out	0
Sutures out	Absorbable sutures used
Off work	1 month

Postoperative care

A scrotal support helps to alleviate discomfort from scrotal swelling or bruising.

OPERATION: RADICAL PROSTATECTOMY

This operation may be performed in the early stages of prostate carcinoma as an alternative to radiotherapy.

Preoperative management

Any urinary infection must be treated. Clotting studies should be performed, since prostatic carcinoma may cause fibrinolysis.

Operation

The prostate is approached either through the retropubic space, via a midline incision or through a perineal incision. The prostate gland and the seminal vesicles are isolated and removed and the bladder outflow refashioned and joined to the membranous urethra using a catheter as a splint. Care is taken not to damage the external urethral sphincter or the nerves.

Codes

Blood	2–4 units
GA/LA	GA
Opn time	2–3 h
Stay	2–3 weeks
Drains out	Retropubic space 5–7 days; catheter 7–10 days
Sutures out	7–10 days
Off work	4–6 weeks

Postoperative care
The main risks with this procedure are of urinary incontinence and impotence.

Acute prostatitis

This is acute inflammation of the prostate gland. It may follow bacteraemia or direct infection after urethral instrumentation. The organisms commonly involved are *Escherichia coli*, *Streptococcus faecalis*, *Staphylococcus aureus* and *Neisseria gonorrhoeae*.

Recognizing the pattern

The patient may be an adult of any age but is usually over 35 years.

The history is of symptoms of general infection including malaise, fever, rigors and muscle pain. There is pain in the perineum and frequency of micturition, dysuria or occasional haematuria. An abscess may cause acute retention or pain on defaecation.

On examination the patient is pyrexial and rectal examination reveals a very tender, swollen, boggy prostate. Occasionally there is an abscess and the prostate is hot, tender and fluctuant and projects into the rectum. Palpate the testicles to exclude epididymo–orchitis.

Proving the diagnosis

An attempt should be made to isolate the causative organism from the urine. The patient is asked to micturate and the first urine passed is collected separately from the rest and examined.

Management

Treatment consists of bed rest and the patient is encouraged to drink as much as possible. Not all antibiotics gain good access to the prostate. The more effective antibiotics include ciprofloxacin (500 mg 12-hourly), trimethoprim (200 mg 12-hourly) and erythromycin (500 mg 6-hourly).

Prostatitis is a difficult infection to eradicate completely so antibiotics are continued for at least 6 weeks.

If an abscess is present, it must be drained. This may either be performed per urethra with a resectoscope or through the perineum.

Chronic prostatitis

This is a condition characterized by recurrent mild episodes of acute inflammation of the prostate gland or by constant pain in the perineum. It may be due to persistent infection, usually with *Chlamydia trachomatis*, or there may be an apparently sterile chronic inflammation.

Recognizing the pattern

The patient is usually middle aged to elderly.

The history is one of persistent episodes of perineal pain varying in severity and frequency and often causing great distress. Other symptoms include low backache, mild bouts of fever and dysuria.

On examination the prostate may be enlarged, firm and irregular. Massage of the prostate will produce a discharge which contains pus cells and may grow organisms such as *Chlamydia*, faecal streptococci, coliforms or anaerobes.

Proving the diagnosis

This is essentially clinical with laboratory confirmation of the infective organism if possible.

Management

Treatment is with antibiotics, especially doxycycline and trimethoprim, but the condition is difficult to eradicate. Resection of the prostate does not usually help. In some patients with refractory chronic prostatitis, treatment with amitriptyline may help to relieve some of the distressing symptoms.

Urethral stricture

This is narrowing of the urethra causing obstruction to urine flow followed by back pressure on the bladder, ureter and kidney. The signs are similar to those discussed under BPH.

It may be caused by inflammation following infection, usually with *Neisseria gonorrhoeae*, or following instrumentation (e.g. transurethral surgery or catheterization). It may also follow traumatic injury to the urethra. Distal stenoses at the meatus are usually caused by condyloma accuminata or by balanitis xerotica obliterans.

Recognizing the pattern

The patient can be of any age and is usually male.

There may be a history of catheterization, prostatectomy, trauma or urethral infection. The patient presents with flow problems including a poor stream and dribbling. The flow can often be increased by abdominal straining (unlike prostatic hypertrophy where the flow is usually worsened by straining). Fibrosis and narrowing may cause painful ejaculation and very occasionally distortion of the erect organ (chordee) which may make intercourse impossible.

On examination the external genitalia should be inspected for meatal stenosis. The urethra should be carefully palpated along its length and the stricture may be felt. Abdominal examination may reveal a palpable bladder.

Proving the diagnosis

The diagnosis is confirmed by the following:

1 Urethrography. This is a radiological technique using contrast medium to outline the urethra.
2 Urethroscopy. This is carried out as part of a general cystoscopy (see p. 473). It is usually not possible to pass the stricture without dividing it.
3 Urinary flow rate. This will demonstrate the reduced flow associated with the stricture.

Management

A stricture is usually a chronic condition requiring regular follow-up. The initial treatment is commonly by internal urethrotomy and this is followed by regular dilatation. A urethroplasty may occasionally be performed for strictures which remain a problem in spite of these measures.

Continued on p. 484

Continued.

Preoperative management

If the urine is infected, antibiotics should be given and bladder washouts performed. Prophylactic antibiotics are given at induction and oral broad-spectrum antibiotics for 5 days postoperatively.

OPERATION: INTERNAL URETHROTOMY

A urethrotome is passed under direct vision. The stricture is viewed and incised to the required depth. This is followed by dilatation.

Codes

Blood	0
GA/LA	GA
Opn time	15–30 min
Stay	3 days
Drains out	Urethral catheter: anything from several days to 4 weeks
Sutures out	0
Off work	1 week

Postoperative care

In larger strictures, if a urethral catheter is required for longer, it is removed after 1–4 weeks. The patient is followed up regularly and usually requires urethroscopy and dilatation on one or two occasions. If the obstruction continues to recur, then dilatation is performed regularly.

OPERATION: URETHRAL DILATATION

This procedure is performed using specific urethral dilators (bougies or urethral sounds). After applying local anaesthetic lubricant gel they are inserted into the urethra and allowed to enter using minimal pressure. Bougies of gradually increasing diameter are passed, the aim being to stretch the urethra without tearing the mucosa.

Codes

Blood	0
GA/LA	GA or LA
Opn time	20 min
Stay	Outpatient
Drains out	0
Sutures out	0
Off work	1–2 days

Postoperative care

Gram-negative bacteraemia is a possible complication and can be very severe. Any patient whose blood pressure remains low and is confused following the operation, perhaps with an abnormally low temperature, requires urgent administration of the appropriate antibiotics.

Other complications include a urethral tear with haematuria and scarring, which may worsen the stricture.

OPERATION: OPEN URETHROPLASTY

There are many types of operation that are performed using skin flaps to enlarge or refashion the urethral lumen. This procedure is used in the treatment of more complex, long or recurrent strictures.

Prevention

Avoidance of excessive instrumentation of the bladder, care at prostatectomy and the use of narrow, soft catheters for as short a time as possible will all help in cutting down the incidence of this condition.

11.3 Male Genitalia

Conditions of the foreskin

The care of the foreskin remains a mystery to most parents.

Generally speaking it should be left alone for the first year or two of life. Thereafter it can be gently but firmly retracted, usually at bath time. Adhesions gradually separate and the glans becomes fully visible. This process is usually complete by the age of 1–5 years.

In young boys the foreskin is often relatively long and the tip tends to be slightly tight causing a groove as it is retracted on to the penile shaft. This will stretch up by natural processes as development occurs. It must be distinguished from a scarred stricture which can result in a paraphimosis, non-retractile foreskin or even a 'pinhole meatus'.

Non-retractile foreskin

Recognizing the pattern

The patient is usually brought along by his parents, who are concerned that the foreskin does not retract. There may be a history of recurrent balanitis.

On examination. The foreskin is adherent. Check how far it can be retracted and whether there is any stricturing at the tip.

Management

There is no need for surgical treatment until after the age of 4 years unless complications such as recurrent balanitis or phimosis occur. Before this time the only management is to reassure the parents and give advice about the care of the foreskin as above. After the age of 4 years examination under an anaesthetic is performed (see below). The preputial adhesions are separated and a circumcision performed only if there is a phimosis.

Balanoposthitis (balanitis)

This is acute inflammation of the glans and foreskin, usually caused by pyogenic organisms (*Staphylococcus*, *Streptococcus* and coliforms) or fungal infection (*Candida*). It occurs commonly in young boys with a non-retractile foreskin. In elderly patients there may be a predisposing cause such as carcinoma or diabetes.

In adults there is a chronic fibrosing condition of the foreskin, called balanitis xerotica et obliterans (p. 483), of unknown aetiology. It is cured by circumcision.

Recognizing the pattern

The patient with acute balanitis may be of any age and presents with either irritation or pain in the penis, and a discharge from beneath the foreskin. Recurrent balanitis may cause a phimosis with disturbance of micturition.

On examination the inflammation is visible.

Management

The management is to give antibiotics and treat the cause. Frequently this means a circumcision once the inflammation has settled down. In older patients the urine should be tested for sugar.

Phimosis

This is a narrowing of the opening of the foreskin. It can follow trauma or recurrent infection. It may be caused by the parents trying to force adhesions apart too early.

Recognizing the pattern

The patient is usually young and there is a history that the foreskin balloons out on micturition, causing a spraying stream. Adults often complain of pain on intercourse.

On examination. The foreskin is usually long with a small, tight opening.

Management

Management is by circumcision (see below).

Paraphimosis

This condition occurs when a tight foreskin is forcibly retracted back off the glans and cannot be pulled forwards again. The tight band causes obstruction of venous return followed by swelling of the distal foreskin and glans. It can occur at any age.

It is especially common in the elderly patient who after catheterization has not had his foreskin pulled forwards again.

Management

Unless reduced quickly the distal foreskin rapidly becomes so swollen that reduction is impossible. The swollen glans and foreskin are wrapped in a swab and squeezed gently to reduce the oedema. This may be facilitated by the application of ice to the glans and by the use of local anaesthetic gel. Once the oedema has reduced, pressure is applied to the glans to push it back through the tight band. This procedure can, if necessary, be carried out with a dorsal penile nerve block. In some cases a dorsal slit may be required to obtain reduction. Circumcision is performed at a later date when the oedema has settled.

Trauma to the foreskin

A torn frenulum is usually seen in young men following intercourse. Occasionally the foreskin may be caught in the zip of trousers resulting in tears or superficial lacerations.

Management

A torn frenulum usually requires no treatment other than reassurance to the patient and advice about intercourse. A catgut stitch may be required if there is bleeding from the torn frenula artery. A lubricant such as KY jelly may be helpful. If the problem becomes recurrent, a circumcision may become indicated.

OPERATION: CIRCUMCISION

The indications for circumcision are as follows:
1 Phimosis
2 Recurrent balanitis
3 Balanitis xerotica et obliterans
4 Carcinoma of the foreskin
5 Religious reasons. Some people or religious groups practise the rite of circumcision and these ritual circumcisions are usually carried out between the ages of 6 months and 1 year.

Preoperative management
Circumcision should not be done in the presence of ammoniacal dermatitis as this can cause ulceration of the meatus.

Balanoposthitis should be treated with antibiotics before surgery.

If there is a phimosis, this is stretched and preputial adhesions are separated.

A dorsal split is made in the foreskin down to the pre-determined level and the foreskin then carefully removed, preserving sufficient epithelium next to the glans (5 mm). Following haemostasis, the preputial layer of skin is sutured to the skin of the penile shaft using absorbable sutures. Care is taken to align the skin correctly. The wound is dressed and some surgeons place a dressing of anaesthetic jelly around the base of the glans. Alternatively, a suprapubic block of the dorsal nerve of the penis using a long-acting anaesthetic, or a caudal nerve block, is effective.

Codes

Blood	0
GA/LA	GA or LA
Opn time	15–30 min
Stay	Day case
Drains out	0
Sutures out	0
Off work	Up to 1 week

Congenital lesions of the male external genitalia

The male external genitalia are formed by the fusion of the external genital folds around the urethra and its surrounding erectile tissue. Failure of this fusion results in a urethra that opens either at the base of the glans or further down the penile shaft, underneath the body of the penis. This condition is known as hypospadias and requires reconstruction of the penis, usually using the skin of the foreskin. This is usually carried out by paediatric or urological surgeons and is not discussed further here.

Rarely the urethra forms a gutter on the upper surface of the penis. This condition is usually associated with major abnormalities in the structure of the bladder and is known as epispadias.

Carcinoma of the penis

This is a squamous cell carcinoma. It is rare in the UK but occurs more frequently in the Far East and Africa.

Carcinoma of the penis is associated almost exclusively with an intact foreskin and may be related to previous infection with the human papilloma virus. It may start as leucoplakia of the glans. Erythroplasia of Queyrat is the name given to carcinoma *in situ* of the penis. It consists of a persistent red, raw area on the glans. This precancerous condition usually responds to local radiotherapy or application of 5-fluorouracil cream.

With advanced disease the whole penis may be engulfed with malignant growth and the urethra may be invaded. Lymphatic spread occurs to the inguinal nodes. Blood-borne spread is late and rare.

Recognizing the pattern

The patient is usually elderly. The presenting complaint is one of a lump or discharge and irritation. Later the discharge becomes bloody and offensive. The foreskin is usually non-retractile. Advanced disease presents with an ulcerated, fungating lesion destroying the whole penis or a mass in the groin. Urethral obstruction with retention of urine is rare.

On examination the lesion is visible if the foreskin can be retracted. If not, it is usually possible to feel it beneath the foreskin. Most commonly it is an indurated ulcer at the base of the glans penis, although it may be a papillary growth. In 60% of cases the nodes in the groin are enlarged but only half of these are malignant. The rest are due to reactive changes secondary to the inflammation and infection.

Proving the diagnosis

The diagnosis is proved by taking a biopsy, and a circumcision may be required to reveal the growth.

A CT scan of the pelvis may be useful to assess lymphatic spread, if block dissection is contemplated.

Management

Even in the presence of enlarged nodes in the groin, it is usual to treat the primary growth first and then only treat the nodes if they are still enlarged after 3–4 weeks.

Radiotherapy is used in early stage disease with no urethral involvement or for palliation. It can be given either by radioactive implants, by external X-rays or as a radioactive mould fitted around the shaft of the penis. The results are good, with a 60–70% 5-year survival rate. Radiotherapy is also used in the treatment of fixed malignant nodes in the groin.

Surgical treatment is used in the following conditions.
1 When the urethra is involved
2 If the growth has failed to respond to radiotherapy
3 If the groin lymph nodes are persistently enlarged 1 month after the surgery, a block dissection or deep X-ray therapy to the inguinal lymph nodes is performed.

OPERATION: PARTIAL AMPUTATION OF THE PENIS

This operation is performed if there is at least 2 cm of uninvolved penile shaft available at the base. The new urethral meatus must be carefully fashioned to avoid ensuing stricture.

Codes

Blood 0
GA/LA .... GA
Opn time .... 1–2 h
Stay .... 7–14 days
Drains out .... Urethral catheter 7–10 days
Sutures out .... 7 days
Off work .... 1 month

Postoperative care

Once the catheter has been removed, regular meatal dilatations may be required. The patient is followed up regularly to assess the inguinal nodes and to look for local recurrence.

OPERATION: COMPLETE AMPUTATION OF THE PENIS

This operation involves complete removal of the penis from the perineal membrane and ischiopubic ramus. The stump of the urethra is brought out through an incision in the perineum behind the scrotum. Occasionally the testicles and scrotum are also removed as they will get in the way of a urethrostomy.

Codes

Blood .... 2–4 units
GA/LA .... GA
Opn time .... 2–3 h
Stay .... 2 weeks
Drains out .... Urethral catheter 7 days
Sutures out .... 7 days
Off work .... 6 weeks

Scrotal conditions

The following conditions in the scrotum commonly present to the general surgeon:

1 Absent testis
2 Lumps in the scrotum
3 Painful testis.

Absent testis (cryptorchidism)

The testis may be absent from the scrotum either because it is undescended or because it is retractile. The testis develops as a retroperitoneal organ at the lower pole of the kidney and during development descends caudally through the inguinal canal and into the scrotum. Its descent may be either incomplete (arrested at any site along the course of its descent) or abnormal. If it is abnormal the testis is ectopic and can lie in a pubic, inguinal, femoral or perineal site.

A retractile testis has descended normally but is pulled up into the inguinal canal by an active cremasteric reflex.

A true undescended testis is frequently abnormal and may never undergo spermatogenesis. There is evidence, however, that bringing the testis down into its correct place early in life can improve the chances of fertility. There is also an increased danger of malignant change in an undescended testis. Neither of these problems occurs with a retractile testis.

It is therefore important to differentiate clinically between these two causes of absent testis.

Retractile testis

In these boys the cremaster is unusually active and the testis readily retracts up into the groin.

Recognizing the pattern

Although the parents may not have seen the testes in the scrotum, close questioning often reveals the fact that the testis does occasionally appear, particularly during a warm bath. Testes may also have been seen in the scrotum earlier in life, during a routine medical examination.

On examination the scrotum is well developed and looks 'as if it could contain a testis'. The clinician must develop a good examining technique to make the diagnosis. Warm hands, a warm examination room and a warm personality all help. One hand is placed in the groin to occlude the inguinal canal and moved down towards the scrotum so as to 'milk' the testis into the external ring. The testis is then gently trapped by the index finger of the other hand as it emerges. Gentle pressure with the finger and thumb can then pull the retractile testis into the scrotum. If the above manoeuvre fails, getting the patient to squat on the examination couch may reveal the testis.

If the testis does descend to the base of the scrotum, its presence there should be demonstrated to the parents. They can be reassured that it will eventually descend normally and nothing further needs to be done. If the testis only comes part of the way down to the scrotum, it probably is undescended and in this case an orchidopexy will be required.

Undescended testis

An undescended testis should be spotted early in life at a routine medical examination. This will enable plans to be made to bring the testis into the scrotum before the age of 2 years. Frequently, however, the condition is first diagnosed later than this. The longer the testis remains undescended, the greater the danger of infertility. There is also an increased risk of malignancy in the undescended testis, though this risk does not appear to be affected by bringing it into the scrotum.

Less common presentations of the undescended testis include torsion and trauma.

Recognizing the pattern

The patient can present at any age from newborn to between 20 and 30 years old, although in the UK boys usually present in infancy.

On examination the scrotum is underdeveloped and flattened. The condition may be unilateral or bilateral and the position of both testes should be determined. The undescended testis may be palpable in the groin or inguinal canal and should be located if possible.

Management

The undescended testis should be brought into the scrotum by performing an orchidopexy, preferably before the age of 2 years. At this age the operation must be undertaken by an expert as damaging the delicate testicular vessels will bring about infertility. This is exactly what the operation is designed to prevent. Orchidopexy ensures optimal conditions for subsequent development of the testis, as well as making it easier to examine in later years, in view of its risk of

Continued on p. 494

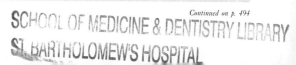

Continued.

malignancy. It also renders it less prone to traumatic injury and torsion.

If the testis is impalpable, it may be located intra-abdominally, or it may be in an inguinal position where it is atrophied and hence impalpable. An ultrasound of the groin may be helpful in locating an undescended testis, as may an abdominal CT scan or laparoscopy. It may be possible to bring an intra-abdominal testis into the scrotum, employing microvascular anastomotic techniques in order to supply it with an adequate blood supply, since the length of the testicular artery will probably be insufficient. If, however, there is a normally sited contralateral testis, then orchidectomy (excision) of the intra-abdominal testis is preferable. This is also the case with an undescended inguinal testis in a male in his late teens and early twenties, as it is unlikely to ever be fertile. Orchidectomy obviates the risk of later malignancy. A prosthesis may be placed in the scrotum at the same operation, for cosmetic appearance.

OPERATION: ORCHIDOPEXY (DARTOS POUCH PROCEDURE)

An incision is made in the groin and the testis found and mobilized together with its vessels. The latter are freed right up into the deep inguinal ring, and further into the abdomen if necessary. They are separated from the processus vaginalis and any small inguinal hernial sac. A subcutaneous pouch is then made in the scrotum between the skin and the dartos muscle. The testis is pulled down through a small hole in the dartos muscle (Fig. 94). Once the bulk of the testis is through this hole it is unable to retract back and hence it becomes fixed in the scrotum. The scrotal and inguinal wounds are closed with a soluble suture.

Codes

Blood	0
GA/LA	GA
Opn time	30 min per side
Stay	Day case
Drains out	0
Sutures out	Absorbable sutures are not removed
Off school or work	2 weeks

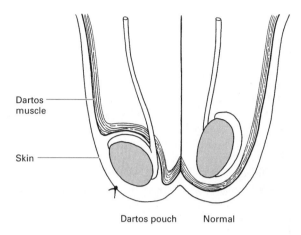

Dartos pouch   Normal

Fig. 94 Dartos pouch orchidopexy.

Postoperative care
The scrotum may be bruised and swollen for a while and the parents may need some reassurance that this will settle down. When a dartos pouch has been made and where the testicular vessels are short the scrotum will he pulled well up into the groin. This should not cause concern providing the testis remains within the scrotal tissues. Apart from these points the postoperative course is usually straightforward.

Lumps in the scrotum

Patients with lumps in the scrotum are common cases in surgical examinations. It is important to develop a disciplined technique for examining them as there is frequently embarrassment on the part of both the patient and the student, making logical thought more difficult.

A routine should be established as follows:

1 Can you get above it? That is to say, is the lump truly scrotal or is it a continuation of a lump in the groin (e.g. an inguinal hernia)?

2 What is its relation to the testis? Which anatomical structure does it arise from?

3 Is the lump tender or not?

4 Does it transilluminate? Scrotal lumps lend themselves to the technique of transillumination. Use a good torch with a narrow beam and observe the other side of the swelling in a darkened environment. A paper tube can be useful for this.

5 Define the characteristics of the lump:
   (a) shape
   (b) size
   (c) surface
   (d) consistency
   (e) mobility.

The features of individual types of lump will be dealt with below.

Hydrocele

A hydrocele is a collection of fluid in the tunica vaginalis. Hydroceles may be either primary or secondary. In the primary type there is no predisposing cause in the scrotum, but there may be a persistent processus vaginalis (congenital or infantile hydrocele, see pp. 617–618).

Secondary hydroceles represent a reaction to some pathology in the testis or its covering (e.g. testicular infections, tumours, torsion of the testis or hydatid of Morgagni). In adults the possibility that a hydrocele is secondary to an impalpable tumour of the testis must always be considered.

Hydrocele of the cord is a condition in which the hydrocele arises in part of the processus vaginalis in the spermatic cord above the testis (see Fig. 123, p. 618). A rounded lump slips up and down the inguinal canal. The abnormality here is that the processus has not closed off fully and the operative repair is the same as for an inguinal hernia in children.

Cysts of the canal of Nuck are a similar condition occurring in females.

Recognizing the pattern

The patient may be of any age. Primary hydroceles are common in young boys; secondary hydroceles are more common in adults.

He usually presents because he has noticed a swelling in the scrotum. Occasionally the hydrocele is large enough to cause discomfort. If it occurs secondary to underlying disease of the testis, there may also be symptoms due to the primary cause such as pain or weight loss.

On examination you can get above the swelling. It has a smooth surface and is of any size. It transilluminates well. The testis is within it and not palpable separately.

Management

Hydroceles in children are treated as a patent processus vaginalis and should be dealt with operatively in the same way as an inguinal hernia (see p. 619).

A hydrocele in an adult may be treated as follows:

1 Conservatively
2 By tapping
3 By operation.

Conservative treatment consists of reassurance and possibly providing the patient with a scrotal support. This may be all that is necessary for a small hydrocele where it is the development of the swelling that usually bothers the patient rather than any symptoms from it. Beware, however, of reassuring a patient who may have a hydrocele secondary to a tumour. If the testis is not palpable through the hydrocele, then it should be visualized by ultrasound. This is also the case if the patient is likely to have to wait for some time before surgery.

Hydroceles may be tapped using a sterile needle and syringe. A sclerosing agent such as tetracycline may be injected after aspiration to prevent reaccumulation of fluid which is common with this procedure. This type of management may be indicated where the patient is not thought fit for surgery.

Operative treatment is indicated where there is doubt about the diagnosis (see secondary hydrocele above), where the hydrocele is very large, or where there are repeated recurrences after tapping.

OPERATION: REMOVAL OF HYDROCELE

An incision is made in the scrotum, and the hydrocoele and its immediate coverings are separated by gentle finger dissection. If this is carried out in the correct layer, very little bleeding occurs. The hydrocele is then delivered out of the scrotum and incised, releasing its fluid. The testis is inspected for abnormalities. The coverings of the tunica fall behind the testis and cord and can be fixed there with sutures. In this way the hydrocele cannot refill. The testis plus the everted coverings are then replaced in the scrotum and the skin is closed over them with absorbable sutures. Accurate haemostasis is essential. A scrotal support may be applied.

Codes
Blood 0
GA/LA .... GA or LA
Opn time .... 15–30 min
Stay .... Day case
Drains out 0
Sutures out .... Absorbable sutures are not removed
Off work .... 1–2 weeks

Postoperative care
The patient should rest quietly for 12–24 h. Haematoma formation is the main complication to be avoided. If a haematoma does occur, convalescence will be prolonged and there is a danger that it may become infected. Large haematomas should be evacuated under sterile conditions in theatre.

Epididymal cysts

Epididymal cysts are very common and often multiple. They may be of any size and contain either clear or milky fluid.

Recognizing the pattern

The patient is usually postpubertal and the condition seems to be more common in the middle aged and elderly.

He has usually noticed a lump which may have become large enough to cause trouble by its size. Occasionally the cyst is painful or the patient may be experiencing pain on direct pressure over it.

On examination it is possible to get above the swelling, which is situated above and behind the testis in the epididymis. The testis is palpable separate from it. Cysts are frequently multiple and several cysts next to each other give rise to a lobulated swelling. The condition is often bilateral. The cysts are fluctuant but only transilluminate if they contain clear fluid.

Management

Conservative management is followed where possible. Patients should be reassured that the cysts are nothing to worry about.

If the cysts are causing trouble because of pain or their size, they can either be tapped (as for hydroceles) or excised. It is important to warn the patient that surgery to excise an epididymal cyst is likely to lead to epididymal dysfunction and impaired sperm transfer on that side, due to postoperative fibrosis.

OPERATION: EXCISION OF EPIDIDYMAL CYST
The testis is exposed within the tunica vaginalis and delivered out of the scrotum. Either the individual cysts or the affected part of the epididymis can then be excised. The epididymis has a good blood supply and a lot of time must be spent securing full haemostasis.

Codes
Blood 0
GA/LA .... GA or LA
Opn time .... 15–30 min
Stay .... Day case
Drains out 0
Sutures out .... Absorbable sutures are not removed
Off work .... 1–2 weeks

Postoperative care
This is much the same as for a hydrocele.

Testicular neoplasms

Ninety-two per cent of testicular neoplasms are malignant but they only account for 1 or 2% of all male malignancies. They are therefore uncommon.

Benign neoplasms are even more rare. Leydig (interstitial) cell tumours account for 7% of testicular tumours and they may secrete androgens. In young boys they may produce early puberty and the 'infant Hercules' syndrome. Sertoli cell adenomas (< 1%) secrete oestrogens and produce feminization.

Malignant neoplasms of the testis are commonly either seminomas (40% of testicular tumours) or teratomas (30%); 15% are of a mixed type. Undescended testes have approximately a 10-fold increased risk of neoplastic change and these patients represent about 8% of those with a malignant testicular tumour.

Seminomas probably arise from the primordial germinal cells in the testicular tubule. This is a solid tumour and tends to be slow growing. It is usually very radiosensitive.

Teratomas may have solid or cystic components and are less radiosensitive than seminomas. Ninety per cent of teratomas will secrete human chorionic gonadotrophin and/or α-fetoprotein, which can be measured in the serum and used as a tumour marker.

The prognosis of seminomas and teratomas depends on the stage of the growth and in the case of a teratoma its degree of differentiation.

Staging of testicular tumours

Stage I: disease confined to the testis.

Stage II: abdominal lymph node involvement.

Stage III: supra- and infradiaphragmatic lymph node involvement.

Stage IV: extralymphatic spread (e.g. lung and liver).

Degree of differentiation of teratomas

TD: teratoma differentiated.

MTI: malignant teratoma intermediate.

MTU: malignant teratoma undifferentiated.

MTT: malignant teratoma trophoblastic.

The less differentiated the teratoma the worse the prognosis.

With the advent of combination chemotherapy 100% 5-year survival can be achieved for stage I or II teratomas. If hepatic metastases are present the 5-year survival falls to 10%. Stage I and II seminomas have a 5-year survival of 90–95%. The overall 5-year survival for stage III seminomas is 50–70%.

Spread of these tumours is usually via the bloodstream and the lymphatics. Local spread to the scrotum is rare. Bloodstream spread occurs earlier in teratomas and metastases appear in the lungs and the liver. Lymphatic spread is common in both seminomas and teratomas. The lymph drainage of the testis follows its arterial supply and spread therefore occurs to the para-aortic lymph nodes at the level of the umbilicus. Inguinal lymph node involvement is rare and occurs when the scrotal skin is invaded.

Lymphomas comprise a further 7% of testicular tumours. They are more common in the elderly and are usually of the non-Hodgkin's type. Treatment is by combination chemotherapy but the overall results are poor.

Recognizing the pattern

Seminomas tend to occur between the ages of 25 and 45 years, whereas teratomas occur in a slightly younger age group, between 15 and 35 years.

The patient or his partner may notice a small painless lump in the testis or that one testis is larger than the other. Alternatively, these findings may be noted at a routine medical examination. Other presenting symptoms are unexplained pain in one testis, haemospermia or the development of a secondary hydrocoele. In up to 30%, however, the first presentation is with an abdominal mass due to enlarged para-aortic lymph nodes, cervical lymphadenopathy or pulmonary metastases.

On examination a hard swelling is felt within the testis, and it is possible to get above it. The tumour does not transilluminate. The examination should include the abdomen, liver, chest and left supraclavicular fossa, feeling for evidence of metastatic spread.

Proving the diagnosis

The tumour may be proved to be solid by an ultrasound examination. However, a mass arising in the testis is a malignant neoplasm until proved otherwise and must be explored and biopsied.

Management

A chest X-ray is performed and blood taken for α-fetoprotein and β-human chorionic gonadotrophin levels before the operation. Other investigations may be performed in the postoperative period. These include a CT scan of the chest, abdomen and pelvis in order to stage the disease.

The patient must be warned of the possibility of an orchidectomy and consent for this obtained. It is worth emphasizing to the patient that fertility ought not to be impaired following orchidectomy, so long as the contralateral testis is normal. It should be explained that the testis will be explored through the groin. Percutaneous biopsy through the scrotal skin should never be carried out because of the risk of seeding along the needle track. The groin is shaved as for a hernia operation.

OPERATION: EXPLORATION OF TESTICULAR MASS/?ORCHIDECTOMY

The groin is explored through an oblique incision as for an inguinal hernia and the spermatic cord isolated. A soft vascular clamp is placed on the cord at the internal ring. This prevents the venous spread of malignant cells while the testis is being manipulated. The testis is delivered into the groin, inspected and if necessary transected to look for a tumour. If it is normal it can be repaired with chromic catgut sutures. If a tumour is found, it may be biopsied to confirm or exclude malignancy, though this is not normally necessary. For removal of the testis, the clamp on the cord is replaced by a tie and the testis plus the spermatic cord are excised. No drains are necessary.

Codes

Blood 0
GA/LA .... GA
Opn time .... 30–60 min
Stay .... 2–3 days
Drains out 0
Sutures out .... 5–7 days
Off work .... Varies according to the need for further
                        treatment

Postoperative care

The patient requires a scrotal support and his recovery is much the same as for an inguinal hernia (see. p. 423). Further treatment then depends on the histology and the clinical staging. Serum tumour markers are measured 1 week postoperatively and if they remain elevated this indicates the presence of metastases. In patients who have had a teratoma excised, the tumour markers should also be measured at 3-monthly intervals, since a rise generally indicates recurrent tumour.

Seminomas. Radiotherapy is given postoperatively to all patients, including those with stage I disease. Those with metastases are also given chemotherapy.

Teratomas. Combination chemotherapy is given postoperatively. Retroperitoneal lymph node dissection may be considered if there is evidence of persistent disease, with elevated tumour markers, following chemotherapy. This operation can be done as an open procedure or by laparoscopy.

Radiotherapy

The dose and field of radiation depend on the histological type and the presence or absence of metastases. Radiotherapy is given over a 5–6-week period. The minimum field includes the retroperitoneal lymphatics, and runs from the scrotum to the tenth thoracic vertebra. Even in the absence of proven secondary deposits, micrometastases are assumed to have occurred. Mediastinal and supraclavicular fields are irradiated in the presence of metastases in these sites. Metastases in the lung are not usually irradiated due to the discomfort and pneumonitis that often results.

Chemotherapy

Chemotherapy is used when there is metastatic disease. The

exception to this is with undifferentiated or trophoblastic teratoma when it is used from the start, whatever the stage of the
disease. Alkylating agents (e.g. cyclophosphamide) are used
against seminoma. Teratoma is usually treated by combination
therapy including bleomycin, etoposide and cisplatin.

Painful testis

A painful testis can follow direct trauma and haematoma formation but in the absence of this history two important diagnoses
must be considered and excluded. One is torsion and the other
is a developing tumour. In the first case the pain is very severe
and in the second it is usually of lower intensity. More often
than not, however, the painful testis turns out to be due to
epididymo-orchitis.

Epididymo-orchitis

Epididymo-orchitis is an inflammation of the epididymis and
testis due to bacterial, chlamydial or viral infection. The most
common viral cause is mumps and it may then be associated
with the characteristic parotitis.

Bacterial infections may be gonococcal or due to other bacteria such as coliforms. Chlamydial infection is becoming more
common. The infection is thought to arise through reflux of
infected urine or prostatic fluid along the vas. It may follow
vasectomy. The epididymis alone may be infected or the inflammation may occasionally spread to involve the testis as well.

Recognizing the pattern

Bacterial infection usually occurs in the elderly whereas viral
infections are more common in the younger age group.

The typical picture is of an acute onset of very severe pain
in the testis. There is swelling of the scrotum and the epididymis
and testis become hard and very tender. The patient is ill with
a fever, and rigors are not uncommon. There may or may not
be associated dysuria and frequency.

Proving the diagnosis

The main differential diagnosis is torsion of the testis. The
presence of a urinary infection, demonstrated by examination
of an MSU, may be helpful, although it does not, of course, rule
out a torsion. In epididymo-orchitis the pain is said to be relieved by elevating the organ where this is not so with a torsion.
The large, hot, swollen testis of epididymo-orchitis is characteristic, as are the systemic signs of infection. When there is

difficulty in deciding whether or not the testis is twisted, the scrotum should be explored. No harm is done by exploring an infection but much harm can follow conservative treatment of a torsion.

Management
The treatment is to give antibiotics, a scrotal support and bed rest. The epididymis frequently remains very hard and indurated for several weeks.

Chronic infections of the testis and epididymis

Two chronic infections, which may affect the epididymis, are tuberculosis and syphilis. Both are now extremely rare due to adequate early antibiotic treatment. Because of this rareness, however, the diagnosis is liable to be missed.

A gumma of the testis may be seen in examinations but fortunately not in clinical practice any more. The treatment of syphilis is penicillin.

Tuberculosis may affect the epididymis as part of an infection involving the urinary tract. The chronically indurated epididymis is not usually painful. The inflammation may slowly progress to sinus formation.

The diagnosis is made either by finding acid-fast bacilli in the urinary tract or by culturing them from sinuses. The treatment is with antituberculous drugs and this may be combined with excision of the affected epididymis.

Torsion of the testis

The testis and epididymis are normally fixed within the scrotum by a 'bare area' which is outside the tunica vaginalis. Part of the epididymis and testis are involved in this 'bare area'. Torsion of the testis can occur when this attachment is minimal and the organ is on a 'mesentery' (Fig. 95). Occasionally the epididymis and testis are more separated than usual and in this case torsion can occur between the two. As these abnormalities are usually bilateral the opposite testis should usually be fixed when torsion has occurred on one side. The actual twist occurs due to the action of the cremaster muscle. The fibres of this muscle run from the inguinal region downwards and medially across the front of the testis. When they contract the testis tends to rotate with its medial side moving forwards, giving rise to the classically described 'bell-clapper' testis. Torsions not infrequently occur at times of excessive strain or exercise or during sexual

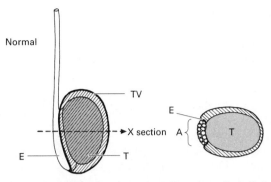

Tunica vaginalis (TV) enveloping testis (T) and anterior half of epididymus (E). Broad bare area (A)

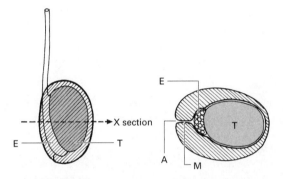

Tunica vaginalis includes epididymis. Small bare area (A) and mesentery (M). Testis prone to torsion

Fig. 95 The anatomy of testicular torsion.

intercourse. Undescended testes have a higher incidence of torsion than those which are fully descended.

Recognizing the pattern

Torsion can occur at any age but is more common between the ages of 10 and 25 years.

There is a sudden onset of very severe scrotal pain, often associated with right iliac fossa pain radiating into the loin. The patient may feel ill and faint and experience nausea and vomiting. He may give a history of previous episodes of testicular pain, which have resolved, when the testis has twisted and untwisted spontaneously.

On examination the patient looks pale and ill and is in pain. The testis is swollen and hard and exquisitely tender. Because of this tenderness the twist in the cord may not be palpable.

However, the testis rides higher than its fellow, and this sign is helpful in making the diagnosis. The contralateral testis may lie horizontally (bell–clapper testis). Elevation of the twisted testis does not relieve the pain in contrast to the findings in epididymo-orchitis.

Proving the diagnosis and management

Where torsion is suspected the scrotum should be explored under a general anaesthetic without delay. Further investigation is inappropriate. If the testis is twisted for more than 4 h irreversible damage is likely to occur. At operation the diagnosis is confirmed by seeing the twist in the spermatic cord.

Preoperative care

The patient or his parents must be warned of the slight possibility of the testis needing to be excised and consent obtained for this, as well as fixation of the contralateral testis.

OPERATION: CORRECTION OF TORSION OF THE TESTIS

The scrotum is incised through the midline septum and the tunica on the affected side is opened. If this is done carefully, the testis is not rotated and the twist may be demonstrated. It is corrected and the colour of the testis observed. It may help to wrap it in a swab soaked in warm water. If the testis is necrotic, it should be removed. For fixation, the tunica is sutured behind the cord, as in a hydrocele. A non-absorbable suture is passed through the upper and lower poles of the testis and it is secured in the scrotum, with its long axis running vertically. The contralateral testis is then approached, via the same incision, and fixed in the same way. The scrotal skin is closed with a soluble suture.

Codes

Blood	0
GA/LA	GA
Opn time	30–60 min
Stay	2–3 days
Drains out	0
Sutures out	Absorbable sutures do not need to be removed
Off work	2 weeks

Torsion of testicular appendage

The testis may have a vestigial appendage, such as a hydatid of
Morgagni, which is the remains of the Müllerian duct. This
arises on a pedicle from the junction of the upper pole of the
testis and the epididymis. Torsion of this pedicle leads to ischaemia and infarction of the appendage.

Recognizing the pattern

The patient may be of any age, although torsion of a testicular
appendage is commoner in preadolescent boys. The presentation is very similar to that of testicular torsion, with acute onset
of severe testicular pain. It may be difficult to distinguish from
testicular torsion on examination, although it may be possible
to palpate the appendage, which will be exquisitely tender.

Proving the diagnosis and management

In view of the fact that the clinical presentation mimics that
of testicular torsion, the diagnosis is usually made at operation, when the scrotum is explored. If a twisted appendage
is found, the pedicle should be ligated and the appendage
excised. There is no need to proceed with fixation of the
testes.

Varicocele

A varicocele is a collection of varicose veins in the pampiniform
plexus of the cord and scrotum. It carries a higher than average
incidence of infertility and this is thought to be due to the
higher scrotal temperature associated with the abnormality.
Varicoceles can be secondary to lesions causing obstruction to
the testicular veins in the abdomen.

Recognizing the pattern

The patient is usually a young adult. The varicocele may have
been spotted at a routine medical examination (e.g. for the
Forces).

The usual complaint is of a dull ache, especially at the end
of the day or after exercise. The varicose veins themselves may
also have been noted and caused the patient concern.

The varicocele is usually plainly visible when the patient stands up. On palpation the typical 'bag of worms' feel is easily recognized. The left side is more commonly affected than the right. The swelling diminishes or even disappears when the patient lies flat.

Management

The patient is reassured that no harm is likely to come from this lesion. Indications for operation are if the pain is persistent in spite of adequate support or if there is associated infertility. An open operation is usually performed, although it may be performed laparoscopically. In some centres, it is possible to embolize the veins by insertion of metal coils via the vena cava under X-ray screening.

OPERATION: FOR VARICOCELE

The cord is explored in the groin and all the veins in the spermatic cord are divided leaving only one to conduct blood from the testis. The artery and vas are also preserved. In the laparoscopic operation the testicular vein is identified in the abdomen, just after it emerges from the internal ring, and clipped.

Codes

Blood	0
GA/LA	GA or LA
Opn time	60 min
Stay	Day case
Drains out	0
Sutures out	Absorbable or 7 days
Off work	2 weeks

Postoperative care

The patient wears a scrotal support and early discharge is the rule.

12 Vascular Surgery

12.1 Assessment of Chronic Ischaemia of the Leg

This section deals with the problems of recognizing and investigating the patient who presents with a chronically ischaemic leg. Leg ischaemia is a result of arterial atherosclerosis in the majority of patients. The management is dealt with in section 12.2.

In the initial assessment five questions have to be answered before decisions about management can be made. These are as follows:

1 Is the leg ischaemic?
2 What is the site of the lesion?
3 How severe is the ischaemia?
4 Which risk factors for atherosclerosis are present?
5 What is the full extent of the atherosclerotic process?

The answers are found first by clinical assessment and then by investigation.

Clinical assessment

Is the leg ischaemic?

Recognizing the pattern

The patient is more often male than female and usually beyond middle age.

The main complaint is of pain in the limb and this may be as follows:

1 Intermittent claudication
2 Rest pain
3 Painful ulceration.

Mild to moderate ischaemia is associated with intermittent claudication, which is a cramp-like pain in the muscles of the leg which occurs on walking a certain distance (known as the claudication distance). It is relieved by rest and recurs on walking again. Intermittent claudication needs to be differentiated from the pain associated with sciatica, cauda equina syndrome and venous claudication.

Rest pain is associated with more severe ischaemia. Typically, it occurs at night when the patient is in bed and affects the toes or the dorsum of the foot and may wake the patient. The pain may be relieved by hanging the leg over the edge of the bed or by walking around the bedroom. Rest pain needs to be differentiated from night cramps and peripheral neuropathy, usually associated with diabetes or nerve entrapment.

Trophic changes are associated with extreme ischaemia. These changes consist of discoloration of the foot with scaly skin, painful ulceration over the pressure points and gangrene. Ulceration and gangrenous changes need to be differentiated from those associated with venous hypertensive disease, neuropathies, infections and malignant ulcers.

On examination the features of ischaemia depend upon its severity and usually include the following:

1 Absent pulses. Feel carefully for the femoral, popliteal and foot pulses. In mild to moderate disease this may be the only abnormal finding. Absent pulses indicate disease at or proximal to the site examined. The presence of blood flow in an artery can be detected with a hand-held Doppler ultrasound probe even when pulses are not palpable.

2 Audible bruits. Auscultate over the aorta, iliac, common femoral and superficial femoral vessels. The presence of a bruit indicates a stenosis at or proximal to the site examined.

3 Cold extremity. Compare the temperature of the good side to the symptomatic side.

4 Postural colour change (Buerger's test). With the patient supine, raise both legs in the air. If the leg is severely ischaemic, there is insufficient pressure to perfuse the elevated limb and the foot becomes pale. After a minute or two, ask the patient to sit up and hang the legs over the edge of the couch. The colour returns slowly to the ischaemic leg and the skin will develop the rubor of reactive hyperaemia.

5 Persistent venous guttering. This sign can be elicited at the same time as postural colour change. As the legs are elevated the foot veins empty. When the legs are placed in the dependent position, the veins remain 'guttered'. The time taken for the venous gutter to fill is an indication of the severity of the ischaemia.

6 Ulcers or gangrene. Ischaemic gangrene is usually dry (may be wet in diabetics) and well demarcated. Arterial ulcers are punched out with pale granulation tissue and show little sign of active healing.

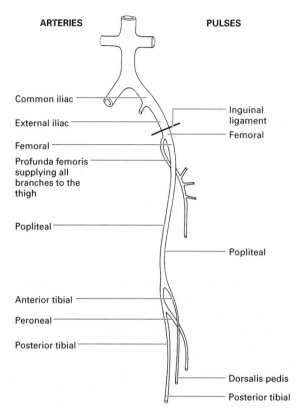

ARTERIES   PULSES

Common iliac

External iliac

Femoral

Profunda femoris
supplying all
branches to the
thigh

Popliteal

Anterior tibial

Peroneal

Posterior tibial

Inguinal
ligament

Femoral

Popliteal

Dorsalis pedis

Posterior tibial

Fig. 96 The arterial supply to the lower leg: the named arteries
and the palpable pulses.

What is the anatomical site of the lesion?

This can usually be diagnosed with accuracy before arteriography is undertaken. A knowledge of the normal anatomy of the vascular tree is necessary (Fig. 96).

Recognizing the pattern

The level of the lesion may be determined from the history. Claudication associated with aortoiliac disease usually starts in the calf, progressing to the thigh and finally involving the buttock. If this occurs bilaterally and is associated with impotence in the male and absent femoral pulses it is known as Leriche's syndrome. External iliac, common femoral or coincident superficial femoral and profunda femoral disease gives rise to calf claudication progressing to the thigh. Superficial femoral, popliteal or crural (calf) vessel disease will give rise to calf claudication only.

In patients with rest pain and or trophic changes, disease is invariably present at more than one level.

On examination the level of the pulse deficit will usually be diagnostic of the level of the block. An absent femoral pulse indicates disease in the iliac system or above, and so on.

The presence of a bruit can tell you if there is a narrowing at or proximal to that site. Proximal bruits are more significant than distal ones.

How severe is the ischaemia?

The severity is determined by the following.

Recognizing the pattern

Intermittent claudication represents the least severe symptom of ischaemia and the longer the claudication distance, the more minor the problem. Rest pain indicates more severe ischaemia. The onset of trophic changes and ulceration are signs that the limb is at risk. Poor cardiac output or the presence of anaemia will exacerbate any symptoms of peripheral vascular disease.

On examination normal appearance of the leg indicates mild ischaemia. The presence of postural colour change and venous guttering indicates a more severe degree of ischaemia. Trophic changes such as ulceration and gangrene indicate that the leg is at risk.

Which risk factors for atherosclerosis are present?

Management of the ischaemic leg depends on risk factor management, therefore it is important to determine the risk factors in each patient.

Recognizing the pattern

Cigarette smoking is the major risk factor for developing atherosclerosis. The patient may be diabetic. The patient may have treated or untreated hypertension. Hyperlipidaemia should be excluded. A strong family history of cardiovascular disease should be noted.

On examination the following should be considered:

1 Nicotine staining of the fingers should be sought
2 Brachial systolic and diastolic blood pressure should be measured
3 Xanthelasmas should be sought
4 Dipstick urinanalysis for glucose should be performed.

What is the full extent of the atherosclerotic process?

Atherosclerosis is a generalized disease process affecting the arteries of the heart and the brain as well as those of the legs.

Recognizing the pattern

Any history of myocardial infarction or angina pectoris should be noted. Recent infarction or unstable angina are significant risk factors if operative intervention is being considered. Look for a previous history of stroke, transient ischaemic attack or amaurosis fugax. Note any history suggestive of mesenteric angina or of deteriorating renal function.

On examination the presence of carotid artery bruits, renal artery bruits and aortic bruits should be noted. An asymptomatic abdominal aortic aneurysm is present in up to 15% of patients presenting with peripheral vascular disease, therefore abdominal palpation is necessary.

Investigations: non-invasive vascular assessment

Clinical assessment as outlined above should give a reasonable indication of the presence, site and severity of leg ischaemia. It should then be possible to confirm the diagnosis of leg ischaemia, locate the haemodynamically significant arterial lesions and plan the intervention (if indicated) using non-invasive vascular assessment. An algorithm for doing this is outlined in Fig. 97.

Ankle brachial pressure index (ABPI)

This gives a good indication of the severity of the disease and forms the baseline for future evaluation of progression of the disease. With the patient supine, a sphygomanometer cuff is placed above the elbow, flow through the brachial artery is detected using a hand-held Doppler ultrasound probe and the cuff is inflated to suprasystolic pressure. The cuff is deflated

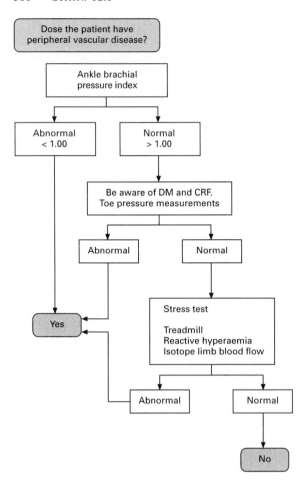

Fig. 97 Algorithm for investigation of patient with chronic leg ischaemia.

slowly and the point at which audible flow is re-established is the brachial systolic pressure. This is repeated on the opposite arm. The cuff is then placed around the leg just above the level of the ankle. Systolic blood pressure is measured in the dorsalis pedis and the posterior tibial arteries using the Doppler in the same manner. The ratio of the highest systolic blood pressure measured at the ankle to the higher brachial systolic pressure, is the ABPI for that leg and is normally greater than 0.95. The ABPI is of limited value in patients with diabetes mellitis or chronic renal failure where artificially high values may be a reflection of the incompressibility of calcified arteries. A normal ABPI does not exclude peripheral vascular disease.

Toe pressure measurements

These may be helpful in patients with diabetes mellitis or chronic renal failure who have ischaemic legs but normal ABPIs due to calcified vessels. The digital vessels are usually spared the calcification process and are therefore compressible. A pneumatic cuff 2.5 cm wide is placed around the base of the digit, usually the great toe. Arterial pulsation is detected with a photoplethysmograph or strain gauge plethysmograph. The cuff is inflated to suprasystolic pressure and then deflated slowly. The point at which pulsation returns is the systolic pressure. The normal toe pressure is at least 60% that of the ankle pressure. If it is less than this then it is indicative of peripheral vascular disease.

Stress testing

If a patient has symptoms typical of intermittent claudication and has a normal ABPI and palpable pulses, they may have peripheral vascular disease which is not haemodynamically significant at rest but becomes so on exercise. It is usually due to a stenosis or narrowing within the arterial tree. There are a number of non-invasive methods to determine if this is the situation.

In exercise treadmill testing the patient's ABPI is measured as outlined above. The patient is placed on a treadmill, which is set at a defined speed and slope, and exercised. The distance at which the patient first complains of pain is the initial claudication distance. The distance at which the pain becomes intolerable is the maximum claudication distance. When this is reached the ABPI is measured again. If there is haemodynamically significant disease present, the ABPI will have fallen after exercise.

Many patients are unable to exercise on a treadmill due to age and coincident infirmity. In these patients it is possible to induce maximal blood flow in the leg using reactive hyperaemia induced by a tourniquet. The ABPI is measured as outlined above. A tourniquet is placed on the leg below the level of the knee and inflated to suprasystolic pressure for 3 min, occluding the circulation. The cuff is deflated and the ABPI remeasured. In patients with haemodynamically significant disease the ABPI will have dropped as inflow is impeded by the stenosis. It is possible to actually measure blood flow in mL/100 mL tissue/min using an isotope modification of this technique.

After performing one or more of these investigations as outlined in Fig. 97, it is possible to confirm with certainty the presence of peripheral vascular disease.

To determine the site or sites of the disease in the chronically ischaemic leg, there are a number of techniques available and these can be used according to Fig. 98.

Segmental pressure measurements

This is a modification of the ABPI technique described above. Blood pressure cuffs are placed above the elbows, around the upper thigh, above the knee, below the knee and above the ankle.

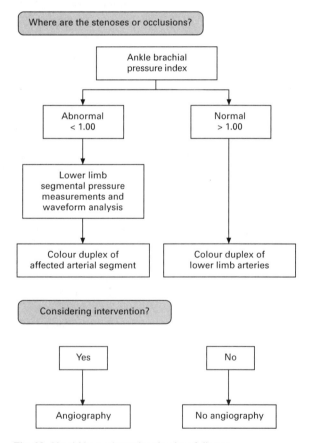

Fig. 98 Algorithim to determine the site of disease.

The ABPI is measured and the vessel with the highest pressure at the ankle is used as the reference vessel. Starting with all the cuffs deflated, the cuffs are inflated and deflated sequentially commencing at the upper thigh and the systolic blood pressure is recorded using the Doppler ultrasound probe at the ankle. This way a series of systolic blood pressures are recorded at these defined levels. The high thigh pressure should be recorded as being at least 20 mmHg higher than the brachial pressure (technical reasons due to the cuff width), if this is not so it indicates significant aortic or iliac disease or alternately coincident superficial femoral and profunda femoris artery disease. If there is a pressure drop of greater than 20 mmHg in the systolic pressure recording between two cuffs, this indicates haemodynamically significant disease in this segment. Thus it is possible to determine the sites at which significant disease occurs.

Colour Doppler imaging (colour Duplex)

This is a combination of B-mode ultrasound imaging with computed colour-coded Doppler ultrasound. It is possible to visualize the vessels using the B-mode imaging component and to focus the ultrasound beam on the vessel lumen to determine the flow velocity through the vessel. The investigation depends on a highly trained individual and it can be time-consuming to visualize the whole arterial tree. Prior segmental pressure measurements can determine the sites of interest in most patients. It is especially important when planning interventional procedures.

Other routine investigations

1 Full blood count — for anaemia, blood dyscrasia
2 Plasma viscosity — for collagen diseases, inflammatory condition
3 Coagulation screen — for coagulopathy
4 Urea and electrolytes and creatinine — for renal disease
5 Blood sugar — for diabetes mellitis
6 Blood lipids — for hyperlipidaemia
7 Electrocardiogram (ECG) — for ischaemic heart disease
8 Ultrasound of aorta — for abdominal aortic aneurysm.

Arteriography

Arteriography should be reserved for those patients in whom surgical or radiological intervention is being considered. There are a number of techniques for obtaining arteriograms. Translumbar aortography is rarely performed now.

Transfemoral arteriography

Under sterile conditions and local anaesthesia, a needle is placed into the femoral artery. A guide wire is passed through the needle into the artery. A dilator covered by a sheath is placed over the guide wire and passed into the lumen of the artery. The guide wire and the dilator are now removed leaving the sheath accessing the arterial lumen. A longer guide wire is now passed through the sheath proximally into the aorta and a fine-bore catheter is passed over the guide wire into the aorta. The guide wire is removed. Radio–opaque contrast material can be injected to acquire the images.

Transbrachial/transaxillary arteriography

The sheath is placed in the brachial artery or the axillary artery. It is usually used when the femoral pulses are impalpable as a result of aortoiliac occlusive disease.

Digital subtraction arteriography

This is a major advance in imaging technology. An initial image is taken and stored in a computer. The contrast material is injected rapidly and a series of images taken in rapid succession and stored on the computer. The initial image with bone and soft tissue shadowing is then subtracted from each of the subsequently obtained images leaving only the contrast material visible. Each of these images is superimposed on one another building up high resolution images of the arteries. The advantages of this technique is that high quality arteriograms are obtained with the minimal use of contrast material. It is possible to inject the contrast material intra-arterially or intravenously. The resolution of the images is not as good using the latter technique.

Magnetic resonance angiography

It is possible to obtain angiographic images of arterial flow using a magnetic resonance technique.

Hazards

There are hazards associated with arteriography. These include haemorrhage, haematoma formation and bruising at the arterial puncture site. False aneurysm formation can also occur.

Intimal dissection may result in detachment of a segment of arterial plaque which embolizes causing distal ischaemia. Thrombosis at the site of puncture or of plaque disruption may also occur resulting in acute ischaemia.

Allergic reaction to the contrast material may also occur. The contrast materials used are nephrotoxic and may cause acute renal failure. In patients with impaired renal function a renal protective regime should be used.

12.2 Management of the Ischaemic Limb

General management

All patients with chronic ischaemia should be advised to stop smoking. The prognosis is worse if they continue. Diabetics should be encouraged to obtain tight control of their diabetes and this should be monitored using glycosylated haemoglobin estimations. Patients with hyperlipidaemias should be encouraged to adopt a lipid-lowering diet and be commenced on lipid-lowering agents if indicated. Hypertension should be controlled, avoiding the use of β-blockers as they may exacerbate the symptoms of ischaemia. Patients who are overweight should be encouraged to lose weight as excess weight requires the leg muscles to do more work, increasing oxygen demand. Foot care is important, and bacterial and fungal infections should be treated. Chiropody should be strongly advised in patients unable to take care of nails, calluses or bunions. Advice on foot hygiene and sensible footwear is important.

Other underlying conditions such as cardiac failure or anaemia should be treated. Atherosclerosis is a generalized disease process and the majority of patients presenting with leg ischaemia will die as a result of coronary or cerebrovascular disease. There is evidence that low dose aspirin (75 mg daily) will decrease the risk of these events and therefore there is an argument for commencing patients on aspirin as long as they are not sensitive to it.

Management of intermittent claudication

The treatment is conservative in the majority of cases. As well as the general measures outlined above, the patient should be advised to commence a walking exercise programme. Ideally this should be supervised with regular monitoring. The patient should be advised to walk at a steady pace until the initial claudication distance is reached, and advised to walk into the pain as far as is possible (ideally 75% of the distance between the initial and the maximal claudication distance) before resting. When the pain has gone the patient should repeat the exercise three or four times, on a daily or twice daily basis if possible. Over a period of time the claudication distance will increase until ultimately the patient will be able to walk as far as they wish without pain. It was initially thought that there was hypertrophy of collateral vessels increasing blood flow but there is no evidence for this. It is now thought that there is an alteration in the metabolic process in the muscle fibres allowing them to function in a state of anaerobic respiration.

Indications for intervention are relative and include the following:

1 Decreasing claudication distance.

2 Short claudication distance (< 100 m and proximal disease).

3 Persisting symptoms which interfere with the patient's work or quality of life to an intolerable degree.

4 The development of rest pain.

5 Low risk for intervention.

Management of rest pain and/or trophic changes

The presence of true rest pain and or ulceration and gangrene is a definitive indication for intervention. After the relevant clinical and non-invasive vascular assessment has been performed and a management plan formulated, an arteriogram is performed. Arterial reconstruction should be considered in terms of risk/benefit to the patient's life and limb. Factors to be considered include the following:

1 The fitness of the patient for the procedure

2 The outcome if the patient does not have the procedure

3 The success/failure rate associated with the procedure. This often depends on the state of the distal arterial tree (run off).

Preoperative care

The preoperative care of the arteriopath is more complex than that of most other surgical patients and includes the following:

1 Assessment of coronary artery disease, diabetes and chronic renal failure are important.

2 Preoperative ABPI measurements are vital in the later assessment of vessel patency.

3 Informed consent.

4 Preoperative marking of the long saphenous vein should be performed if it is being considered for use as a bypass

Continued on p. 524

Continued.

conduit. Formal mapping using colour Doppler imaging of the vein is useful as the size of the vein can be assessed, and the branches and main trunk marked.

5 If the long saphenous vein is not suitable or has been stripped previously, the vein on the opposite leg should be marked. If this is absent the cephalic or basilic veins of the arm should be mapped. It must be considered that this may be necessary when the patient is admitted and one arm spared the attentions of the phlebotomist.

6 Prophylactic antibiotics should be given with the premedication or at the time of anaesthetic induction in theatre.

7 Deep venous thrombosis prophylaxis using subcutaneous heparin should be used; antiembolic compression stockings are contraindicated in patients with chronic ischaemia.

8 A renal protective regime may be necessary especially in patients undergoing endovascular procedures.

9 All patients should undergo shaving of the area to be operated upon.

Endovascular techniques

Angioplasty. The treatment of patients with lower limb ischaemia has been revolutionized by the development of angioplasty. Using angiographic techniques a guide wire is passed across the lesion to be treated. A fine-bore catheter with a balloon at the tip is passed into the artery and positioned across the lesion. The balloon is inflated dilating the stricture.

Stent deployment. Re-stenosis may occur at the site of angioplasty. It is possible to place and expand a metal stent at the site of angioplasty to decrease this possibility. It is also possible to deploy a stent in an area of intimal flap dissection after angioplasty, thus preventing thrombosis.

Stent grafting. A further advance is the use of a stent covered with prosthetic material (Dacron or polytetrafluorethylene [PTFE]) which is introduced into the artery using the same technique but when expanded forms an uninterrupted tube graft within the artery. This technique is under development.

Limitations

These techniques have limitations. Long-term success is greater in proximal vessels such as the iliacs and the superficial femoral arteries. Stenoses greater than 10 cm long or occlusions greater than 5 cm have poor results. Diseased distal vessels also lower the success rates.

Codes

Blood	Group and save
GA/LA	LA
Opn time	30–120 min
Stay	Day case/overnight
Drains out	0
Sutures out	0
Off work	1 week

Operative techniques

There are a number of operative techniques available to help patients with chronic ischaemia.

Endarterectomy. The atheromatous lining of the narrowed artery is cored out. This procedure is particularly suitable for short stenoses in the larger vessels proximal to the superficial femoral artery and also for the removal of plaques in the internal carotid arteries in patients with transient ischaemic attacks. It is usually associated with a vein patch angioplasty which prevents narrowing of the artery when it is being closed.

Bypass. Using this technique a new conduit is anastomosed above and below the blockage. The conduit of choice is the patient's own long saphenous vein but because of its size this is only suitable for bypass procedures below the inguinal ligament or for renal artery bypass. If a vein is not available, synthetic grafts are used but the results with these are not as good as they are prone to thrombosis. They are much more successful above the inguinal ligament as the vessels are larger and higher flow rates decrease the risk of thrombosis.

Replacement. The diseased artery is taken out of the circulation and replaced by a prosthetic graft. The technique is used particularly in the replacement of aortic and other aneurysms.

Sympathectomy. Division of the sympathetic nerves supplying the limb results in the dilation of the vessels in the skin. It cannot increase the flow of blood to the limb, and therefore its use is limited to patients who have disease of the small vessels such as Buerger's disease. It may also be of benefit in patients with Raynaud's phenomenon. Sympathectomies can be performed by operation or injection.

Postoperative care of these procedures

Postoperative observations of pulse rate, blood pressure, respiratory rate, temperature and urinary output are invaluable. Central venous pressure monitoring is valuable in patients with cardiac failure. Low cardiac output or hypotension may precipitate thrombosis. The distal pulses should be recorded at the end of any arterial operation and should be checked regularly thereafter. If the pulses disappear the surgeon should be informed immediately. If a bypass graft occludes in the postoperative period, it may be possible to unblock it if the situation is detected early.

All patients should be commenced on aspirin (if there are no contraindications), as this decreases the risk of graft failure.

Patients should be entered in a graft surveillance programme using colour Doppler imaging. This will pick up 'at risk' grafts which can be modified to improve long-term patency.

Types of procedure

Each vascular operation is tailor made for each patient using one or a combination of the techniques described above. The procedure may be named by the proximal and distal vessels to be dealt with, e.g. aortobifemoral bypass, femoroanterior tibial bypass, common femoral endarterectomy and patch angioplasty. Some of the commoner types of procedure are described below.

OPERATION: AORTOFEMORAL BYPASS

In this operation, disease of the aorta or iliac arteries which is not amenable to angioplasty or stenting, is bypassed. The aorta is exposed transperitoneally or retroperitoneally. The femoral arteries are exposed through vertical groin incisions and a prosthetic bypass graft is placed retroperitoneally and anastomosed to one or both femoral arteries.

Codes

Blood .... 6 units (Cell saver if available)

GA/LA .... GA

Opn time .... 2–4 h

Stay .... 8–10 days

Drains out .... 48 h

Sutures out .... 7–10 days

Off work .... 4–6 weeks

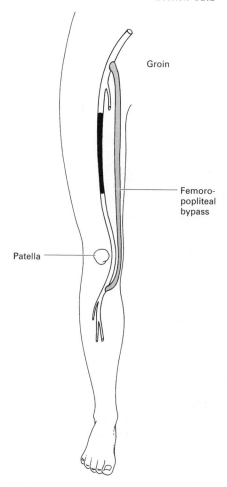

Fig. 99 Femoropopliteal bypass.

OPERATION: FEMOROPOPLITEAL BYPASS/
FEMORODISTAL BYPASS (Fig. 99)

In this operation the femoral artery is exposed in the groin
and the popliteal artery is exposed in the popliteal fossa or
one of the distal leg vessels exposed in the calf. The long
saphenous vein is excised along its length in the thigh,
reversed so that the valves do not disrupt flow, and used to
bypass the blocked femoral artery. Sometimes the vein is left
in its bed ('*in situ* bypass') and the valves destroyed with a
special instrument called a valvulotome. If a vein is not
available it is possible to use prosthetic material usually a
Teflon (PTFE) graft.

Codes

Blood .... 4 units
GA/LA .... GA/LA
Opn time .... 2–5 h
Stay .... 6–10 days
Drains out .... 48 h
Sutures out .... 7–10 days
Off work .... 4–6 weeks

OPERATION: PROFUNDOPLASTY

This operation is performed if the commencement of the profunda femoris artery is narrowed. It is sometimes combined with an endarterectomy. A vertical incision is made along the narrowed area and a gusset patch of long saphenous vein or prosthetic material is inserted to widen the narrowed artery.

Codes

Blood .... 2 units
GA/LA .... LA or GA
Opn time .... 1–2 h
Stay .... 5–7 days
Drains out .... 48 h
Sutures out .... 7 days
Off work .... 3–6 weeks

OPERATION: AXILLOFEMORAL/
AXILLOBIFEMORAL BYPASS

These operations are used to bring blood to ischaemic lower limbs in patients with an aortic occlusion who are not fit for an aortofemoral procedure. Also, it can be used in patients with an infected aortic graft. A long prosthetic graft is anastomosed to the axillary artery under the clavicle and tunnelled subcutaneously to the common femoral artery in the groin. If both legs are ischaemic an inverted Y graft may be used to bring blood to both femoral arteries.

Codes

Blood .... 4 units
GA/LA .... GA
Opn time .... 1–3 h
Stay .... 7–10 days
Drains out .... 48 h
Sutures out .... 7–10 days
Off work .... 4–6 weeks

OPERATION: ILEOFEMORAL/FEMOROFEMORAL CROSS-OVER BYPASS

This is usually performed where there is an iliac blockage on one side which is not treatable by angioplasty or stenting and the patient is not fit for a more major procedure. A prosthetic graft is sutured from the normal iliac artery or the common femoral artery on the good side and tunnelled preperitoneally (from the iliac) or subcutaneously (from the femoral artery) to the common femoral artery on the diseased side.

Codes

Blood	4 units
GA/LA	GA or spinal
Opn time	2 h
Stay	7–10 days
Drains out	24 h
Sutures out	7–10 days
Off work	4–6 weeks

OPERATION: LUMBAR SYMPATHECTOMY

The lumbar sympathetic chain is approached retroperitoneally through an anterior flank incision. The lower lumbar ganglia are identified and excised. This operation can also be carried out endoscopically.

Codes

Blood	2 units
GA/LA	GA
Opn time	60–90 min
Stay	5–7 days
Drains out	24 h
Sutures out	7 days
Off work	4–6 weeks

OPERATION: INJECTION LUMBAR SYMPATHECTOMY

A needle is passed through the back under radiographic control. Its position is confirmed by injecting contrast medium and phenol is then injected to destroy the lower lumbar sympathetic chain. This can be carried out under local or general anaesthesia.

Amputation

When all attempts to save an ischaemic limb have failed or the patient presents with gangrene, amputation may be necessary to relieve the symptoms. The level of the amputation will have to be high enough to ensure adequate healing of the stump.

Preoperative management
The option of amputation should be given to the patient against the background of failure or unavailability of other options. It should not be seen as a purely negative option as it gives excellent pain relief and mobility is good with modern prosthetic limbs. Always leave the final decision to the patient and their family. There is some evidence that preoperative insertion of an epidural anaesthetic for 24 h may decrease the risk of phantom limb pain after major amputation, and it will give the patient preoperative pain relief.

OPERATION: ABOVE-KNEE AMPUTATION
The bone is divided approximately 40 cm from the greater trochanter. Equal sized anterior and posterior skin flaps are formed 5 cm beyond this. Once the bone has been divided the muscles are closed over the cut end and the skin flaps closed with loose sutures. The wound is drained and the stump bandaged.

Codes

Blood	2 units
GA/LA	GA or spinal
Opn time	90 min
Stay	2–3 weeks
Drains out	48 h
Sutures out	10–14 days
Off work	Variable

OPERATION: BELOW-KNEE AMPUTATION
The blood supply to the tissues of the lower leg is better posteriorly than anteriorly. This amputation is designed to use a long posterior flap of muscle and overlying skin to close the wound. The tibia is divided 10 cm below the tibial tuberosity and the fibula 2.5 cm proximally. The skin and

muscle of the long posterior flap is folded forward over the divided bone and sutured to the skin anteriorly. This amputation has the advantage of preserving the knee joint, making rehabilitation easier.

Codes
As on p. 530.

OPERATION: RAY AMPUTATION
Where there is necrosis of a digit accompanied by necrosis or infection of the muscles of the foot, a ray amputation of the toe and its metatarsal may be necessary. The incisions extend from the interdigital clefts at either side of the affected toe to the base of the relevant metatarsals. The wound is left open and dressed daily. The overall effect is to narrow the forefoot.

Codes

Blood	Group and save
GA/LA	GA or spinal
Opn time	30–60 min
Stay	10–14 days weeks
Drains out	0
Sutures out	0
Off work	Variable

OPERATION: TRANSMETATARSAL AMPUTATION
In this operation the forefoot is amputated. The sole of the forefoot is preserved as a flap which is sutured to the skin of the dorsum of the remaining foot.

Codes

Blood	Group and save
GA/LA	GA or spinal
Opn time	30–60 min
Stay	2–3 weeks
Drains out	48 h
Sutures out	10–14 days
Off work	Variable

OPERATION: AMPUTATION OF TOE

The toe is amputated with the head of the metatarsal, as exposed cartilage will impair healing. It is usually performed with a racquet-shaped incision, circumferential around the toe with the 'handle' extending onto the dorsum of the foot. The skin is closed with a number of loose sutures.

Codes

Blood .... Group and save
GA/LA .... GA or spinal
Opn time .... 30–60 min
Stay .... 7–10 days
Drains out 0
Sutures out .... 10–14 days
Off work .... Variable

Postoperative care

In the case of above- or below-knee amputation check that the bandages are not too tight after 8 h. Drains should be removed, without disturbing the dressings. Gentle physiotherapy should be commenced after 48 h to prevent development of contractures at the hip or knee joints. Liaise with limb fitting and rehabilitation services at an early stage. Patients with trans-metatarsal and ray amputations may need orthotic shoe implants to aid them walking.

12.3 Aneurysms, Acute Ischaemia and Arteriovenous Fistulae

Arterial aneurysms

An aneurysm is an abnormal dilatation of a blood vessel, usually caused by atherosclerosis, which results in weakening of the arterial wall. The aneurysm occurs most commonly in the aorta below the level of the renal arteries, followed by the popliteal and femoral arteries, but may occur in any artery including the thoracic aorta.

Other causes

1 Congenital. The best example is the berry aneurysm in the cerebral arteries.

2 Traumatic. The arterial wall may be damaged during arteriography, surgery or by penetrating trauma with a sharp object or gunshot injury.

3 Inflammatory. Non-specific inflammatory aneurysms can occur, but mycotic aneurysms associated with specific bacterial infection can also occur. Syphilitic aneurysms are the best known but thankfully are now rare.

4 Cystic medial necrosis is a degenerative condition of the arterial media and may occur as part of Marfan's syndrome.

Aortic aneurysm

Aortic aneurysms usually arise below the renal arteries and may extend into the iliac arteries. When small, aneurysms are usually asymptomatic As the wall weakens they get progressively larger. Although an aneurysm may rupture at any size, it is unusual for this to occur if the maximum diameter is less than 5 cm. The risk of rupture is related to size and this is in the order of 20% per year for aneurysms greater than 5 cm. If the aneurysm is repaired as an elective procedure in a good centre the mortality should be in the order of 5%. However, if the aneurysm ruptures, the likelihood is that the patient will die immediately. Even if they survive and undergo emergency surgery the perioperative mortality is in the order of 50%. Therefore the aneurysm should be repaired before it ruptures. Aortic aneurysms may be lined with thrombus, some of which may break off and embolize to the smaller vessels of the legs causing acute ischaemia. Patients with aortic aneurysms may have aneurysms at other sites (e.g. iliac, femoral, popliteal).

Recognizing the pattern

The patient is usually over 50 years of age and males are more frequently affected than females. There may be associated atheromatous disease such as a history of myocardial infarction or angina or stroke.

They sometimes notice an abdominal mass or prominent pulsation. They may complain of back pain or epigastric discomfort as the aneurysm enlarges. There may be a sudden onset of pain and discoloration in the toes of one or both feet ('blue toe syndrome') which is caused by embolization of thrombus. Frequently the aneurysm is detected as an incidental finding at clinical assessment or during ultrasound examination.

On examination the pulsatile swelling is usually felt in the epigastrium and central abdomen. Palpation from side to side confirms that the pulsation is true and not transmitted. In thin elderly patients with a prominent lordosis the normal aorta is easily palpable and if somewhat tortuous may feel like an aneurysm. Careful bimanual palpation of its lateral and medial margins should demonstrate that it is not widened. It is important to examine for aneurysms at other locations especially in the femoral and popliteal arteries and also to assess distal pulses.

Proving the diagnosis

The best method of diagnosing an aneurysm is using ultrasound, which is non-invasive. Computed tomography (CT) scanning is the most accurate method of measuring the size and extent of the aneurysm and determining whether it contains thrombus or not. Spiral CT scanning and magnetic resonance imaging (MRI) are expensive and time-consuming but give excellent detail on the size and configuration of the aneurysm. A plain abdominal X-ray may show the characteristic curved line of calcification of the aneurysm wall and a lateral view may help define its size. Arteriography is not useful in the diagnosis of aortic aneurysm. However, it can give information with respect to the relationship of the renal vessels to the aneurysm and with newer methods of treatment, calibrated angiography to measure exact length of the aneurysm and the angulation of its 'neck' is important.

Management

The indications for repair are as follows:

1 An aneurysm greater than 5 cm maximum diameter
2 An aneurysm giving rise to emboli
3 An expanding aneurysm
4 The onset of symptoms of abdominal or back pain as these may herald impending rupture.

If an aneurysm is less than 5 cm in diameter at presentation and is asymptomatic, its size should be observed every 3 months using ultrasound, to determine whether it is enlarging.

Preoperative management

The patient and their relatives should be informed about the risks and benefits of surgery and the dangers of an untreated aneurysm. They should also be informed of the necessity of inserting a prosthetic graft to replace it. The patient's cardiac, respiratory and renal status should be assessed and optimized preoperatively. If the patient is having an endovascular repair of the aneurysm, the results of their spiral CT scan and calibrated angiogram should be available. Prophylactic antibiotics are given with the premedication or at induction of anaesthesia. Deep venous thrombosis prophylaxis using subcutaneous heparin should be used. Antiembolic stockings may be used if the patient does not have chronic ischaemia and ABPI is normal. The patient should have a urinary catheter inserted preoperatively to measure urinary output during and after the procedure.

Endovascular repair of aortic aneurysm is undergoing clinical assessment at present. It requires a proximal and distal neck of suitable configuration to hold a stent attached to the graft. A tube graft or bifurcated graft may be inserted. Only 50% of aneurysms have a suitable configuration for this procedure to be used at present.

OPERATION: ENDOVASCULAR REPAIR OF AORTIC ANEURYSM

The femoral vessels are exposed and controlled through a groin incision. A guide wire is passed proximally into the aorta and a catheter passed over the guide wire. A preoperative angiogram is performed. A graft previously prepared from the calibrated angiogram and attached to stents at its proxi-

Continued on p. 536

Continued.

mal and distal extent is loaded into a delivery system and passed through an incision in the femoral artery into the aorta. The delivery system is withdrawn and the upper stent expanded in the proximal neck using an angioplasty balloon. The balloon is withdrawn and reinflated in the distal stent anchoring it in the distal neck. The distal neck may be in the aorta or iliac artery. Bifurcated grafts may be inserted into the iliac arteries using this technology. If one iliac artery is aneurysmal in addition to the aorta it is possible to insert an aortic uni-iliac graft, occlude the opposite iliac endovascularly and perform a femorofemoral cross-over graft.

Codes

Blood	6 units
GA/LA	LA or GA
Opn time	2–4 h
Stay	2–5 days
Drains out	0
Sutures out	7–10 days
Off work	4–6 weeks

OPERATION: CONVENTIONAL REPAIR OF AORTIC ANEURYSM

The aorta is exposed and the extent of the aneurysm confirmed. An aneurysm lying between the renal arteries and the aortic bifurcation may easily be replaced by a straight tube graft. If it extends into the iliac arteries it may be necessary to insert a bifurcated graft to the bifurcation of the iliac arteries or even to the femoral arteries in the groin. Once the aneurysm has been controlled proximally and distally, the lumbar vessels are suture ligated from within. The Dacron prosthesis is then sewn into the upper aorta and a similar anastomosis is made at the aortic bifurcation, iliac arteries or femoral arteries as indicated. The aneurysm wall is then wrapped around the graft.

Codes

Blood	6 units (Cell saver if available)
GA/LA	GA
Opn time	2–4 h
Stay	8–10 days
Drains out	Abdomen 0; groin 24 h
Sutures out	7–10 days
Off work	About 4–6 weeks

Postoperative care

Thrombus lining the aneurysm may become dislodged during the operation. The presence of palpable pulses should be assessed before the patient is taken off the operating table. If previously palpable pulses are absent it is an indication for embolectomy. Haemodynamic monitoring is vital (see section 1.11) as hypotension, tachycardia and oliguria may indicate bleeding and the surgeon should be informed. Dopamine infusion to maintain renal output may be valuable especially in patients with impaired renal function, but must be used only when the patient is haemodynamically stable.

The patient is mobilized on the third or fourth day postoperatively and may commence oral intake once the postoperative ileus has settled.

Follow-up of patients undergoing endovascular repair of aneurysms is vital as the long-term outlook is unknown. Patients undergoing standard operative repair need not be followed up although there is the possibility of developing graft infection or aortoenteric fistula where a loop of bowel becomes adherent and the graft fistulates into the bowel.

Ruptured aortic aneurysm

This is one of the most dramatic conditions which faces the surgical team. The initial rupture is temporarily controlled by the surrounding tissues, in patients who survive long enough to be admitted to hospital. This gives a short time interval for the operation to be organized as the patient will die unless the aorta can be replaced before they exsanguinate. Rapid intervention is needed for the patient to survive.

Recognizing the pattern

The patient usually complains of sudden onset severe pain in the abdomen, back or flank, sometimes associated with collapse. The pain is more commonly on the left than the right. They may feel faint, cold and sweaty. Occasionally the presentation is less dramatic.

On examination the patient is pale and shocked with hypotension and tachycardia. The aneurysm is tender. Avoid palpating it more than is necessary. Note the presence or absence of distal pulses for future reference.

Proving the diagnosis

Time should not be wasted on investigations if the patient is shocked. A tender aneurysm in a shocked patient is an indication for surgery. If the situation is less acute, the diagnosis is in doubt and the patient is haemodynamically stable, a CT scan will confirm the presence of an aneurysm and show whether it is leaking.

Management

Warn the surgeon, anaesthetist and theatre as soon as possible that a patient with a leaking aneurysm has been admitted. Take blood for cross-matching (10 units) and baseline investigations (full blood count, urea and electrolytes and coagulation screen). Set up two large-bore intravenous lines and transfer the patient to theatre. If the patient is hypotensive, do not attempt to bring the blood pressure up at this stage as it may precipitate intraperitoneal rupture.

Prior to induction of anaesthesia pass a urinary catheter and give prophylactic antibiotics. Reassess the situation in the anaesthetic room if the patient is haemodynamically stable. Check how long it would be until the blood is available.

The patient will usually be induced on the operating table in theatre once the surgeon and the rest of the team are ready to start operating. The relaxation of the abdominal muscles associated with anaesthesia, results in the loss of the tamponading effect and frequently precipitates major blood loss.

OPERATION: REPAIR OF RUPTURED AORTIC ANEURYSM

The abdomen is opened and a massive retroperitoneal haematoma is usually present. The aorta above the rupture and the iliac arteries are controlled. Once this is done the haemorrhage is controlled. The aneurysm is opened and a Dacron graft is sewn inside it as in an elective procedure (p. 536).

Codes

Blood .... 10 units (Cell saver if available)
GA/LA .... GA
Opn time .... 2–5 h
Stay .... 8–21 days
Drains out .... Abdomen 0; groin 24 h
Sutures out .... 7–10 days
Off work .... Variable, 8–12 weeks

Postoperative care
This is as for an elective aneurysm repair and is described on p. 537. There is, however, a more prolonged period of intensive care as the patient has almost certainly been hypotensive for a period of time. Acute renal failure may occur in the postoperative period because of this. The patient will have a prolonged ileus because of the retroperitoneal haematoma and nutritional support may have to be considered. As the haematoma breaks down the patient may develop haemolytic jaundice which should resolve spontaneously.

Femoral aneurysms

These may present with acute thrombosis or embolization to the feet; they rarely rupture. They require resection or replacement with a graft if they are symptomatic or enlarge markedly.

Popliteal aneurysms

These frequently thrombose causing acute limb ischaemia. The presence of a popliteal aneurysm is therefore an indication for surgery. The aneurysm may be tied off and a saphenous vein bypass graft inserted.

Acute arterial occlusion

This condition results in an acutely ischaemic limb, which has a high risk of limb loss unless intervention is swift. The causes are as follows:

1 Acute arterial embolism. In this condition there is an acute blockage of an artery due to an embolus arising from thrombus formed proximally. Sources of emboli include the following:
   (a) atrial fibrillation
   (b) myocardial infarction with mural thrombus
   (c) subacute bacterial endocarditis
   (d) thrombus formation on an ulcerated atheromatous plaque
   (e) thrombus formation within an aneurysm.

2 Acute thrombosis of chronic peripheral vascular disease. In this condition the patient has significant narrowing in an artery which thromboses when the flow through it decreases.

3 Acute thrombosis of a previous bypass graft. In this condition the patient has had a previous bypass graft which occludes, usually as a result of stenosis within the graft or a progression of the atheromatous process above or below the graft.

Recognizing the pattern

Arterial emboli can occur in either sex and at any age but are more common in the elderly. Arterial thrombosis occurs in arteriopaths, typically middle-aged or elderly male smokers. Graft occlusion can occur in anybody who has undergone a previous bypass graft.

Symptoms which occur in the affected limb are characterized by the following:

1 Pain
2 Pallor
3 Paralysis
4 Paraesthesia.

The history of embolism is characterized by sudden onset of these symptoms. If there is a previous history of intermittent claudication, the possibility of acute thrombosis should be considered. A history of previous vascular surgery is significant. The paraesthesia and paralysis are later symptoms and are due to ischaemia of the nerves. They are indicative that early intervention is indicated.

On examination the limb is pale, cold and immobile. Distal pulses are absent. There may be loss of pin-prick and light touch sensation in a stocking distribution over the distal leg. The pulse may be irregular and the patient may have other signs suggesting a source of embolus (e.g. a heart murmur, an aortic aneurysm or a localized arterial bruit).

Proving the diagnosis

Acute arterial embolism must be distinguished from thrombus on a previously existing atheromatous plaque or an occluded graft. The history and examination is a reliable guide. Arteriography is the definitive investigation.

Management

The treatment of acute ischaemia is urgent intervention to remove the blockage and restore the circulation. Blood is taken for group and cross-match and baseline heamatological investigations (full blood count, urea and electrolytes and coagulation screen). Heparin infusion is commenced if there are no contraindications.

The treatments available to unblock the arteries include surgery and thrombolysis.

Thrombolysis is performed when there is limb-threatening acute arterial occlusion of short duration. It is contraindicated in patients with bleeding disorders, gastrointestinal bleeding, stroke, recent surgery or allergy to thrombolytic agents. It should not be considered in patients with paraesthesia and paralysis as the time taken to lyse the thrombus may result in irreversible ischaemia and limb loss. It is especially valuable in reopening occluded bypass grafts.

Surgery is indicated when thrombolysis is not possible or has failed.

OPERATION: INTRA-ARTERIAL CATHETER-DIRECTED THROMBOLYSIS

The radiologist should be aware that thrombolysis is being considered as the approach will probably be different if a diagnostic arteriogram is being performed. A catheter is placed in the artery percutaneously and an angiogram performed. The catheter is directed into the embolus or thrombus and a bolus of thrombolytic agent injected through the catheter directly into the clot. There are three thrombolytic agents in common usage, streptokinase, urokinase and tissue plasminogen activator. An infusion of thrombolytic agent is then commenced and the patient returned to the ward with the infusion running. A repeat arteriogram is performed at set intervals to assess clot dissolution. If the clot does not dissolve in 12 h surgery should be considered.

If the procedure is successful, an angioplasty of the lesion causing thrombosis is indicated.

Codes

Blood	4 units
GA/LA	LA
Opn time	2–12 h
Stay	2–5 days
Drains out	0
Sutures out	0
Off work	2–4 weeks

OPERATION: CATHETER EMBOLECTOMY

The vessel where the embolus has lodged is isolated and controlled (commonly the femoral, occasionally the popliteal). An arteriotomy is made and visible clot extracted. The inflow of blood to the limb is checked. A Fogarty balloon

Continued on p. 542

Continued.

catheter is passed down the arterial lumen. This is a thin catheter with a balloon at its tip. Once beyond the clot the balloon is dilated and gently pulled back towards the arteriotomy, extracting the clot. Once all the clot is extracted the arteriotomy is closed with a patch if necessary. Great care must be taken not to overinflate the balloon as this may cause damage to the vessel wall, with resultant stricture formation and permanent obstruction to the blood flow.

Codes

Blood	4 units
GA/LA	LA or GA
Opn time	1–2 h
Stay	3–10 days
Drains out	48 h
Sutures out	7 days
Off work	Variable

Postoperative care

This is similar to that following other arterial operations. The possibility of compartment syndrome, due to swelling of revascularized ischaemic muscles, must be considered if the patient develops pain or swelling of the leg after successful treatment. This is an emergency and the patient may require fasciotomies.

Arteriovenous fistulae

An arteriovenous fistula is a condition in which there is an abnormal connection between the arterial and the venous circulations. The common causes are as follows:

1 Congenital — often associated with haemangioma or hamartoma formation.

2 Post-traumatic — arteriovenous fistulae may follow penetrating injury or damage done to vessels during operation.

3 Iatrogenic — arteriovenous shunts are created, usually in the forearm, as a route of access to the circulation for those on dialysis (Cimino fistula).

The high pressure and increased flow causes the vein to dilate and become tortuous. There may be an increased cardiac output and a high pulse pressure if the shunt is large.

Recognizing the pattern

Arteriovenous fistulae are rare but can occur at any age from birth onwards.

The patient may have noticed prominent pulsatile veins, the mass of a haemangioma or the appearance of a 'throbbing' swelling at the site of previous trauma. Occasionally they complain of 'buzzing' associated with the flow disturbance. Rarely they present with high output cardiac failure.

Superficial fistulae are usually associated with dilated pulsatile veins. Subcutaneous fistulae present as a swelling beneath the skin, possibly associated with a scar suggestive of an old wound. On palpation there is an expansile pulsation. The characteristic sign is that of an audible 'machinery murmur' over the lesion present in both systole and diastole. It may be abolished by proximal arterial compression. There may be a palpable 'thrill'. Limb enlargement may be associated with congenital arteriovenous malformations.

Proving the diagnosis

Colour Doppler imaging will prove the diagnosis. Arteriography is required in planning appropriate therapy.

Management

Small arteriovenous fistulae may not require treatment. If there are dilated veins associated with the fistula, a graduated compression stocking or sleeve may be beneficial. Larger arteriovenous fistulae may be treated by embolization or surgery.

Embolization. The radiologist performs an angiogram to identify the vessels forming the fistula. These are selectively cannulated and a thrombogenic substance is injected via the catheter, blocking the vessels and occluding the fistula.

Surgery. In this case the feeding vessels are defined by preoperative arteriography, isolated and ligated.

OPERATION FOR ARTERIOVENOUS FISTULA

The feeding vessels are dissected out and tied off and the fistula excised. There may be multiple feeding vessels especially in congenital arteriovenous fistulae and blood loss may be high. For this reason embolization is the preferred treatment.

Codes

Blood	4–6 units (Cell saver if available)
GA/LA	GA
Opn time	2–5 h
Stay	7–14 days
Drains out	2–3 days
Sutures out	7 days
Off work	4–6 weeks

12.4 Other Arterial Conditions

Carotid artery disease

The brain is supplied by four major arteries, the two internal carotid arteries and the two vertebral arteries. These interconnect within the cranial cavity through the circle of Willis.

An atheromatous plaque in the carotid artery may affect the blood supply to the brain. Plaques are commonly formed at the bifurcation of the carotid arteries or at the origin of the internal carotid artery. Although reduction in cerebral blood flow is unusual because of the excellent collateral circulation through the circle of Willis, the plaque may undergo ulceration, thrombus formation and distal embolization resulting in a transient ischaemic attack or a stroke. A transient ischaemic attack is a focal neurological deficit lasting less than 24 h (usually lasting only a few minutes) with complete recovery. The symptoms depend upon the region supplied by the vessel in which the embolus lodges. Approximately one-third of patients who suffer from a transient ischaemic attack will have no further symptoms, another third will have further transient ischaemic attacks and the final third will progress to stroke. Acute, total occlusion of a carotid artery may cause a stroke resulting in a complete hemiparesis. This is often, but not always, preceded by transient ischaemic attacks.

The ophthalmic artery is the first branch of the internal carotid artery after it enters the skull. An embolus to this artery may lodge in the retinal artery giving rise to transient monoocular blindness or amaurosis fugax. The embolus usually breaks up with full restoration of vision. If this does not occur the patient will suffer a retinal infarct in the area supplied by that branch of the retinal artery.

The unpredictability of the situation has made choosing which patients benefit from intervention difficult, but the indications for surgery are becoming clearer.

Recognizing the pattern

The patient is usually an arteriopath, middle aged or elderly, a smoker and hypertensive. They may have had previous peripheral or coronary arterial problems.

There may be a history of a single or multiple transient ischaemic attacks or an established stroke. These will affect the cerebral cortex on the same side as the carotid lesion and will result in a weakness or paraesthesia of the arm and leg on the opposite side of the body and possibly a speech disturbance. Amaurosis fugax will present as a transient blindness which the patient describes as a shutter coming down over the eye involved.

There may be nothing to find on examination but a localized bruit over the lateral side of the neck which may arise from a narrowed carotid artery. The neurological and eye signs may be transient. Examination of the visual fields may reveal defects and fundoscopy may reveal evidence of previous emboli.

Proving the diagnosis

To confirm carotid artery disease, bilateral colour Doppler ultrasound imaging (Duplex) of the carotid arteries should be performed. This is a very accurate method of diagnosing carotid artery stenosis. On the basis of recognized blood velocity criteria, the degree of narrowing can be assessed as < 20%, 20–49%, 50–69% and 70–99%. Its limitation is in the differentiation of a very tight stenosis and an occlusion of the artery where operation is contraindicated. In this situation arteriography is helpful.

Magnetic resonance angiography is non-invasive but at present its availability is limited to certain centres. It can confirm blood flow in the carotid arteries and simultaneously give information about the brain.

Conventional arteriography and intra-arterial digital subtraction arteriography give better images of the arteries, but there is a risk of causing a stroke when they are performed.

CT of the brain is useful to rule out other pathology (if an MRI study has not been performed).

Patients with suspected carotid artery disease should have the same risk factor assessment as those presenting with peripheral vascular disease.

Management

All patients should undergo risk factor modification to decrease the risk of disease progression. There are two approaches to treatment.

1 The use of antiplatelet medication, such as aspirin or dipyridamole and/or anticoagulants such as warfarin.

2 Surgical endarterectomy to remove the plaque.

The decision over which treatment to use depends upon the symptomatic status of the patient and the degree of narrowing of the carotid arteries.

Asymptomatic bruit

Where a bruit is found in the neck but the patient has no symptoms, a Doppler imaging study should be requested. If there is a less than 70% narrowing of the carotid artery the patient should be commenced on low-dose aspirin (75 mg daily) to reduce the risk of stroke. If there is a 70–99% stenosis, most clinicians would treat the patient conservatively although there are ongoing clinical trials to determine whether surgery would be beneficial.

Transient ischaemic attacks

If a patient presents with transient ischaemic attacks and carotid Doppler studies show a narrowing of < 20%, treatment should be with aspirin or some other antiplatelet agent. If the patient has a 20–69% stenosis, most surgeons would treat the patient conservatively with aspirin although there are ongoing studies to determine if surgery would be of benefit to these patients. If there is a stenosis of 70–99% surgery is indicated and is of definite benefit in preventing a stroke. If the carotid artery is occluded, surgery is not indicated. Antiplatelet therapy should be prescribed postoperatively in all patients.

Preoperative management

The patient should be fully informed of the nature of the operation and of the risks of developing a stroke if surgery is not performed. They should be warned about the possibility of developing a stroke during or immediately after the operation. Such occurrences are thankfully rare and usually transient. The neck should be shaved on the relevant side. Medications should be reviewed preoperatively and the surgeon should be asked about continuing anticoagulants and antiplatelet agents preoperatively.

OPERATION: CAROTID ENDARTERECTOMY

The common, internal and external carotid arteries are exposed and controlled through an incision along the anterior border of the sternomastoid muscle. The patient is heparinized and the arteries clamped. A longitudinal incision is made in the common carotid artery extending into the internal carotid artery. The surgeon may decide to use a shunt. This is a tube placed in the common and internal carotid arteries to carry blood to the brain during the procedure. The localized plaque is removed by endarterectomy. The artery is closed and a vein patch or a Dacron prosthetic patch may be used to prevent narrowing.

Codes

Blood	2 units
GA/LA	GA/LA
Opn time	2 h
Stay	3–7 days
Drains out	24 h
Sutures out	5 days
Off work	4–6 weeks

Postoperative care

Patients should undergo neurological observation in addition to the routine haemodynamic observations.

Maintaining the blood pressure between 100 and 180 mmHg systolic is important. With hypertension there is a risk of bleeding from the arterial suture line and possibly a haemorrhagic stroke. Hypotension may result in thrombosis of the endarterectomy site resulting in stroke. Any neurological deficit should be reported to the surgeon immediately. Tongue deviation to the side of operation on protrusion indicates a hypoglossal nerve lesion, the majority of which recover. The patient may complain of headache which is due to cerebral reperfusion and is an indication that the operation was successful. The patient should be reassured and given adequate analgesia. It usually settles within days but the patient should be observed until it does so.

Raynaud's phenomenon

This is a clinical condition characterized by a sequence of colour changes in the digits on exposure to cold or emotional stress. The colour changes result from intense vasospasm of the digital vessels which cause the fingers (or toes) to go white initially, then cyanosed as the spasm relaxes in the arterioles but not in the venules and then red with reactive hyperaemia as there is complete relaxation of the spasm. The spasm may be due to a normal vasoconstrictive response to cold in diseased arteries or an excessive response to cold in normal vessels. The latter occurs more frequently and is called Raynaud's disease. It is a disease of unknown aetiology.

Secondary Raynaud's phenomenon usually occurs in diseased vessels and is seen in scleroderma, systemic lupus erythematosus and other connective tissue diseases. Other conditions which can cause stenoses in the arteries include cervical rib, atherosclerosis, Buerger's disease, cryoglobinaemia and certain drugs (e.g. the contraceptive pill). Certain occupational hazards such as working with vibrating tools, exposure to vinyl chloride and heavy metals may also cause it.

Recognizing the pattern

The patient is usually a woman in her late twenties or early thirties.

There is a history of colour changes following exposure to cold as described above. In Raynaud's disease the changes usually occur in all the fingers or toes and are symmetrical. In secondary Raynaud's phenomenon, the changes may be asymmetrical. There is usually numbness or pain associated with the attacks.

During an attack the characteristic sequence of colour changes are evident. Between attacks the hands may appear normal. The skin of the fingers may be dry and fissured or there may be ulceration and gangrene at the tips of the fingers in extreme cases. Peripheral pulses are usually normal. It is important to rule out a cervical rib.

Proving the diagnosis

The diagnosis of Raynaud's disease is based on the history and exclusion of underlying causes. Delayed or abnormal hand rewarming after cold provocation can be measured using thermography or thermocouples applied to the skin. This will confirm a vasospastic tendency. Upper limb and digital pressure measurements will rule out occlusive disease in the arteries of the upper limb. Haematological investigations should be performed to rule out other underlying causes. These should include full blood count, plasma viscosity, liver function test, Thyroid function tests (TFTs), rheumatoid factor, antinuclear antibodies and cryoglobulins.

Management

Conservative measures are the mainstay of treatment. Keeping the extremities warm (gloves and socks) and the avoidance of sudden exposure to cold. Battery-heated gloves are available for patients with frequent attacks. Skin care with moisturizing creams should be advised. It is important to maintain the central body core temperature and not just concentrate on the hands. Ulcers or infection should be treated with antibiotics as indicated. Patients should be

Continued on p. 550

Continued.

advised to stop smoking as nicotine is a powerful vaso-constrictor.

Medications used include the calcium–channel blockers nifedipine and nicardipine, and the α-adrenergic blockers prazosin and thymoxamine. Response to medication is variable.

If symptoms are severe or trophic changes are present cervical sympathectomy may be indicated. This is effective in only 50–75% of cases and the benefit may be short-lived.

OPERATION: CERVICAL SYMPATHECTOMY

The anaesthetist must be informed whether the procedure is unilateral (which side) or bilateral.

This operation is best performed thoracoscopically (see p. 599). In the open operation the sympathetic chain may be approached using a supraclavicular incision or by an axillary incision, where access to the chest is gained by resecting a portion of the third rib. The second and third cervical ganglia are exposed and resected or destroyed. Chest drains may be used if a bilateral procedure is performed.

Codes

Blood	Group and save
GA/LA	GA
Opn time	1–2 h
Stay	2–7 days
Drains out	24 h (if inserted)
Sutures out	4–7 days
Off work	1–2 weeks

Postoperative care

A chest X-ray is performed in the recovery room to rule out pneumothorax. As well as routine haemodynamic observations, oxygen saturation should be assessed by oximetry. Chest infection or atelectasis are recognized complications of a thoracotomy. Horner's syndrome may occur especially after supraclavicular cervical sympathectomy and is usually transient.

12.5   Venous Disorders

Varicose veins

Varicose veins are elongated, dilated and tortuous veins which usually occur in skin of the lower limb. The veins in the leg may be divided into the skin veins and the deep veins. They are connected by 'perforator' veins which cross the deep fascia of the leg and drain blood from the superficial veins into the deep veins. The deep veins tend to lie within the muscle mass of the calf and thigh. When these muscles contract they act as an auxiliary pump to aid venous return. Valves in the perforating veins prevent blood flowing into the skin veins under normal circumstances. During muscle relaxation, reverse flow of blood is prevented within the deep veins by valves.

If the valves in the connecting veins become incompetent, pressure will be transmitted from the deep veins into the skin veins resulting in the formation of varicose veins (Fig. 100).

Common sites for incompetent valves to occur are as follows:
1   Where the long saphenous vein joins the femoral vein in the groin.

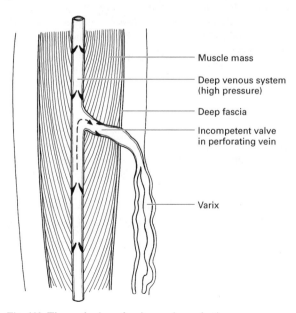

- Muscle mass
- Deep venous system (high pressure)
- Deep fascia
- Incompetent valve in perforating vein
- Varix

Fig. 100 The mechanism of varicose vein production.

2 Where the short saphenous vein joins the popliteal vein in the popliteal fossa.

3 Where there are perforator veins in the medial aspect of the mid-thigh.

4 Where calf perforators connect the deep veins and the skin veins behind the medial border of the tibia.

Making the diagnosis

The clinician's task is to determine if the patient's symptoms are due to the varicosities and to determine the site of reflux from the deep to the superficial system.

Patients are usually female in their twenties or thirties but may be either sex or any age.

A history of previous deep venous thrombosis should be sought. Symptoms which may be associated with varicose veins include the following:

1 Cosmetic. The patient is upset about the appearance.

2 Pain. Varicose veins characteristically give rise to ache in the leg especially after prolonged standing. It is relieved by leg elevation and support stockings.

3 Itching. This often occurs over the varicosities, is worse in warm weather or after a hot bath and may occur in the presence of eczema.

4 Symptoms. These include, due to the complications of varicose veins oedema or leg swelling (worse at the end of the day), pigmentation and thickening of the skin in the region of the medial malleolus, eczema and even ulceration.

On examination the site of reflux through an incompetent perforator or perforators should be sought.

Inspection and palpation

The presence of varicosities are self evident and different patterns of visible varicosities are outlined in Fig. 101. A dilated saphenofemoral junction presenting as a 'lump in the groin' is a saphena varix. The presence of complications of varicose veins should be sought. Peripheral pulses should be palpated. Palpable defects in the deep fascia on the medial aspect of the calf may be indicative of calf perforator incompetence.

Trendelenburg test

With the patient lying supine, the leg is elevated and the veins emptied. A tourniquet is applied to the high thigh below the saphenofemoral junction. The patient is asked to stand. If the

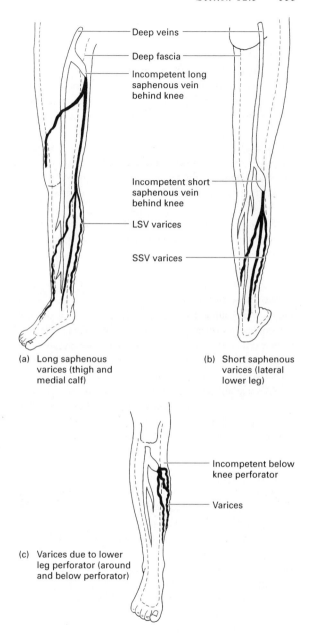

(a) Long saphenous varices (thigh and medial calf)

(b) Short saphenous varices (lateral lower leg)

(c) Varices due to lower leg perforator (around and below perforator)

Deep veins

Deep fascia

Incompetent long saphenous vein behind knee

Incompetent short saphenous vein behind knee

LSV varices

SSV varices

Incompetent below knee perforator

Varices

Fig. 101 (a–c) The three examples of varicose veins due to incompetent perforating veins.

tourniquet prevents the varices reappearing then the reflux occurs above the level of the tourniquet (Fig. 101a). It is possible to repeat the test with the tourniquet lower down the leg until the site at which the veins are prevented from refilling by the tourniquet occurs, indicating the level of perforator incompetence. The varices in Fig. 101(c) for instance will be controlled by a below-knee tourniquet, not one above the knee.

Hand-held Doppler assessment
It is possible to confirm reflux using a hand-held Doppler. With the patient standing, the saphenofemoral junction is identified (medial to the femoral artery) and the probe placed over it. The patients calf is squeezed and an augmentation of blood flow is heard. On release of the calf normally nothing is audible, but in patients with saphenofemoral junction incompetence, sustained reverse flow is heard. The saphenopopliteal junction can be assessed in a similar manner.

Proving the diagnosis
The results of surgery depend on the accuracy of the diagnosis of the site of valvular incompetence. Colour Doppler imaging of the veins may be helpful in the accurate localization of sites of reflux as the veins can be visualized and the direction of flow can be assessed simultaneously.

Ascending phlebography may occasionally be useful in localizing calf perforator incompetence but only in selected cases.

Assessing venous refill times using photoplethysmography without and with a tourniquet may be helpful.

Management
The indications for intervention are severe disfiguring varices, aching or pain, the presence of skin changes or ulceration. Intervention may be contraindicated if there is any evidence of deep venous occlusion (usually after deep venous thrombosis). Conservative treatment is advised if the varices are not very severe or if intervention is contraindicated. Loosing weight, skin care and graduated compression hosiery are the mainstay of conservative treatment. Hosiery should be renewed every 4–6 months as it tends to lose its elasticity. Active treatments are injection sclerotherapy or surgery.

Injection sclerotherapy

This is suitable treatment for patients with isolated, residual (after surgery) or recurrent varicose veins where there is no reflux of blood from the deep to the superficial system.

It is performed in the outpatient department. A sclerosant is injected into the superficial veins and compression bandaging immediately applied and maintained for 6 weeks. The patient is advised to walk frequently to decrease the risk of deep venous thrombosis. It has been used for treating incompetent calf perforators, but has been superseded by surgery in many centres.

OPERATION: FOR VARICOSE VEINS

Operation is the treatment of choice in patients with reflux of blood from the deep to the superficial system, especially into the long saphenous and short saphenous veins.

Preoperative management

Increasingly, varicose vein surgery is being carried out as a day-case procedure. If this is the case it may be better to operate on one leg at a time to encourage postoperative mobility.

The patient is measured for a full length graduated compression stocking. With the patient standing, the veins are marked as they are difficult to localize when the patient is supine. The sites of reflux are also marked. If saphenopopliteal junction reflux is present the saphenopopliteal junction may be marked preoperatively using colour Doppler imaging as there is anatomical variation in the level of the saphenopopliteal junction. This should be done by the operating surgeon. Deep venous thrombosis prophylaxis is given.

There are a number of operations performed for varicose veins surgery. The technique involves ligating the site of reflux from the deep to the superficial venous systems and removing the varicose veins.

HIGH TIE OF THE LONG SAPHENOUS VEIN

The long saphenous vein is ligated at its origin flush with the saphenofemoral junction. This is synonymous with flush ligation. All its branches in the groin should be ligated.

STRIPPING

The long saphenous vein may be removed by passing a wire with a metal 'olive' attached at one end, down through its lumen. The vein is tied around the wire and the 'olive' strips the vein when the wire is pulled. This procedure is done to disconnect the vein from its branches and from mid-thigh perforators. The long saphenous vein used to be stripped to the ankle but a high incidence of saphenous nerve damage was associated so now the vein is only stripped to knee level. It has been shown to decrease the risk of recurrence.

MULTIPLE AVULSIONS

The actual varicosities are avulsed through small incisions over the vein.

SAPHENOPOPLITEAL JUNCTION LIGATION

The short saphenous vein is ligated at its junction with the popliteal vein behind the knee. The short saphenous vein is rarely stripped because of the risk of damage to the sural nerve which is intimately related to it.

SUBFASCIAL LIGATION

Subfascial endoscopic perforator surgery (SEPS) has supplanted Cockett's operation where an extensive incision was made in the skin and deep fascia of the lower leg and the calf perforators ligated. The endoscopic technique involves a small incision in the skin and deep fascia, and the passage of an endoscope between the deep fascia and the calf muscle, before clipping the identified perforators. This way damaged or ulcerated skin is subjected to minimal dissection.

Codes

Blood	0
GA/LA	GA
Opn time	1–2 h
Stay	Day case or overnight stay
Drains out	0
Sutures out	7 days
Off work	1–2 weeks

Postoperative care

The patient's leg is bandaged in theatre and they are discharged later that day on appropriate analgesics. Patients are encouraged to mobilize the following day. After a week the bandages are removed and the graduate compression stocking which has been fitted preoperatively is worn for a further 5 weeks. At that stage the patient is reviewed in the outpatients and discharged if all is well, or scheduled for surgery on the other leg if this is indicated.

Venous ulceration

Chronic venous hypertension leads to damaged capillaries, oedema and induration, red cells leaking out of the capillaries are broken down in the interstitial tissue resulting in haemosiderin deposition and brownish discoloration of the leg. The nutrition to the skin is impaired which leads to eczema and ulceration.

Venous ulceration is ultimately a complication of chronic venous hypertension following valvular damage in the deep system after deep venous thrombosis or in the superficial system following chronic varicose veins. It is important to recognize that there may be an arterial component to the ulceration in up to 15% of patients.

Recognizing the pattern

Women are more commonly affected and usually present over the age of 40 years.

There is chronic painful reddening or discoloration of the skin above the medial malleolus. The ulcer is commonly precipitated by minor trauma. The ulcer is frequently painless but any discomfort is exacerbated when the leg is dependent. There is often a previous history of deep venous thrombosis.

The typical site for a venous ulcer is the lower third of the calf on the medial aspect. There may be slough on the ulcer surface or a seropurulent discharge. The base is covered with granulation tissue and never penetrates the deep fascia. There is usually an irregular shelving edge which is usually a dark blue colour. The surrounding skin is usually pigmented, dry and flaky but there may be cellulitis present. Varicose veins are invariably present and the sites of valvular incompetence should be sought. Peripheral pulses should be sought and documented and the ABPI should be measured prior to treatment.

Proving the diagnosis

The ABPI will confirm or rule out the presence of peripheral vascular disease. In cases where the diagnosis is uncertain, full blood count and plasma viscosity (PV), culture of the ulcer, TPHA and Mantoux tests may be indicated. If an ulcer is chronic, biopsy of the edge is indicated to rule out malignant change (Marjolin's ulcer). The underlying sites of venous reflux can be confirmed using colour Doppler imaging or phlebography.

Management

There are three aspects to the management of venous ulceration.

1 The prevention of ulceration in patients with the pre-ulcerative changes associated with venous hypertensive disease and the prevention of recurrent ulceration in patients who have a healed ulcer.

2 Healing an established ulcer.

3 Prevention.

Prevention of ulceration

Skin care. Patients who have thickened dry skin benefit from having an emollient in their bath water and in applying unperfumed oil to their skin after bathing. Patients with eczema may benefit from local application of a steroid ointment. Cellulitis should be treated with systemic antibiotics; locally applied antibiotics are of no benefit and may induce sensitivity.

Compression. Graduated compression hosiery (class II, pressure 18–24 mmHg or class III, pressure 25–35 mmHg), below knee, above knee or tights should be prescribed. Two pairs should be prescribed at a time as the patient should always wear one set when the other is being washed. These should be replaced every 4–6 months as they tend to lose their elasticity over time. It is important that the patient is satisfied as compliance is vital.

Surgery. Surgical correction of underlying sites of valvular incompetence must be corrected if possible to prevent ulceration.

Treatment of established ulceration

Patients with venous ulceration need to have an ABPI measurement prior to treatment. If the ABPI measurement is less than 0.8 an arterial assessment should be performed as improvement in arterial blood flow may be required to heal the ulcer. A culture swab should be taken from the ulcer if it is infected and the skin care measures outlined above should be commenced.

If ABPI is above 0.8, four-layer compression bandaging should be applied. The ulcer is cleaned with saline and a non-adhesive dressing applied. A layer of padding bandage is applied from the level of the metatarsal heads to the tibial tuberosity. A light crêpe bandage is then applied to smooth the contour of the limb. A light compression bandage is then applied and finally an elasticated cohesive bandage. The dressing is changed weekly in patients with clean ulcers or twice weekly in those with sloughy ulcers. Using this technique it is possible to heal 75% of venous ulcers in 12 weeks.

If the deep venous system is normal, then surgical correction of the underlying venous disorder may accelerate healing and prevent recurrence. If the deep system is not functioning correctly, patients need to wear support stockings for the rest of their life to prevent ulcer recurrence.

Prophylaxis

Anyone who develops a deep venous thrombosis should wear 'blue line' elastic bandages until the tendency to swelling is controlled. They should then be encouraged to wear good supportive stockings until all tendency to oedema formation has disappeared. If the tissues are adequately supported in this way (for 3–6 months) induration can be prevented and ulceration avoided. Tubigrip elastic supports are not adequate (see p. 561).

12.6 Lymphoedema

Fluid and a small quantity of protein normally leaks out of the capillaries into the interstitial space to form interstitial fluid. Most of the fluid is resorbed at the venous end of the capillaries but some, together with the protein is collected in the lymphatic channels and returned to the circulation after being filtered through the lymph nodes. Obstruction to the flow of lymph produces chronic oedema. Causes may be grouped as follows:

1 Primary. This is a rare condition affecting 1 in 33 000 of the population. It is due to absent, hypoplastic or hyperplastic (dilated) lymphatics with absent valves.

2 Secondary. The lymphatics are blocked due to external causes such as:

    (a) fibrosis, e.g. following infection or radiotherapy

    (b) infestation, e.g. filariasis

    (c) infiltration by neoplasm, e.g. malignant melanoma

    (d) trauma, e.g. following block dissection of the groin or axilla.

Recognizing the pattern

Primary lymphoedema frequently affects females. It may present at birth (Milroy's disease) but usually presents in the teens or at any time up to middle age. Secondary lymphoedema can occur at any age.

The patient notices painless swelling of one or both limbs which is worse at the end of the day. Primary lymphoedema always presents in the legs, secondary lymphoedema may occur in the arms or legs, depending on the underlying cause. Occasionally, the patient presents with cellulitis in which case the limb will be painful.

On examination in early cases, the oedema is of the pitting type, however, in chronic cases the oedema is brawny and non-pitting. The quality of the skin should be noted and the size of the limb measured (circumferential measurements at recorded points from bony landmarks) and recorded.

Proving the diagnosis

It is necessary to exclude other causes of limb oedema such as cardiac failure, venous hypertensive disease, hypoproteinaemia, renal failure, hepatic impairment, and hypothyroidism.

A positive diagnosis of lymphoedema can be obtained by a lymphoscintogram. Technetium^{m99} labelled sulphur colloid is injected into a web space of the foot and its clearance is monitored by a gamma camera.

Lymphangiograms may also demonstrate hypoplastic or hyperplastic lymphatics or abnormalities in the proximal lymphatics.

Management
The management is conservative and surgery is rarely indicated.

Conservative treatment
Initial therapy. The aim of initial therapy is to treat any infections, heal any ulcers and reduce the size of the limb. Cellulitis occurring in patients with lymphoedema is a serious condition and needs admission and treatment with intravenous antibiotics. Skin care with moisturizing creams or lotions is important to improve the quality of the skin and decrease the risk of infection. Limb volume reduction methods include, elevation, manual lymphatic drainage (a physiotherapy technique), external elastic compression bandaging, and external pneumatic compression. These treatments can be provided on an out-patient basis.

Maintenance therapy. Once the limb volume has been reduced, continued skin care is required. The patient should be fitted with fully supported graduated compression hosiery as for chronic venous insufficiency. Tubigrip is contraindicated as it applies constant pressure through out its length and impedes lymphatic drainage from the foot. If the patient suffers from recurrent cellulitis, long-term, low-dose penicillin may be required. Diuretics are rarely of value.

Operative treatment
Most surgical treatments for lymphoedema are experimental. The patient should be informed that there are no effective methods of restoring lost lymphatic channels. Two operations have been performed in the past but are rarely performed now. The operations are performed under tourniquet control to reduce blood loss and the leg is elevated and supported during the operation using a Kirschner wire through the calcaneum.

HOMANS' OPERATION

An area of skin with a wider area of subcutaneous tissue is excised from the medial aspect of the lower leg, reducing its bulk. A similar procedure may be carried out on the lateral aspect, usually at a later date.

CHARLES' OPERATION

A circumferential excision of all the skin and subcutaneous tissue from the knee to the ankle is excised and skin grafts applied to the defect.

13 Skin Surgery

13.1 Benign Lesions of the Skin

Skin lumps

Much differing pathology presents as lumps in the skin. Skin 'lumps and bumps' are therefore popular in examinations. Your examination technique for these should include determination of the following:

1 Shape — rounded, irregular, elliptical, etc.
2 Size — in centimetres, including depth, width and length
3 Surface — smooth, nodular, irregular, ill defined
4 Consistency — hard, soft, fluctuant
5 Colour
6 Edge — well defined, ill defined
7 Fixation — to superficial layers of skin or deep to the muscle or fascia
8 Transillumination
9 Pulsation — ?present
10 Bruit — ?present.

Make a habit of running through each of these headings each time that you encounter a lump in the skin.

Papilloma (syn. skin tag, fibroepithelial polyp)

This is a benign overgrowth of normal skin. It consists of a core of connective tissue and blood vessels covered by epidermis. Intradermal naevi and neurofibromas can produce a similar appearance.

Recognizing the pattern

Papillomas occur at any age but are more common in the elderly. Patients request removal for cosmetic reasons or because they catch on clothing or have been traumatized

Papillomas occur at any site and occur in all shapes and sizes. They are either soft and compressible, or solid smooth pedunculated nodules. There may be surface ulceration due to trauma. Multiple tiny tags are common around the neck and axilla.

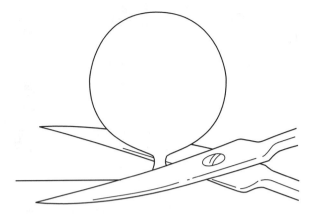

Fig. 102 Snip excision of fibroepithelial polyp.

OPERATION: REMOVAL OF SKIN PAPILLOMA
Small tags (1–5 mm diameter) can be snipped off with scissors without using anaesthetic (Fig. 102). Bleeding will stop spontaneously. When larger tags are snipped off anaesthetic is required mainly to enable cautery to be used for haemostasis. In both instances the wound will heal spontaneously providing it is kept clean. Alternatively, the papilloma pedicle can be removed using an elliptical excision. The ellipse direction should follow the skin crease lines. The wound is closed with monofilament nylon sutures. All papillomas should be sent for histology.

Codes
Blood 0
GA/LA .... LA
Opn time .... 15 min
Stay .... Outpatient
Drains out 0
Suture out .... 3–7 days
                                     (depending on site of wound)
Off work .... Less than 24 h

Seborrhoeic keratosis (syn. seborrhoeic wart, basal cell papilloma)
This is a benign overgrowth of the basal cells of the epidermis.

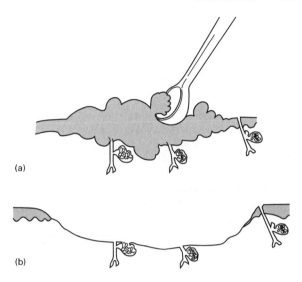

Fig. 103 (a) Curettage of seborrhoeic wart, (b) eroded surface remaining with retained hair follicles and sweat ducts after curettage.

Recognizing the pattern

The patient is usually elderly and concerned because the lesion is unsightly, itchy or slowly getting bigger.

On examination it is a flattened well-defined, greasy, tan or dark brown warty plaque that appears to be 'stuck onto' the skin rather than an integral part of it. Any site can be affected. Multiple warts are commonly present on the trunk, head and neck.

Management

Reassurance is usually sufficient. Seborrhoeic warts can be removed by curettage (Fig. 103) or destroyed by cryotherapy. Lesions that do not curette off easily may be warty pigment naevi and these have to be excised. In general elliptical excision of seborrhoeic warts is unnecessary and produces an inferior cosmetic result. Any seborrhoeic wart removed should be sent for histology.

Infective warts

Common warts are the result of a human papilloma virus infection. They are thus contagious and common on children's

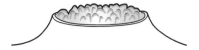

Fig. 104 Viral wart with typical 'acorn cup' appearance.

hands. Immunity to the virus is conferred by previous infection so that viral warts are uncommon in older immunocompetent people. On the sole of the foot, pressure pushes the wart into the skin producing the characteristic verruca.

Recognizing the pattern

It is a slow-growing nodular lesion of the skin which eventually regresses spontaneously. Many warts last for more than 2 years. Warts may bleed on trauma, become painful particularly if infected, but are principally social embarrassments.

Without repeated injury, e.g. on the face, a wart will develop multiple frond-like surface growths. At sites exposed to regular minor trauma, e.g. fingers and feet, these frond-like growths are worn away leaving a hard keratinized papule with a warty or irregular surface. This is characteristically surrounded by an acorn-cup like rim of normal skin (Fig. 104).

> **Management**
> Treatment is not necessary. Reassurance that warts regress spontaneously is usually sufficient. Regression can be hastened by topical keratolytics (salicylic acid and lactic acid), curettage or cryotherapy. Because warts are infectious none of these treatments are definitively curative.

Keloid

In a keloid the overgrowth of fibrous tissue spreads beyond the original scar boundaries and never resolves spontaneously. By contrast in a hypertrophic scar the thickening remains localized to the original scar and eventually softens and flattens (Fig. 105).

Recognizing the pattern

Keloids are common in Afro-Caribbeans and young people.

The lump is slow growing, tender or itchy. There is usually a history of previous trauma or surgery although keloids may form after minimal trauma (e.g. acne scarring).

On examination red–brown or purple firm scar tissue is heaped up above the level of the skin and it may even become pedun-

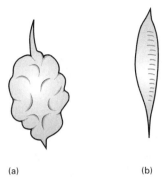

(a)   (b)

Fig. 105 Comparison of (a) a keloid, and (b) a hypertrophic scar.

culated. Keloids can occur at any site but are commonest at keloid-prone sites (central chest, upper back and shoulders). The whole or part of the scar may be involved.

Management

Keloids are difficult to manage. No treatment is uniquely effective. The surgeon should avoid the temptation to excise a keloid as it is almost certain to recur. Repeated injection of steroids into the keloid (triamcinolone 10–40 mg/ml) will reduce scar thickness. Silicone gel sheeting is useful for large hypertrophic scars. Radiotherapy should be avoided because of the risk of inducing tumour formation. Excision of keloids that are easy to excise (e.g. ear lobe) is advocated with intra-operative and postoperative intralesional steroid injection. Hypertrophic scars, by contrast, will improve spontane-ously. Intralesional steroids will hasten this outcome but, as with keloids, there is the risk of perilesional steroid atrophy.

Lipoma

This is a benign tumour composed of fat cells divided into large lobules by loose fibrous septa. Lipomas are frequently multiple. Painful lipomas are actually angiolipomas.

Recognizing the pattern

The patient is usually an adult. The lesion is rare in children.

The lump takes several years to reach the size of a walnut. Advice is usually sought when the lump becomes unsightly. There may be a family history of similar lesions.

Lipomas occur anywhere there is adipose tissue but are com-moner on the upper limb and trunk. They may be of any size

from a few millimetres to several centimetres in diameter.
Occasionally a lipoma arises in the muscle or close to the deep
fascia, in which case it appears to be attached to the muscle. The
tumour has a smooth, lobulated surface with a well-defined
edge. It is usually soft although small lipomas may be quite
firm. It often lies in the subcutis, and the skin can then be moved
over it.

Management
If the lipoma is causing trouble it should be removed.

OPERATION: REMOVAL OF LIPOMA
An incision is made over the lipoma in the direction of the
skin creases and deepened until the lipoma is reached. The
lipoma is then gently freed from the surrounding skin. Soft
lipomas can be squeezed out through the incision. If a large
lipoma has been removed the cavity may be need to be
drained.

Codes
Blood 0
GA/LA .... LA or GA (depending on size)
Opn time .... 10–30 min
Stay .... Outpatient or 24 h
Drains out .... 0–24 h
Sutures out .... 5–7 days
Off work .... 1–2 days

Epidermoid cyst (syn. sebaceous cysts, steatoma, epithelial cyst)

The term epidermoid cyst causes great confusion. Epidermoid
cysts are lined with stratified squamous epithelium which produces keratin; this slowly accumulates to form a foul smelling
cheesy material. Epidermoid cysts are not derived from sebaceous glands. Most cysts arise spontaneously. When they appear
on the face and back some are the result of old acne scarring
blocking a hair follicle. Epidermoid cysts characteristically have
a punctum through which the contents can be expressed and
via which infections sometimes enter.

Implantation dermoid. This is an acquired condition due to
implantation of epidermis into the subcutaneous tissue. The
epidermis continues to grow and forms a cyst that is lined with

stratified squamous epithelium. The patient may be a gardener or manual worker likely to suffer hand injuries.

Pilar cysts (syn. sebaceous cyst, trichilemmal cyst). These are very similar except that they mainly occur on the scalp, do not have punctum, are lined by a non-stratified epithelium and are much thinner walled and thus burst more easily during removal. They contain more watery contents than an epidermoid cyst. Both types of cyst can be treated in the same way. Rarely a pilar cyst can develop into a proliferating pilar (trichilemmal) cyst which may be confused with a squamous cell carcinoma of the scalp.

Recognizing the pattern

Epidermoid cysts occur at any age but are rare in children. They may be multiple. The patient presents because they are unsightly, infected or discharging. On examination the lump is a spherical, smooth, well-defined swelling of variable size, which may be visible as a white cyst through the overlying stretched skin. A punctum is frequently visible. Epidermoid cysts are common on the scalp, face and upper back.

Management

An infected epidermoid cyst must first be drained and excised later. Inflamed epidermoid cysts are not invariably infected. If the cyst wall bursts, usually because of injudicious squeezing by the patient, the keratin leaks out into the surrounding tissues and provokes a brisk foreign-body reaction. Inflamed or infected cysts are best left to settle with antibiotics before removal is attempted because the tissues are friable and excision is difficult. A non-infected cyst can be removed under a local anaesthetic.

OPERATION: EXCISION OF EPIDERMOID CYST

On a hair-bearing site adjacent hair should be shaved off. Lignocaine 1% plus adrenaline (1 : 200 000) should be infiltrated around and immediately above the cyst so as to partly separate the skin and the cyst wall. The punctum should be excised with the cyst using an ellipse centred on the punctum (Fig. 106). Alternatively, large cysts can be incised, the contents expressed and the cyst lining grasped with artery forceps and enucleated. Removal of the intact cyst is a surer way of guaranteeing complete removal because retained wall fragments will cause recurrence. Pressure should

Continued on p. 572

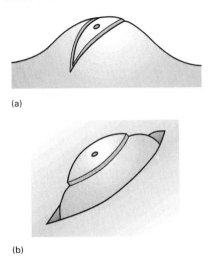

(a)

(b)

Fig. 106 Excision of an epidermoid cyst. (a) The ellipse should be centred on the punctum. (b) The cyst can be removed intact using the ellipse to manoeuvre the cyst.

Continued.

be applied to occlude the remaining dead space and the skin closed with a monofilament nylon suture. If the cyst has previously ruptured or been infected, the cyst plus the surrounding fibrotic tissue should be removed.

Codes

Blood	0
GA/LA	LA
Opn time	15–30 min
Stay	Outpatient
Drains out	0
Sutures out	5–7 days
Off work	1–2 h

Dermoid cysts

Dermoid cysts are different. These are rare developmental abnormalities developing at embryological lines of skin fusion when a piece of epidermis comes to lie beneath the skin's surface. Seventy per cent present in children as soft nodules on the midline of the head and neck, or outer third of the eyebrow (external angle dermoid). Surgery is potentially complicated because a proportion have deeper attachments to bone or periosteum. Preoperative computed tomography (CT) scanning may therefore be required.

Ganglion

The cause of ganglia is not established. Ganglia may arise from the leakage of synovial fluid secondary to myxomatous degeneration occurring in fibrous tissue close to a joint capsule or tendon sheath. The cystic lesion contains glairy, sticky, clear fluid. On the finger a similar lesion, called a myxoid cyst, results from leakage of synovial fluid from the distal interphalangeal joint into the posterior nailfold.

Recognizing the pattern

The patient is usually an adult who presents with a disfiguring, painful or movement-restricting lump.

The lump is commonly around the hand or wrist or on the foot, close to the joints. The swelling is lobulated with a smooth surface and a well-defined edge. It may be of any size and consistency. It often becomes more tense when the joint is flexed or extended. It is attached deeply but not to the skin.

Management

A ganglion can sometimes be dispersed by pressure (being hit with the family bible) or by aspiration with a needle, but tends to recur. The favoured method of treatment is excision.

OPERATION: REMOVAL OF A GANGLION

It is usually possible to remove the ganglion under a local anaesthetic but, at difficult sites or in a young patient, a general anaesthetic is preferred. An exsanguinating tourniquet is used where possible. Ganglia are often intimately related to tendons, arteries and nerves and must be dissected out with great care.

Codes

Blood	0
GA/LA	LA or GA
Opn time	30 min
Stay	Outpatient
Drains out	0
Sutures out	5–7 days
Off work	Depends on occupation: a typist/computer operator with a ganglion on the wrist may be advised to stay off work for a week, otherwise about 24 h

Neurofibroma

These are benign tumours arising from both the nerve sheath and neural tissue. In neurofibroma the whole nerve is therefore involved and complete removal inevitably results in removal of the nerve. Neurofibromas may arise from unnamed small nerve radicals, larger nerve branches, individual major nerves and dorsal nerve roots in the paraspinal region.

Neurilemmomas (syn. schwannoma) by contrast arise from the myelin-producing Schwann's cells only and have a true capsule. Whilst they may press on the nerve axon they do not involve it. A neurilemmoma can therefore be carefully dissected out without damage to the nerve function (Fig. 107).

Multiple neurofibromatosis (syn. von Recklinghausen's disease, neurofibromatosis type 1 or NF1, peripheral neurofibromatosis) is caused by an autosomal dominant gene on chromosome 17. Patients have multiple neurofibromas, café-au-lait patches, axillary freckling, Lisch nodules (brown specks) in the iris, optic gliomas, skeletal and endocrine abnormalities including phaeochromocytoma. Neurofibromatosis type 2 (NF2) patients (syn: central neurofibromatosis) also have multiple neurofibroma but in association with bilateral acoustic neuromas and other neural tumours but none of the other skin or skeletal changes and different eye abnormalities. The abnormal autosomal dominant gene is on chromosome 22.

Recognizing the pattern

The patient may present at any age but is usually adult. When taking a history ask about other affected family members. A neurofibroma is often asymptomatic but is occasionally painful. It may be disfiguring or rarely cause paraesthesiae or motor weakness in the distribution of the nerve involved. Rapid size increase and pain may be caused by haemorrhage into the neurofibroma or malignant transformation.

On examination three types of neurofibromas are recognized.
1 Discrete cutaneous neurofibromas that move when the skin is moved. These are soft, lilac or flesh coloured, pedunculated or sessile, cutaneous or subcutaneous tumours.
2 Subcutaneous neurofibromas that are not attached to the skin and appear as a firm, possibly tender, subcutaneous oval swelling. These may be attached to a large nerve and consequently are relatively fixed in the direction of the nerve but mobile at right angles to the nerve trunk. Pressure on it may cause tingling in the nerve distribution.

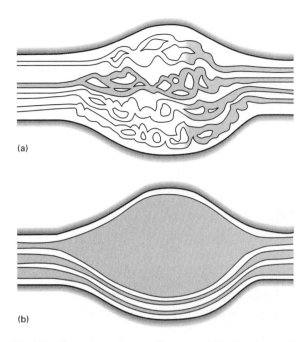

(a)

(b)

Fig. 107. Comparison of a neurofibroma in which (a) both neural tissue and nerve sheath are involved, with (b) a neurilemmoma in which just the neural sheath is affected.

3 Plexiform neurofibroma arise from larger nerves and may be very large and infiltrate into adjacent structures. All types may undergo sarcomatous change although this is more likely in plexiform neurofibromas.

Management

Neurofibromas need only be removed if they interfere with normal function, or are disfiguring, excessively big or painful. Complete removal may be difficult because some cutaneous neurofibromas are diffuse and difficult to excise. Large, proximally based, neurofibromas may be associated with potentially serious loss of function due to nerve damage during removal. If this is suspected thorough investigation of the potential for sensory or motor loss should be carried out before surgery and the patient warned. Sarcoma formation occurs in approximately 5% of multiple neurofibromatosis patients and is characterized by increasing pain and size of the neurofibroma. The diagnosis should be confirmed by incisional biopsy and excision thereafter.

OPERATION: EXCISION OF A NEUROFIBROMA
An attempt should be made to excise the neurofibroma fully.
The nerve ends may need to be resutured if the function
supplied is vital. The risk of sarcomatous change is not
increased by incomplete excision.

Codes
Blood 0
GA/LA .... LA or GA
Opn time .... 30 min
Stay .... Inpatient/outpatient
Drains out 0
Sutures out .... 5–7 days
Off work .... Variable, 24 h for a small cutaneous
lesion

Postoperative care
The patient may occasionally need admitting and the limb
immobilizing to protect a nerve anastomosis.

Keratoacanthoma (molluscum sebaceum)

This is a self-healing tumour of keratinocytes that arises on sun-
damaged sites. It is easily confused, both clinically and
histologically, with squamous cell carcinoma and if there is
doubt about the diagnosis it should be treated as a squamous
cell carcinoma.

Recognizing the pattern

The patient is usually elderly and complains of a rapidly expanding lesion with a dark central core. The nodule should

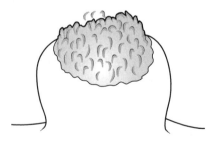

Fig. 108 Characteristic appearance of a keratoacanthoma with a
symmetrical shape and shoulder of normal skin expanded by the
enclosed tumour.

reach its maximum size by 3 months and begin to regress in size thereafter.

Keratoacanthomas arise on chronically sun-exposed skin as a round symmetrical nodule with a smooth shoulder of stretched skin. The central keratin horn (Fig. 108) becomes necrotic in older lesions.

Management

A clinical diagnosis of keratoacanthoma should only be made if there is a history of a rapidly growing lesion that starts to spontaneously decrease in size after 3 months. The lesion should be symmetrical with an edge of normal skin rather than tumour. If a confident clinical diagnosis is made the lesion can be allowed to resolve spontaneously leaving a small crateriform scar. If removal is required this can be done by excision, curettage or radiotherapy. If there is doubt about the diagnosis the lesion should be managed as a squamous cell carcinoma by wide local excision.

13.2 Pigmented Naevi and Malignant Skin Conditions

Moles (pigmented naevi)

Terminology

Moles commonly appear in the first two decades of life. An average adult in their late twenties will have 20–30 naevi. There are several normal variants of benign naevi. Moles evolve and therefore change in appearance with time.

Benign naevi evolve through three stages (Fig. 109) and these changes are characteristically best seen on facial naevi. Initially they appear as flat brown moles. Histologically these are junctional naevi with clumps of melanocytes centred around the

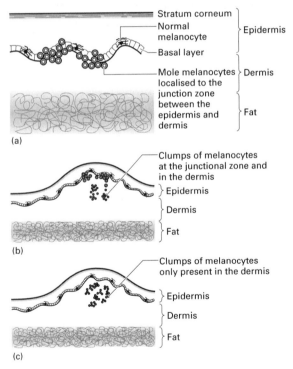

Fig. 109 Stages in the development of a normal mole. (a) These start as a flat brown junctional naevus. (b) Then become raised brown compound naevi and (c) finally raised flesh-coloured intradermal naevi.

junction between the epidermis and dermis. This evolves into a compound naevus when some melanocytes move deeper into the dermis whilst others remain at the junction. These appear as raised brown moles. Finally all the naevus cells move into the dermis to create a papular, flesh-coloured, often hairy intradermal naevus.

Normal variants of benign naevi include the following:

1 Congenital naevi are moles present at birth or that appear in the first few months of life. Giant congenital naevi have greater risk of melanoma transformation. There is debate about whether the commoner small congenital naevus have similar higher frequency of malignant transformation.

2 A blue naevus is slatey grey or blue in colour. The striking colour is produced by melanin deposited by melanocytes that remain deep in the dermis.

3 Spitz naevus (juvenile melanoma). These appear as red facial papules in children and brownish red papules on limbs in adults. They are clinically and histologically distinct from malignant melanoma.

4 Halo naevus. Some naevi disappear spontaneously. The first indication of this is a white halo appearing around the pigmented papule.

5 Dysplastic naevus. Clinically they may have features suggestive of a melanoma (pigment and edge irregularity) but histologically they are benign. Patients with multiple dysplastic naevi or a family history of melanoma have a greater risk of developing melanoma.

Benign naevus

A benign mole has uniform colour (i.e. all brown, all tan, and so on), a regular margin, is usually symmetrical about one axis and sometimes hairy. Moles on the scrotum, palms and soles are no more likely to turn malignant than moles elsewhere.

Management

A benign naevus that is causing no symptoms can be left alone. The lesion is usually excised either because it is cosmetically unattractive, or because it is showing some features suggestive of malignant change.

OPERATION: SHAVE EXCISION OF BENIGN PAPULAR NAEVI

Removal of benign papular pink naevi for cosmetic reasons is usually best done by shave excision because this simple

Continued on p. 580

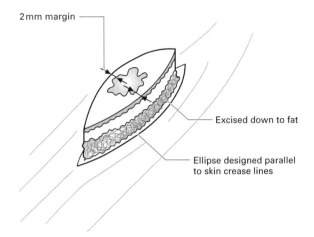

2mm margin

Excised down to fat

Ellipse designed parallel
to skin crease lines

Fig. 110 Excision of a suspect mole or staging excision of a
malignant melanoma.

Continued.

procedure produces a good cosmetic result. Pigment and
hair will remain in 25% of brown or hairy naevi. If this is
unacceptable an elliptical excision is appropriate. Anaesthetic is injected into the mole to stiffen the tissue and make
is easier to shave off. The protruding part of the mole is
shaved off flush with the skin. Bleeding is stopped using
cautery and the wound allowed to heal spontaneously.

OPERATION: REMOVAL OF A
SUSPICIOUS NAEVUS
Removal of suspect moles should be done under a local
anaesthetic using an elliptical incision, parallel to skin crease
lines, down to fat, taking a 2 mm margin on either side of
the edge of the mole (Fig. 110). The wound should be
sutured using absorbable and nylon surface sutures. The
specimen should always be sent for histology. If this shows
evidence of malignant change, the scar will need to be re-
excised.

Malignant melanoma

Approximately 50% of malignant melanomas arise in an existing naevus. The remainder develop spontaneously. Five
clinicopathological types are recognized. In all these types the
best guide to prognosis is the depth (Breslow thickness) to
which malignant melanocytes have penetrated at the time of
excision (Fig. 111).

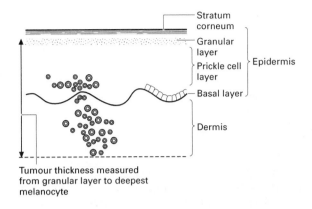

Fig. 111 Measurement of melanoma thickness by the Breslow method.

1 Lentigo maligna (Hutchinson's melanotic freckle). This is a completely flat brown or black macule usually on the face. Malignant melanocytes are only present in the basal layer of the epidermis. Solid melanomas (lentigo maligna melanoma) develop in approximately 25% of cases.

2 Superficial spreading melanoma. The malignant melanocytes grow laterally through the epidermis for some time before clumping together and growing downwards into the dermis. This type occurs at any site as a just-palpable irregularly pigmented lesion.

3 Nodular melanoma. The malignant melanocytes invade deeply into the dermis from the start. These appear as raised pigmented nodules at any site.

4 Amelanotic melanoma. These melanomas do not produce sufficient pigment to make them change colour. They are usually misdiagnosed as squamous cell carcinomas. Because of the potential delay in diagnosis amelanotic melanomas may present late. They are, however, no more likely to metastasize than a pigmented melanoma of similar thickness.

5 Acral lentiginous melanoma. This type develops around nails and on the feet. They present with nail destruction, pigment streaks or solitary nail dystrophy. They are commonly misdiagnosed as ingrown toenail, fungal infections, etc.

Tumour staging

The stage of a melanoma refers to its extent of spread and gives some indication of prognosis. There are three clinical stages.

Stage 1: confined to the primary lesion (including satellite lesions within a radius of 5 cm). The prognosis depends on tumour thickness (Fig. 111).

Stage 2: involvement of the first single group of regional lymph nodes and cutaneous secondaries in this course.

Stage 3: involvement of two or more groups of lymph nodes with visceral metastases particularly to the liver, lungs and brain.

Recognizing the pattern

Malignant melanoma usually occurs after adolescence. Melanomas in prepubertal children that have not developed from giant congenital naevi are extremely rare. Melanoma is commoner in white-skinned people exposed to the sun. It occurs in approximately 10 : 100 000 individuals in Europe (a male to female ratio of 1 : 2) and 40 : 100 000 in Australia.

There may be a positive family history. The patient usually presents because the mole has changed or a new pigmented lesion has appeared.

The malignant lesion can occur anywhere but is more common on the limbs, head and neck. Signs suggestive of malignant change are as follows:

1 Colour change. Melanomas have pigments of different hues in the same lesion, e.g. red and black, grey and brown.

2 Change in shape. Melanomas are asymmetrical. Extensions or margin irregularities (knotching) are characteristic.

3 Increasing size. Most melanomas are greater than 7 mm.

Bleeding and itching are not specific. Ulceration is a late feature. Benign moles may be traumatized accidentally or because they are itchy.

Examine the adjacent skin for satellite nodules around the melanoma and examine draining lymph nodes. Systemic symptoms of weight loss or metastasis to other organs may be present.

Management

OPERATION: EXCISION OF MALIGNANT MELANOMA

A staging excisional biopsy down to fat with a 2 mm margin of normal skin is done to confirm the diagnosis and establish the tumour thickness. Tumours less than 1 mm thick require a 10 mm margin of excision. Narrower margins may be as effective but studies to confirm this have not been completed. Tumours 1–2 mm thick can be excised with a 10–20 mm margin and tumours thicker than 3 mm are normally excised with a 30 mm margin. In all cases excision should be carried down to, but not including, the deep fascia. The defect can be closed directly, or using a skin graft. A split-skin graft should be taken from the opposite limb to avoid transferring a metastasis *in situ*.

Pretreatment liver function tests and a chest X-ray are commonly done to exclude distant metastasis in thicker melanoma.

Codes

Blood	0
GA/LA	LA/GA
Opn time	1–2 h (depending on site)
Stay	Day case or 5–7 days
Drains out	0
Sutures out	7–10 days
Off work	6 weeks

OPERATION: BLOCK DISSECTION OF THE GROIN

There is no established role for elective node dissection in melanoma. However, if there is evidence of spread to the regional nodes, a block dissection may be performed.

A frozen section biopsy of the enlarged node is taken. If tumour is present, all the groin nodes are excised. The long saphenous vein is tied lower down the thigh and a block of tissue removed from the front of the femoral vein and artery. The upper end of the saphenous vein is again divided as it enters the femoral vein. The block may be continued up under the inguinal ligament to remove nodes in the iliac region.

Codes

Blood	2 units
GA/LA	GA
Opn time	2–3 h
Stay	7–10 days
Drains out	2–5 days
Sutures out	7–14 days
Off work	4–6 weeks

Postoperative care

The leg will swell due to lymphoedema. It is important to keep it elevated postoperatively and to apply heavy-duty elastic bandages before the patient is mobilized. The patient should continue to have the foot of the bed raised for 2 or 3 months after the procedure until the tendency to oedema has subsided. The oedema may be permanent.

Palliative and adjuvant therapy

Patients with thick (> 1.5 mm) melanomas may benefit from inclusion in on-going trials. Seek the advice of the local melanoma study group. Other treatments include the following:

1 Radiotherapy. This is useful for the treatment of bone pain or cerebral metastases.

2 Chemotherapy. This can occasionally be helpful in advanced disease. The effective agents are the following:

    (a) melphalan — especially when used for isolated cytotoxic hyperthermic limb perfusion

    (b) combination chemotherapy — various combinations are undergoing trials, e.g. VBM (vindesine, bleomycin, metho-trexate) or BOLD (bleomycin, vincristine, 1-(2-chloroethyl)-3-cyclohexyl-1-nitrosourea, 5-(3, 3-dimethyl-1-triazino)-imidazole-4-carboxamide). Toxicity of these regimes is significant

    (c) interferon-a_{2b} has been shown to reduce the risk of metastasis in high-risk patients with thick tumours.

Other malignant skin conditions

Squamous cell carcinoma *in situ* (Bowen's disease)

This is carcinoma of the skin limited to the epidermis. Approximately 5% of cases develop into an invasive squamous cell carcinoma.

Recognizing the pattern

Bowen's disease occurs on sun-exposed sites, particularly the lower legs in elderly women. Previous arsenic ingestion, in the form of 'tonics', predisposes to Bowen's disease.

    The lesion is painless, slowly enlarging and patients complain of the appearance. It can be distinguished from psoriasis because lesions are solitary, crusted rather than scaly and have an irregular edge. Biopsy will confirm the diagnosis.

Management

Lesions can be treated by topical 5-fluorouracil application, curettage, cryotherapy, excision or radiotherapy.

Squamous cell carcinoma

This is a malignant keratinizing tumour of stratified squamous epithelium. It is locally invasive and also metastasizes via the lymphatics and the blood stream.

Recognizing the pattern

Squamous cell carcinoma occurs on chronically sun-exposed sites particularly in elderly men. Characteristic sites include the lower lip, top of the ear, back of the hand and other head and neck sites. The tumour can arise in immunosuppressed younger patients, particularly following organ transplantation.

Most patients give a history of previous regular excess exposure to sunlight. Other carcinogenic factors include coal tar exposure (road workers) and tobacco (lip tumours). The lesion enlarges slowly and has usually been present for several months before presentation. Squamous cell carcinomas are sometimes painful.

The nodule is hard, irregular in outline, and usually has a keratin- and crust-covered surface or a central necrotic ulcer and everted edge. There may be evidence of local or distant metastases. It is important to examine draining lymph nodes.

Management

The lesion can either be excised or treated with radiotherapy.

Basal cell carcinoma (BCC, basal cell epithelioma, rodent ulcer)

This is a locally malignant condition arising from basal epidermal cells. BCCs grow into surrounding tissues and can cause extensive local destruction but only exceptionally metastasize.

Recognizing the pattern

The patient is usually elderly but BCC also occurs in the 20+ age group. The condition is more common in white-skinned people with a history of repeated sun exposure.

The tumour is painless and slow growing. Patients sometimes notice the enlarging nodule or an ulcer that does not heal, occasionally bleeds, scabs over and then reulcerates.

An early nodular BCC is a smooth pearly papule. As the tumour enlarges the centre becomes necrotic, ulcerates and crusted. At this stage only the edge is raised (rolled) and pearly white in colour; this feature is best seen if the skin is stretched. The lack of keratin formation and the presence of the characteristic pearly-coloured edge distinguish BCC from squamous cell carcinoma. BCCs may also be scarring (morphoeic), superficial (plaque-like patch on the trunk) or pigmented.

Management

BCCs can be treated by cryotherapy, curettage, radiotherapy or excision.

OPERATION: EXCISION OF BASAL CELL CARCINOMA

The excision margin depends on the tumour characteristics. Small (< 2 cm), well-defined tumours can be excised with a 3–4 mm margin. Large (> 2 cm), recurrent or ill-defined tumours are more likely to recur using this excision margin. These tumours can be treated by wide (10 mm) local excision or using histological control to confirm the adequacy of excision (Mohs surgical technique). The defect is closed either directly, using local flaps or with a skin graft.

Codes

Blood 0

GA/LA .... LA, occasionally GA

Opn time .... Depends on size and need to skin graft, 30–90 min

Stay .... Day case or 24–48 h

Drains out 0

Sutures out .... 4–7 days (skin graft 10 days)

Off work .... 1 day or more depending on size of lesion

Skin metastases

Metastases from visceral carcinoma can present as a swelling or ulceration in the skin. They are particularly common on the scalp. The treatment consists of chemotherapy or radiotherapy appropriate to the original primary tumour. The diagnosis is made by biopsy to help identify the primary malignancy.

13.3   Skin Infections and Hyperhidrosis

Skin infections

Skin abscess

This is the result of a *Staphylococcus aureus* infection producing a collection of pus surrounded by granulation tissue in the subcutaneous tissues or dermis.

Recognizing the pattern

There is a painful swelling. The pain is throbbing and characteristically worse at night or if the affected part is dependent. It may have discharged pus.

On examination there is a localized swelling which is warm, red and tender. It is initially firm but as suppuration occurs it becomes softer, spherical and fluctuant. It may later discharge. The patient is usually pyrexial and the regional lymph nodes become enlarged and tender.

Management

The abscess must be drained unless it ruptures spontaneously. A swab should be sent for culture and sensitivity.

OPERATION: INCISION AND DRAINAGE OF ABSCESS

An incision is made over the most fluctuant area. A closed haemostat is inserted into the cavity and then opened. A drain is inserted.

Codes

Blood	0
GA/LA	LA
Opn time	15 min
Stay	Outpatient
Drains out	48 h
Sutures out	0
Off work	1–2 days

Postoperative care

Any predisposing cause should be treated. Antibiotics are only appropriate if there is associated cellulitis or constitutional disturbance.

Hidradenitis suppurativa

This is a troublesome recurrent infection of apocrine sweat glands and characteristically affects the axillae, groins and perineum. Mild cases respond to antibiotics according to sensitivities. Oral oestrogens or antiandrogens can also be used in females. Surgery may be the only effective treatment in resistant cases. Sinus tracts may need to be laid open and allowed to granulate as described for pilonidal sinus. Eventually areas of recurrent sepsis may need to be fully excised.

Pilonidal sinus

In this condition broken-off hairs come to lie in a subcutaneous sinus. Lesions characteristically occur over the sacrum in the gluteal cleft. It can also occur in the hands, axillae or umbilicus.

The lesion in the sacral area probably starts as a preformed congenital pit. Hairs break off the head and back and tend to gravitate towards the cleft. It seems likely that the barbed surface of the hair results in it working its way under the skin once its tip has become lodged in the pit. Several hairs follow down the sinus, which then becomes infected. The patient complains of recurrent abscesses in this area. The abscess usually points to the skin at the side of the midline. Pilonidal sinuses also occur in barbers and in this case the sinus lies between the fingers. The hairs are derived from the customer rather than the sufferer.

Recognizing the pattern

The patient is typically male with thick black hair. The condition is more common between the ages of 15 and 40 years.

There are recurrent episodes of pain and sepsis, often with several months between each episode. As the sinus becomes larger, the episodes become more frequent.

On careful inspection the pit is seen in the midline. There may be several such pits. The abscess is visible and palpable laterally.

Management

A small sinus may settle with antibiotic treatment but once the condition has become recurrent surgery is required. An acutely inflamed abscess will need to be drained.

Three operative procedures are described. The sinus may be incised and laid open, it may be completely excised or it may be curetted and injected with phenol.

OPERATION: FOR PILONIDAL SINUS

When the lesion is laid open, a probe is passed along the track and an incision is made onto it from above. Granulation tissue in the base of the sinus is preserved but the hairs and debris are removed. Any lateral extensions into an abscess cavity are also laid open.

If the sinus is excised, the skin is closed directly over the wound.

Codes

Blood 0
GA/LA .... GA or LA, depending on size
Opn time .... 30–45 min
Stay .... 3–7 days depending on size
Drains out 0
Sutures out .... If present 7–10 days
Off work .... About 3 weeks depending on size of sinus and occupation of patient

Postoperative care

If the sinus has been excised, and if the wound heals by primary intention, the postoperative care is uncomplicated. If the wound breaks down due to tension or infection it can be allowed to heal by secondary intention.

If the sinus has been laid open, it is dressed daily by inserting a plug of tulle gras or silastic foam. As the wound granulates and the epithelium grows in from the edges, the bulk of the dressing is reduced. It is important to make certain that no 'bridging' of the skin edges occurs as this will lead to renewed pit formation and a recurrent sinus. Similarly, the hairs around the wound must be shaved regularly to prevent them sticking into the granulation tissue and reforming a sinus.

OPERATION: PHENOL INJECTION OF
PILONIDAL SINUS

The surrounding skin is carefully protected using petroleum jelly. Phenol (80%) is injected and left in the sinus for 1 min. This is repeated three times. The sinus is then gently curetted and the hairs removed. A small drain may be inserted.

Codes

Blood	0
GA/LA	GA
Opn time	10 min
Stay	24 h
Drains out	0 or 24 h
Sutures out	0
Off work	48 h

> *Postoperative care*
> After phenol injection the area remains painless as the phenol destroys local nerves. Occasionally a sterile abscess develops, which requires drainage. The recurrence rate is about 17% if the sinus has fewer than three openings.

Boil (furuncle) and carbuncle

A boil is a small abscess developing in an infected hair follicle. A carbuncle is an infection of a group of adjacent follicles. In both instances *Staphylococcus aureus* is the infecting organism. Necrosis of the skin between the follicles is a common associated feature. This results in the formation of a large ulcer, which slowly heals to leave a substantial scar. Infections are more common in diabetics, the malnourished and patients on long-term steroid therapy.

Recognizing the pattern

The presentation is initially similar to a skin abscess. There is a spreading, very painful lesion of the skin with constitutional disturbances.

The neck is the most common site affected. The lesion is diffuse, hard and reddened with a central area of slough surrounded by multiple sinuses extruding pus.

> ### Management
> The initial management is conservative with regular cleaning and dressing. Culture the pus and prescribe antibiotics to control the infection. The necrotic central area of skin may need to be excised. Check for predisposing causes such as diabetes.

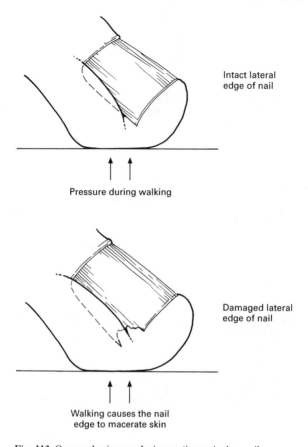

Intact lateral
edge of nail

Pressure during walking

Damaged lateral
edge of nail

Walking causes the nail
edge to macerate skin

Fig. 112 One mechanism producing an 'ingrowing' toenail.

Conditions of the nails

Ingrowing toenail

Ingrown toenails are caused by incorrectly cutting the toenails, bad footwear, trauma and congenital nail abnormalities.

Toenails should be cut transversely so that the corners of the free nail edge protrude beyond the lateral nailfolds. If the nail corners are trimmed further back the cut may not quite reach the lateral edge of the nail leaving a spicule of nail. This grows into and finally penetrates the lateral nailfold (Fig. 112). The resulting foreign-body reaction and secondary infection produce the symptoms.

Footwear should allow the toes to spread adequately. High heels that cause the toes to be forced into a narrow pointed shoe

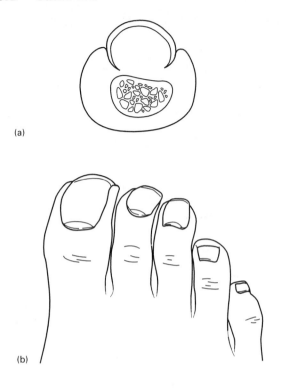

(a)

(b)

Fig. 113 Congenital malformations of the toenails producing (a) a
pincer toe, and (b) congenital malalignment of the great toe.

may also force the lateral nail margin into the nailfold. Trauma
may split the side of the nail and the sharp edge may grow into
the nailfold.

Congenital abnormalities that predispose to ingrowing toenails should be distinguished (Fig. 113). These include over-
curvature of the nail (pincer nails) and malalignment of the big
toenails. All the toenails are affected although symptoms are
most frequent in the great toe. In pincer nails the deformed
nailplate grips the nailbed like a claw and the lateral and medial
nail borders need to be removed. Malaligned nails should be
realigned rather than destroyed.

Recognizing the pattern
The patient may present at any age though the condition is
unusual before the age of 5 years.

The usual complaint is of a painful big toe, which is swollen, red and intermittently discharges pus. Attempt to establish the likely cause in acquired disease.

On examination the nailfolds are affected to a variable extent on one or both sides of the nail. Identify congenital abnormalities that predispose to ingrowing toenail.

Management

Conservative management of acquired ingrowing toenail

1 Prevent secondary infection and reduce pain: keep the feet dry, use oral antibiotics if required and avoid tight shoes or socks.

2 Reduce granulation tissue formation. Potent topical steroid (clobetasol proprinate) application or cryotherapy will reduce inflammation and granulation tissue.

3 Redirection of nail growth. Pack cotton wool pledglets moistened with surgical spirit or tincture of iodine under the corner of the nail so that the free edge of the nail grows out without puncturing the lateral nailfold.

4 Prevent recurrence. Teach the patient how to cut their nails correctly (Fig. 114). Advise on the need for correct size and shape of shoe. Minimize the consequences of excessive foot sweating. Generally improve foot hygiene.

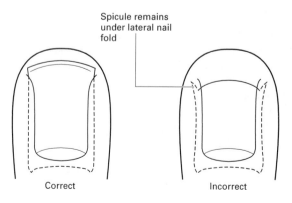

Spicule remains under lateral nail fold

Correct   Incorrect

Fig. 114 Correct method of cutting toenails.

OPERATION: AVULSION OF THE BIG TOENAIL

The toe is anaesthetized by digital nerve block. If a tourniquet is applied this should be as wide as possible to prevent digital nerve damage and left on for no longer than 20 min. A haemostat is passed under one edge of the nail, the nail is grasped and twisted off to the other side. The toe is dressed with paraffin gauze, a gauze pad and then a bandage. The foot should be kept elevated overnight and the toe redressed within 48 h.

Simple avulsion of the nail removes the source of infection and pain. If it is not followed by preventative measures it will usually be followed by recurrence. Recurrence after conservative treatment can be managed by excision (Zadik's operation) or destruction (phenol matricectomy) of the whole nail matrix and hence the entire nail. Alternatively, only one side of the matrix and hence nail can be excised (wedge excision) or destroyed (lateral nailfold phenol matricectomy).

OPERATION: ZADIK'S OPERATION (NAIL MATRIX EXCISION)

The nail is removed and the skin is incised diagonally from the corners of the posterior nailfold and folded back. The exposed nail matrix is then excised down to bone taking care to include the lateral horns of the matrix (Fig. 115). The skin edges are then stitched loosely together and a dressing applied and changed at 24 h. Avoid operating if there is active infection because of the risk of osteomyelitis in the distal phalanx.

Codes

Blood	0
GA/LA	LA
Opn time	30 min
Stay	Outpatient
Drains out	0
Sutures out	7 days
Off work	2–5 days

OPERATION: WEDGE EXCISION

This is similar to the Zadik's procedure except that only the side of the nail matrix is removed. It is performed for recurrent ingrowing toenail where only one nailfold is involved. The resulting nail is narrow but patients may prefer this outcome for functional and cosmetic reasons.

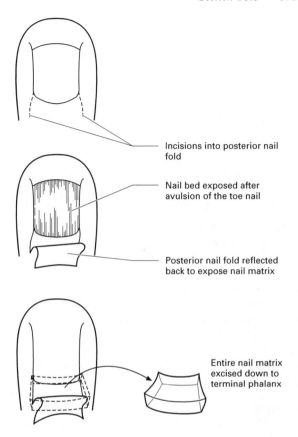

Incisions into posterior nail fold

Nail bed exposed after avulsion of the toe nail

Posterior nail fold reflected back to expose nail matrix

Entire nail matrix excised down to terminal phalanx

Fig. 115 Zadik's procedure for surgical removal of the nail matrix.

Phenol matricectomy

Phenol can be used to destroy part, or the entire, nail matrix. This procedure is simpler, results in less pain postoperatively and in skilled hands produces better functional and cosmetic results than surgical matricectomy.

> OPERATION: PHENOL MATRICECTOMY OF INGROWN TOENAIL
>
> An exsanguinating tourniquet is applied because phenol is neutralized by blood and bleeding will reduce its effectiveness. If the complete nail matrix is to be destroyed the entire nail is avulsed. A cotton wool bud dipped in phenol (90% in water) is placed beneath the proximal nailfold and rolled from side to side and into the lateral horns of the matrix.

Continued on p. 596

Continued.

Three 1-min phenol applications are required. There is little postoperative pain. The patient should change dressings daily for the first week.

Only one side of the nail matrix can be destroyed if required. The side of the nail is separated from the nailbed and lateral nailfold using a nail elevator. A piece of nail approximately 4–5 mm wide is then trimmed off down to the base of the nail using nail splitters. The phenol-tipped applicator is then inserted into the gap created under the posterior nailfold and into the lateral nail matrix horn (Fig. 116). Two 1-min phenol applications are required.

Acute paronychia

Paronychia is a soft tissue infection of the lateral and posterior nailfolds. Acute paronychia is usually caused by *Staphylococcus aureus* and may require surgery. Herpes simplex infections around the nail, or herpetic whitlow (particularly common in nurses and doctors), should be distinguished and treated medically. Chronic paronychia (usually due to *Candida albicans*) occurs in persons whose hands are regularly in water, rarely follows acute paronychia and is relatively painless. Surgical removal of part of the posterior nailfold is occasionally used in recalcitrant chronic paronychia.

Recognizing the pattern

Acute paronychia is very painful and there is erythema, swelling, tenderness and possibly visible pus in the nailfold. If pus has spread under the nail, pressure over the nail will be painful. Advanced infection may spread to the pulp space.

Management

In the first 48 h the infection may resolve with antibiotic therapy. Splinting the finger and elevation of the limb will reduce pain. Once pus has formed it must be drained.

OPERATION: INCISION AND DRAINAGE OF A PARONYCHIA

Under digital nerve block and with a tourniquet applied, the skin is incised at one or both proximal corners of the nailfold and a flap raised to release the pus. The entire slough must be excised. If pus is trapped beneath the nail, that part of the nail must also be removed. The finger is dressed with paraffin gauze. Inadequate primary treatment may result in nail dystrophy or destruction.

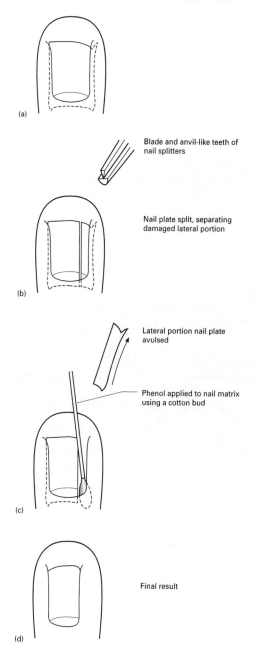

Blade and anvil-like teeth of nail splitters

Nail plate split, separating damaged lateral portion

Lateral portion nail plate avulsed

Phenol applied to nail matrix using a cotton bud

Final result

Fig. 116 Phenol wedge matricectomy for unilateral ingrown toenail. (a) The problem. (b) The sliver of nail snipped off, and (c) a phenol-tipped cotton bud inserted into the space under the posterior nailfold and into the lateral horn of the matrix. (d) Final result.

Codes

Blood 0

GA/LA ....LA

Opn time ....10 min

Stay ....Outpatient

Drains out 0

Sutures out 0

Off work ....1–2 days

Postoperative care
The dressing is changed daily until the finger heals.

Subungual haematoma

This is a collection of blood beneath the nail following a crushing injury to the fingertip. It is painful because the rigid nailplate prevents the inflamed tissue from expanding.

Recognizing the pattern

The patient presents following trauma with a very painful finger and a collection of blood beneath the nail.

Management

The digit must be X-rayed to exclude fracture of the phalanx. The blood is released by burning a hole in the nail over the clot with the end of a red-hot paper clip. This procedure is surprisingly painless.

A fracture of the phalanx beneath does not usually require manipulation and the nail provides sufficient splintage. However, a finger splint and elevation of the arm in a sling for 24–48 h will help to ease the pain.

Hyperhidrosis

Excessive sweating usually affects the axillae, hands and feet. This causes social embarrassment and the sweat may damage paper, shoes and clothing.

Management

Medical management is not very effective. Twenty per cent aluminium chloride applied at night helps axillary hyperhidrosis. One per cent formaldehyde soaks can be used on the feet and iontophoresis tried at any site.

When conservative measures fail, hyperhidrosis of the hands can be treated by transthoracic cervical sympathectomy. Lumbar sympathectomy may help foot sweating but is a radical procedure for a relatively minor problem (p. 529). Quadrilateral sympathectomy is not advisable as it produces postural hypertension.

Preoperative management
Check there is no history of chest trauma or infection as these may be associated with pleural adhesions. Warn the patient of the possibility of Horner's syndrome, compensatory sweating and the very slight chance of the need for a thorocotomy or a persistent chest drain. Horner's syndrome is due to inadvertent damage to the sympathetic supply to the eye resulting in a small pupil and drooping eyelid (ptosis) on the side of the lesion. It is rare with transthoracic sympathectomy. Look for and note any pre-existing ptosis. Compensatory sweating is a postoperative increase in sweating from other areas of the body. Usually it is not a problem with unilateral sympathectomy but is more pronounced after bilateral or extensive sympathectomies.

OPERATION: TRANSTHORACIC ENDOSCOPIC CERVICAL SYMPATHECTOMY
Two axillary ports may be required, one for the telescope (5 or 10 mm) and one for a diathermy hook (5 mm). An excellent view of the sympathetic chain is obtained. The lung is deflated either by using a double-lumen endotracheal tube and blocking off one bronchus, or by insufflating the chest with a low pressure of CO_2. The chain is destroyed from the lower edge of the stellate ganglion to the third thoracic ganglion to denervate the hand. Progressing distally may denervate the axilla. The pleura is emptied of any gas by inserting a drain at the end of the procedure.

Axillary hyperhidrosis is best treated by local excision of the sweat glands. The disadvantage of this approach is the large scar produced and general poor healing due to wound tension. Alternatively, only part of the axillary skin is excised and the sweat glands in the remainder are damaged or removed by curettage, extensive undermining (Hurley–Shelley procedure) or liposuction.

Continued on p. 600

OPERATION: EXCISION OF AXILLARY SWEAT
GLANDS

Preoperative management
The day before operation the sweat gland area is mapped out
using either a starch iodine reaction or quinizarin both of
which change colour when moist. Alternatively, just the hair-
bearing portion of the axilla can be excised and the wound
closed with suction drainage to the subcutaneous space.

Codes
Blood 0
GA/LA .... LA/GA
Opn time .... 1 h
Stay .... Day case or 3–5 days
Drains out .... 48 h
Sutures out .... 10 days
Off work .... 2 weeks

Postoperative care
After the wound has healed active shoulder exercises with
or without physiotherapy may be required to restore full arm
movements.

14 Surgery of Children

14.1 Surgical conditions of neonates
Neonatal intestinal obstruction
Oesophageal atresia
Small bowel atresia
Malrotation
Meconium ileus
Hirschsprung's disease
Anorectal malformations
Necrotizing enterocolitis
Paralytic ileus

14.2 Surgical conditions of children
Congenital hypertrophic pyloric stenosis
Intussusception
Inguinal hernia and hydrocoele
Umbilical hernia
Umbilical discharge
Rectal bleeding in children
Constipation in children
Urinary tract infection in children

14.3 General management of the paediatric patient
Environment
Nursing
Fluids
Analgesia
Electrolytes

14.1 Surgical Conditions of Neonates

Neonatal intestinal obstruction

Vomiting in the first week after birth is common and usually of little significance, settling on symptomatic treatment. Where the vomit is bile-stained and persistent it may indicate a serious problem.

Obstruction may be due to defects such as atresia, stenosis or a web. Other causes of obstruction include compression from outside by bands, volvulus or malrotation. The lumen may be obstructed by inspissated meconium as in cystic fibrosis. The bowel wall itself is abnormal in Hirschsprung's disease. It is important not to miss an inguinal hernia strangulating a loop of small bowel. Necrotizing enterocolitis and adynamic ileus should be borne in mind.

Recognizing the pattern

Neonatal problems can be anticipated during pregnancy if there is a family history of congenital defects, polyhydramnios or abnormality on antenatal ultrasound. After birth the child will present with vomiting. Depending on the level of obstruction, this may be bile-stained and associated with abdominal distension. Passage of meconium is delayed (normally it is passed within the first 24 h).

Proving the diagnosis

An erect abdominal X-ray will show dilated bowel loops and fluid levels. It may reveal the level of obstruction.

Management

The baby must be rehydrated. A nasogastric tube is passed to reduce the risk of aspiration. Definitive treatment depends on the underlying pathology.

Oesophageal atresia

In development the trachea buds on the oesophagus and atresia at this site often results in a fistula between the two. In 85% of cases the proximal oesophagus ends as a blind pouch, with the distal oesophagus arising from the trachea (Fig. 117).

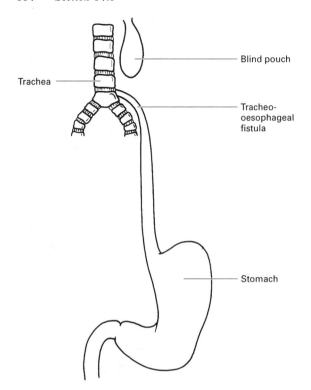

Fig. 117 The most common form of oesophageal atresia.

Recognizing the pattern
The baby continuously froths, as it is unable to swallow saliva.
If fed, it coughs and becomes cyanosed.

Proving the diagnosis
Gentle attempts to pass a nasogastric tube reveal the blockage.
Abdominal X-ray shows bowel gas only if there is a tracheo-oesophageal fistula.

Management
Place a tube in the oesophageal stump and aspirate secretions.

OPERATION: REPAIR OF OESOPHAGEAL ATRESIA
A right thoracotomy gives good access. Any tracheo-oesophageal fistula is ligated and divided. The ends of the oesophagus

can then usually be anastomosed directly. With a long defect it may be necessary to raise a feeding gastrostomy and bridge the gap at a later date with a stomach, colon or small bowel interposition graft.

Codes
Blood .... 1 unit
GA/LA .... GA
Opn time .... 2 h
Stay .... 1 week (longer for difficult cases)
Drains out .... Pleura 1–2 days
Nasogastric tube .... 5 days
Sutures out .... 5–7 days

Small bowel atresia

An atresia is a missing segment of bowel, occasionally with a fibrous cord joining the two ends. Obstruction is complete, resulting in gross dilation proximally and distal atrophy. Related problems include stenosis (a narrowing where obstruction may be only partial) and luminal web (a mucosal barrier which may be complete or perforated).

Recognizing the pattern

The patient presents with bile-stained vomiting. Meconium has never been passed. Abdominal distension is greater if obstruction is distal.

Proving the diagnosis

Abdominal X-ray shows dilated proximal bowel. In duodenal atresia a typical 'double bubble' is seen in the upper abdomen (Fig. 118). A similar double bubble can result from an annular pancreas encircling the duodenum. A barium enema will show a hypoplastic colon as a result of disuse.

Management

OPERATION: FOR SMALL BOWEL ATRESIA
A laparotomy is performed via a transverse incision. The affected segment is resected and an end-to-end anastomosis performed. A side-to-side anastomosis is required for duodenal atresia.

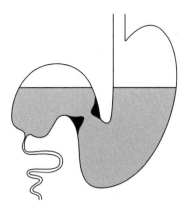

(a)

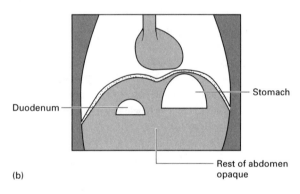

(b)

Fig. 118 (a) Duodenal atresia, (b) the double bubble seen on erect X-ray.

Codes
Blood .... 1 unit
GA/LA .... GA
Opn time .... 60–90 min
Stay .... 1–3 weeks, depending on duration of ileus
Drains out 0
Sutures out .... 7 days

Postoperative care
It can take days or even weeks for the hypoplastic segment to achieve normal function and during this period intravenous feeding is required. A transanastomotic feeding tube can be placed peroperatively if the distal bowel is very hypoplastic.

Malrotation

During development the gut is normally a midline structure. As it elongates it herniates through the abdominal wall (Fig. 119). At 10 weeks *in utero* it returns to the abdominal cavity, rotating 270 degrees anticlockwise about the axis of the superior mesenteric artery as it does so. This places the caecum in the right iliac fossa. If the process is not fully completed the caecum may lie in the right hypochondrium, where its peritoneal attachments ('Ladd's bands') can obstruct the duodenum. There is also an increased risk of midgut volvulus, as the close proximity of caecum and duodenojejunal flexure result in a mesentery with a very short base.

Recognizing the pattern

Presentation is with small bowel obstruction and may be at any age, most often during the first year (50% during the first week). Diagnosis can be difficult, since obstruction is often incomplete and partial. A volvulus presents with severe acute obstruction in an extremely ill patient.

Proving the diagnosis

Abdominal X-ray may show a double bubble similar to that in duodenal atresia if Ladd's bands are present, but with gas in the

Lateral view

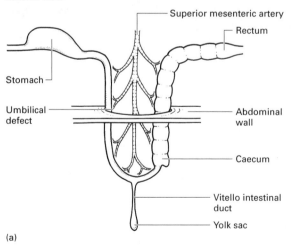

(a)

Fig. 119 (a) Normal development of the gut: lateral view. The midgut is originally a midline structure protruding through the umbilical defect.

Continued on p. 608

Ventral view

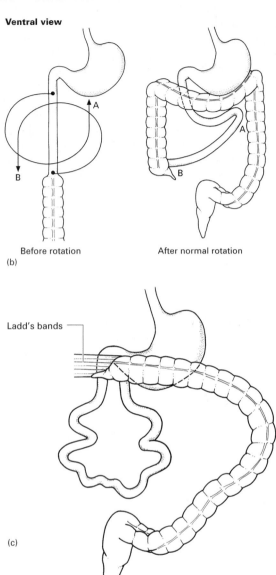

Before rotation   After normal rotation
(b)

Ladd's bands

(c)

Fig. 119 *Cont.* (b) Normal development of the gut: ventral view,
before and after normal rotation. Points A and B rotate 300°
anticlockwise to achieve the adult position of the gut. The colon
comes to lie over the proximal gut. (c) Malrotation: the caecum lies
over the duodenum. The duodenojejunal junction is close to the
ileocaecal valve.

distal bowel. Barium enema confirms the abnormal position of the caecum.

Management

OPERATION: FOR MALROTATION
If there is a volvulus present, this is reduced and any necrotic bowel resected. If Ladd's bands are obstructing the duodenum, they are divided. Before closing the abdomen the bowel is unrotated by placing the large bowel on the left and the small bowel on the right. This is a more stable arrangement that reduces the risk of future volvulus, even though it differs from the normal anatomical layout.

Codes

Blood .... 1 unit
GA/LA .... GA
Opn time .... 90–120 min
Stay .... 1–2 weeks
Drains out 0
Sutures out .... 7 days

Meconium ileus

Deficient pancreatic function results in inspissated meconium, causing complete obstruction. This occurs in 15% of patients with cystic fibrosis (mucoviscidosis), a familial condition due to a recessive gene.

Recognizing the pattern

The baby vomits bile and may have a distended abdomen with palpable loops of bowel.

Proving the diagnosis

Abdominal X-ray shows dense meconium pellets resembling ground glass. If perforation occurs it results in widespread peritoneal calcification. A sweat test will confirm cystic fibrosis.

Management

In stable cases a gastrografin enema may help shift the meconium. Intravenous infusion is necessary as hypovolaemia can rapidly be precipitated by this procedure.

OPERATION: FOR OBSTRUCTION DUE TO
MECONIUM ILEUS
Resection of the massively dilated loop may be necessary,
with washout of the distal inspissated meconium. A loop
ileostomy allows distal washout to be continued
postoperatively.

Postoperative care
Respiratory complications are common, requiring treatment
with oxygen, physiotherapy and antibiotics. Long-term care
is a specialist area. Pancreatic enzyme supplements will be
required.

Hirschsprung's disease

Absence of intramural ganglia in the distal bowel results in a
functional obstruction due to lack of peristalsis and tonic contraction of smooth muscle. The rectum is involved in all cases.
In 70% the lower sigmoid is involved as well, and in 15% the
whole colon. The bowel proximal to the affected segment is
grossly dilated (megacolon).

Recognizing the pattern

It causes obstruction in 1 : 5000 live births, with gross distension and bile-stained vomiting. There is a significant risk of
fulminating enterocolitis. Rectal examination causes dramatic
deflation and improvement, but this is only temporary. Short
segment disease may cause chronic constipation with spurious
diarrhoea later in childhood.

Proving the diagnosis

Barium enema shows a dilated proximal bowel and narrowed
distal segment. Suction biopsy with acetylcholinesterase staining confirms the absence of ganglia, but requires an experienced
pathologist.

Management
Obstructed neonates are managed initially with colostomy
or an ileostomy, taking care to ensure the stoma is proximal
to the affected segment (frozen section may be required).
The aganglionic segment is resected later and the normal
bowel anastomosed to the anus by one of several alternative
techniques, e.g. Duhamel or Soave.

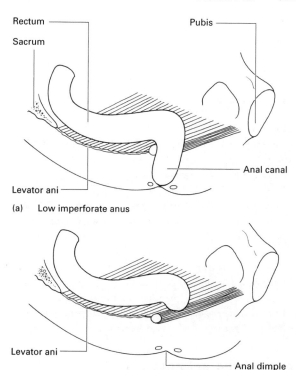

(a)   Low imperforate anus

(b)   High imperforate anus

Fig. 120 (a,b) Two forms of rectal agenesis (imperforate anus).

Anorectal malformations

Anorectal malformations are classified into high or low types according to the relation to the levator ani and puborectalis sling (Fig. 120). In the low type the anus is closed by a membrane or stenosed, commonly with a fistula passing to the base of the scrotum or into the vagina. In the high type, the rectum ends as a blind pouch and there is no sphincter mechanism. There are often associated congenital malformations and a fistula may pass to any cloacal structure, resulting in frequent urinary tract infections.

Making the diagnosis

The absent anus is usually noted at birth. Untreated the baby will fail to pass meconium and become increasingly distended. An abdominal X-ray is taken with the baby inverted and with a ball-bearing to mark the anal dimple. It is taken after 24 h so that air has time to reach the distal bowel. If the pouch is above a line joining the pubis to the coccyx on a lateral view the abnormality is a high one. Ultrasound may also be used to assess the type.

Management

Low anorectal malformations
The membrane is perforated and the stenosed anus dilated. Dilation needs to be repeated. In general the child should achieve normal continence at a normal age.

High anorectal malformations
In the immediate postnatal period a colostomy is required. Between 6 months and 1 year of age the descending colon is brought through the levator ani and anastomosed to the skin. The colostomy is closed 1 month later. The lower rectum may require regular dilatation for many months. Results are often disappointing and continence cannot always be achieved, mainly because of the deficient sphincter. A permanent stoma may then be necessary.

Necrotizing enterocolitis

This condition may occur in any baby, but is most common in the premature, or babies asphyxiated during birth. Umbilical catheters may be a risk factor. The aetiology is not known, but it may result from ischaemia of the mucosa during an episode of stress.

Making the diagnosis
Bloody or mucous stools are passed. The baby is ill, hypothermic and distended. Abdominal X-ray may show gas in the bowel wall. Free air will be seen if there is perforation.

Management
Feeds are withheld and intravenous fluids are given. Nasogastric suction should be considered. Broad-spectrum antibiotics are given, including cover for anaerobes (especially clostridia). Abdominal X-rays are taken every 8 h to assess progress. In the event of perforation, laparotomy is required to resect the affected segment and raise a stoma. Second-look operations may be required. Those babies managed conservatively may develop strictures which need resection later.

Paralytic ileus

The bowel is atonic and fails to peristalse. Infections are a common cause; the baby is characteristically floppy and may be hypothermic, but external signs of infection may be minimal. Features of obstruction in the absence of infection or mechanical cause may be seen in premature or stressed babies. Drugs used during pregnancy, especially antihypertensives, may be responsible.

Investigation

A full septic screen is required, looking especially for ear or throat infections, pneumonia, urinary tract infection, meningitis and umbilical stump infection.

Management

Infections are treated with appropriate antibiotics and careful fluid balance. Idiopathic functional obstruction usually resolves on conservative management.

14.2   Surgical Conditions of Children

Congenital hypertrophic pyloric stenosis

There is obstruction of the outlet of the stomach by hyperplasia of the circular muscle of the pylorus. The aetiology is not known. There is a slight male predominance and a family history is common.

Recognizing the pattern

Presentation is typically between the ages of 3 and 6 weeks, but may occur any time from birth to 5 months. There is projectile vomiting of non–bile-stained vomit, following which the baby is eager for further feed. The baby fails to gain weight and is often dehydrated. After a test feed, an olive-like 'tumour' may be palpable in the right hypochondrium.

Proving the diagnosis

If a tumour is not felt, ultrasound should be requested to exclude rare problems such as annular pancreas or a partial luminal web.

Management

Vomiting results in dehydration and potassium depletion, which must be corrected preoperatively.

OPERATION: RAMSTEDT'S PYLOROMYOTOMY

The 'tumour' is delivered through a transverse incision and the muscle layer is split until the mucosa pouts through. Care is taken to avoid perforating the mucosa. Some paediatric surgeons do this operation using a mini-laparoscope.

Codes

Blood	0
GA/LA	GA
Opn time	30–60 min
Stay	2 days
Drains out	0
Sutures out	5 days

Intussusception

A segment of proximal bowel is passed distally along the lumen
as a result of peristalsis (Fig. 121). Five per cent of cases result
from a lead point such as a polyp or Meckel's diverticulum.

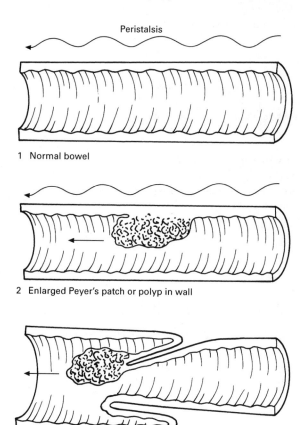

Peristalsis

1   Normal bowel

2   Enlarged Peyer's patch or polyp in wall

3   Formation of intussusception

Fig. 121 The production of an intussusception.

Idiopathic cases may follow mild upper respiratory infections, perhaps as a result of enlargement of Peyer's patches. The commonest site is ileocaecal, while ileoileal or colocolic are comparatively rare.

Recognizing the pattern

Presentation may be at any age. Idiopathic cases often present between the ages of 5 and 9 months. Cases with causative lesions are usually older. There is a classic triad of symptoms.

1 Pain. A healthy child suffers recurrent spasms of pain, which may be so severe as to cause screaming. The legs are drawn up and a squatting position may be adopted. Between spasms the child is normal.

2 Vomiting. Initial vomiting is due to pain. This settles, but recurs as obstruction becomes established.

3 Bleeding per rectum. Blood-stained mucus resembling red-currant jelly is passed. Obstruction occurs later.

On examination a tender, sausage-like mass may be felt in the right hypochondrium. The right iliac fossa feels 'empty'. The apex of the intussusceptum may be felt (or even seen) per rectum.

Proving the diagnosis

Abdominal X-ray shows intestinal obstruction and an empty right iliac fossa. Barium enema shows a 'coiled spring' appearance.

Management

Rehydration and blood transfusion may be necessary before reduction.

Reduction of intussusception by barium enema

The hydrostatic pressure generated by a 1-m column of barium may reduce an intussusception if attempted within 24 h of the onset of symptoms. It is important to achieve complete reduction, including observation of barium in the ileum.

OPERATION: REDUCTION OF
INTUSSUSCEPTION
A transverse incision is used and the intussusception reduced by 'milking' (not by traction). Any gangrenous bowel or causative lesion is resected. About 3% of cases recur.

Codes

Blood .... Group and save serum
GA/LA .... GA
Opn time .... 1 h (longer if resection required)
Stay .... 3–5 days
Drains out 0
Sutures out .... 7 days

Inguinal hernia and hydrocele

Inguinal hernia is the commonest paediatric surgical referral and is much more common in boys. It results from failure of closure of the processus vaginalis, a peritoneal pouch related to the testis during its descent into the scrotum (Fig. 122). Hydrocoeles arise from the same structure (Fig. 123).

Recognizing the pattern

Most childhood hernias occur in the first year of life. The incidence in boys is 1 in 50 and in girls is 1 in 500. They are more common in premature babies where there is a high risk of small bowel strangulation. The history is of an intermittent swelling in the groin, especially on crying or straining. Incar-

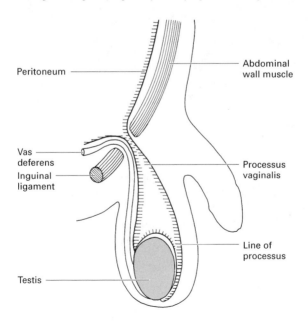

Fig. 122 The processus vaginalis.

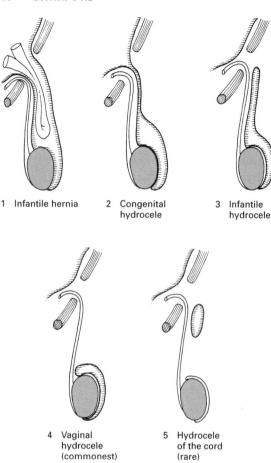

1 Infantile hernia   2 Congenital   3 Infantile
                          hydrocele   hydrocele

4 Vaginal   5 Hydrocele
   hydrocele   of the cord
   (commonest)   (rare)

Fig. 123 Types of inguinal hernias and hydrocoeles.

ceration is not uncommon, resulting in emergency presentation. On examination the swelling may or may not be visible. In girls a sliding hernia containing an ovary results in a firm 1 cm lump in the inguinal canal.

Hydrocoeles present as a swelling of the testis. Occasionally a swelling proximal to the testis may result from an encysted hydrocoele of the cord.

Proving the diagnosis
The diagnosis is proved by feeling the swelling. If no swelling is present, the characteristic history of intermittent groin swelling is virtually diagnostic.

Management

Operation is required. All babies less than 6 months, or children who have had an episode of strangulation should have their operation on the next available list. The presence of both testes in the scrotum should be checked.

OPERATION: HERNIOTOMY IN CHILDREN

The spermatic cord (or round ligament in girls) is exposed through a transverse groin incision. The hernia sac is separated from the cord structures, to which it is closely related, and ligated at the level of the internal ring. At the end of the operation the testis must be at the base of the scrotum, since, if it is in the groin, it may be fixed there by postoperative fibrosis.

Codes

Blood 0
GA/LA .... GA
Opn time .... 15–40 min
Stay .... Day case or 24 h
Drains out 0
Sutures out .... 5 days
Off school .... 1–2 weeks

Umbilical hernia

Umbilical hernias in children are of two types.

1 Central. This results from failure of fusion of the abdominal wall. Closure usually occurs spontaneously at any age up to 3 years.

2 Paraumbilical. This is a true defect in the linea alba close to the umbilicus. This type of hernia does not close spontaneously.

Recognizing the pattern

There is a bulge in the region of the umbilicus, which has often been present from birth. There may be tenderness, as the defect is often very small compared with the size of the hernia. Strangulation almost never occurs in central hernias and is rare in paraumbilical hernias in children.

Management

A central umbilical hernia should be followed up to ensure that it closes. If it does not do so by the age of 3 years, operative closure is appropriate before school age. Para-umbilical hernias should be repaired at the same age.

OPERATION: REPAIR OF UMBILICAL HERNIA
The defect is closed through a small semilunar incision.

Codes

Blood	Group and save
GA/LA	GA
Opn time	1–2 h
Stay	2–7 days
Drains out	24 h (if inserted)
Sutures out	4–7 days
Off school	1–2 weeks

Umbilical discharge

Infection of the stump of the umbilical cord can occur in the first few days of life. If it persists a granuloma can result. A swab should be taken and antibiotics given. Cauterization with a silver nitrate stick will speed resolution.

A more profuse, persistent discharge may indicate a congenital fistula or sinus. A persistent vitellointestinal duct results from failure of the endodermal communication between gut and yolk sac to close. Partial failure of closure results in a Meckel's diverticulum. A patent urachus arises when the communication between umbilicus and bladder fails to close. The same structure can give rise to a urachal cyst.

Proving the diagnosis

X-ray contrast can be injected into any obvious opening. A small bowel barium study or a cystogram may also help. Ultrasound will reveal any urachal cyst.

Management

OPERATION: CLOSURE OF UMBILICAL FISTULA
Through a transverse incision the umbilicus is mobilized. A fine probe is used to define the fistula, which is isolated, ligated and divided. Any associated urachal cyst or Meckel's diverticulum is excised.

Codes

Blood	Group and save serum
GA/LA	GA
Opn time	60 min
Stay	2–3 days
Drains out	2–3 days
Sutures out	7 days

Rectal bleeding in children

Most cases are mild and result from straining. The stool should be examined, as worms may be responsible. Piles are extremely rare in children. Stool softeners are used to ease passage of motions and the child is prevented from staying on the potty for long, as this causes venous congestion.

An anal fissure causes pain and bleeding. Constipation results, as the child is frightened to pass motions, which compounds the problem. Stool softeners are given if the child is constipated, a high-fibre diet if not. An examination under anaesthetic may be necessary if there is no improvement after 3 months.

Intermittent passage of blood and mucus may be due to a benign rectal polyp or prolapse. A polyp can be ligated at its base and will slough off painlessly a few days later. Prolapse usually affects the mucosa only and may be observed by the mother when the child strains. It results from a lack of sacral spinal curvature, which normally develops at 2 years of age. Treatment is reassurance and administration of stool softeners. If it persists beyond 2 years, submucosal injections of phenol in almond oil under general anaesthetic may be required.

Massive haemorrhage is most often due to a Meckel's diverticulum. Peptic ulcer, intussusception, blood dyscrasias, intestinal duplications and angiomas should all be considered.

The incidence of inflammatory bowel disease in children is increasing and should be remembered in a child with cramping pains and passage of bloody mucus.

Rectal prolapse in children

Rectal prolapse in children is associated with a lack of the sacral spinal curvature which develops about the age of 2 as the child begins to walk upright. The condition is usually a mucosal prolapse rather than a complete prolapse (p. 401).

Recognizing the pattern

The child is usually in the first year of life and the mother either notices rectal bleeding or the strawberry-coloured prolapse during defaecation. She is often extremely alarmed by this. Where no prolapse has been seen, there may be a history of excessive staining by the child. The prolapse usually reduces spontaneously.

Proving the diagnosis

If you are lucky enough to see the prolapse, there is no problem. Otherwise the diagnosis can only be made on the mother's history. It is important for the clinician to have this condition in mind.

Management

The management is to reassure the mother and to take no further action apart from making sure the stools are kept soft. This can be achieved by giving extra roughage in the diet and making sure the child has enough fluid to drink.

The mother should be told that a prolapse is not uncommon in the first year of life and that it should settle as the baby begins to adopt the upright posture. The child is followed up at 3–6-monthly intervals and in most cases the condition resolves spontaneously.

If the prolapse persists, injections may be required.

OPERATION: INJECTION OF RECTAL PROLAPSE IN CHILDREN

The child is given a general anaestietic and the anal canal inspected. A nasal speculum can be useful for this. Submucosal injections of phenol in almond oil are inserted.

Codes

Blood	0
GA/LA	GA
Opn time	15 minutes
Stay	24 hours
Drains out	0
Sutures out	0

Constipation in children

This is infrequent passage of stools. The passage of hard stools, sometimes referred to as constipation, is usually the result of a low-residue diet and is treated with high fibre and high fluid intake. Transient constipation may result from dietary changes.

Chronic constipation may have an organic cause such as neurological deficits or anal stenosis. Alternatively, it may be precipitated by pain, as occurs with an anal fissure. It can result in acquired megarectum due to incomplete emptying, and the consequent impaction of faeces causes spurious diarrhoea and soiling.

Management
Management is difficult and often prolonged, requiring specialized nursing. An impacted mass is removed by daily irrigation, or sometimes under general anaesthetic. Stimulant laxatives and habit training are then continued until a normal habit is achieved.

Urinary tract infection in children
Urinary tract infection in children must be taken seriously as long-term complications are likely unless properly treated.

Recognizing the pattern
Infants may present with abdominal pain, vomiting, pyrexia or failure to thrive. Older children may present with wetting by day, having previously been fully continent. Only a minority present with loin pain, rigors and dysuria.

Making the diagnosis
At least two 'clean catch' midstream urine specimens are required. They should be cultured rapidly, or refrigerated if delay is unavoidable, to avoid growth of contaminants. Confirmed infections require ultrasound, to assess the kidneys and ureters. A micturating cystourethrogram is required, since vesicoureteric reflux is commonly responsible. Nuclear isotope scans (MAG3, DTPA, DMSA) are used to assess renal function and structure. Cystoscopy is performed if no cause is found on other investigations.

Management
Initial infections are treated with antibiotics. All cases then require investigation to determine the cause and long-term follow-up. Precise treatment protocols are a specialist area beyond the scope of this book.

14.3   General Management of the Paediatric Patient

Environment
Babies less than 28 days old have a high surface to volume ratio and immature temperature regulating mechanisms. It is therefore important to maintain them in a thermoneutral environment to minimize metabolic demands. The use of radiant heaters is helpful, and dry Gamgee dressings are useful for covering exposed areas.

Nursing
The gag reflex is poor, so there is increased risk of aspiration. Ideally the baby should be nursed on its side, with suction readily to hand.

Fluids
Fluid overload is a significant risk, especially in neonates. A 1-day-old baby should be given no more than 60 ml/kg/24 h intravenously. This can be increased by increments of 10 ml/kg/24 h each day up to a maximum of 120 ml/kg/24 h. Postoperative requirements are reduced because of high levels of antidiuretic hormone. For oral fluid intake the maximum is 150 ml/kg/24 h.

For older children, maintenance fluid requirements can be calculated from the following:
1   Give 100 ml/kg/24 h for each of the first 10 kg
2   Give 50 ml/kg/24 h for each of the next 10 kg
3   Give 20 ml/kg/24 h for each kilogram above 20 kg.

For example, a 22-kg child requires 1.54 L/24 h (64 ml/h) for ordinary maintenance.

Dextrose saline (0.18% sodium chloride, 4% dextrose) is suitable. Daily weighing provides a useful guide to fluid balance. Loss of fluid above the norm must be compensated for additionally, aiming for a urine output of about 1 ml/kg/h. A child that is peripherally shut down and has a low urine output can be given a repeatable 'challenge' of 10–15 ml/kg of albumin 4%.

Analgesia
See Table 25.

Table 25

Drug	Dose	Frequency
Paracetamol[†]	12 mg/kg p.o.	4–6 hourly
	15 mg/kg p.r.	Max. 80 mg/kg/day
Ibuprofen	4–10 mg/kg p.o.	6–8 hourly
		Max. 20 mg/kg/day
Diclofenac	0.5–1 mg/kg p.o./p.r.	8–12 hourly
		Max. 3 mg/kg/day
Codeine phosphate[*]	3 mg/kg/day p.o.	In divided doses
	1 mg/kg i.m.	Max. 4 mg/kg i.m.
Pethidine[*]	0.5–2 mg/kg p.o./i.m.	4–6-hourly
	0.5–1 mg/kg i.v.	
Morphine[*†]	0.2–0.5 mg/kg p.o.	4-hourly
	0.15–0.2 mg/kg s.c./i.m.	Max. 2.5 mg/kg/day
	0.1–0.2 mg/kg i.v.	
	0.05–0.1 mg/kg i.v.	Neonatal dose

[*]Opiates should be used with caution in infants (< 1 year) due to increased susceptibility to respiratory depression.
[†]Suitable for neonates (up to 1 month).
Avoid the intramuscular route in children where possible.

Age	Weight (kg)	Age (years)	Weight (kg)
Newborn (full term)	3.5	7	23
2 months	4.5	10	30
4 months	6.5	12	39
1 year	10	14	50
3 years	15	16	58

Electrolytes

As with adults, hypokalaemia can result from diarrhoea or vomiting and must be considered in any intravenous fluid regime.

Hypocalcaemia can cause collapse or fits. Initial treatment is with intravenous calcium gluconate 10%. If this fails to raise the calcium level, check for low magnesium levels.

The poor glycogen reserves of the neonate result in a risk of rapid onset hypoglycaemia. BM-stix testing is routinely done 6-hourly postoperatively, and corrective action taken if the level falls below 3 mmol/L.

15 Trauma Surgery

15.1 Dealing with a Major Accident

General principles

The principles of management of the trauma victim are taught on the Advanced Trauma Life Support (ATLS) course. This is essential for all doctors who, following their house year will be involved in the management of trauma.

When a major trauma case arrives in hospital, there may be many people involved in the initial assessment and resuscitation. There is often great danger for the patient and urgent decisions need to be made. Good organization is imperative, and action, however, rapid, has to be methodical and thoughtful. Priorities must be decided and one doctor should assume overall control and assess the progress of resuscitation without being too embroiled in the action.

Accurate notes are important, particularly for victims of assault, road accidents or industrial injuries. Legal action may be taken many months after the injury when the actual details have been forgotten.

How do you cope when the victim of a major accident suddenly comes under your care? The following is a basic plan, which may be helpful. There are seven overall steps.

1 Assess vital functions — primary survey

2 Resuscitation

In practice these two steps are virtually simultaneous. The motto is 'treat as you find'.

3 Secondary survey — a full history and examination

4 X-ray

5 Special investigations

6 Decide on priorities for management

7 Treatment.

Assess vital functions — primary survey

The principles of initial assessment are embodied in the primary survey A (airway), B (breathing), C (circulation), D (disability) and E (exposure).

Airway and breathing

1 Check the airway. Is it clear?

2 Is the patient breathing? Is mechanical ventilation effective?

3 Is there adequate gaseous exchange, i.e. is the patient cyanosed or adequately oxygenated?

4 Check whether there is any injury to the chest that may embarrass respiration.
5 Does the patient have a pneumothorax or haemothorax?

Circulation

1 Check the blood pressure and pulse.
2 Stop any external bleeding and beware of bleeding into cavities.

Disability

1 Check the basic level of consciousness. Is the patient Alert, or responding to Voice, Pain, or Unresponsive (AVPU)?
2 Look at the pupils and limbs for evidence of extradural haemorrhage (see p. 642).

Exposure

Ensure the patient is completely undressed. Do a log roll and rectal examination. Insert a urinary catheter (see p. 664) and nasogastric tube. Test the urine for blood.

Resuscitation

1 Order a portable series of X-rays (lateral cervical spine, chest and pelvis) in the resus' room.
2 Action on:
  (a) airway and breathing
  (b) circulation.

Airway and breathing

Clear the airway of all potential obstruction, including broken teeth, debris, vomit, etc. The airway may need frequent aspiration. Give the patient oxygen. If the patient is still not breathing adequately and remains cyanosed, consider intubation and ventilation. Severe maxillary facial injuries are also an indication for intubation.

Treat any life-threatening injury of the chest immediately, e.g. tension pneumothorax or haemothorax (see pp. 649–650). Beware an injury to the cervical spine and ensure that at all times the cervical spine is prevented from being moved until this injury is excluded.

Circulation

Put up at least two good intravenous lines with large cannulae. You should use this opportunity to take blood for cross-matching and investigations. Request 8 units. Treat any hypo-volaemia by plasma expanders such as Haemaccel, plasma or blood. O negative blood can be used if blood is needed before the cross-match is completed. The longer the delay in instituting such therapy, the more collapsed are the veins and therefore the more difficult intravenous cannulation will be. Expect hypotension where there is multi-focal injury. Monitor the patient's response to your resuscitation.

Stop any external bleeding with external pressure. By now there should be adequate cerebral perfusion of oxygenated blood, and a fuller assessment of all the injuries can begin.

Secondary survey — a full history and examination

A full history and examination are undertaken together with documentation of the injuries. The exact order in which this is done will be governed by events. However, it must be thorough and, if urgent treatment interrupts it, it must be completed at the earliest opportunity. Patients have, for instance, had a fractured finger left untreated because in the excitement of the initial effort to save life, no one has had time to examine the digits. Monitor vital functions during this.

The history

Try to determine exactly what happened and how long ago. Obtain a detailed account of the time and nature of the accident including the mechanism and direction of injury. This may be obtained from the patient, ambulance personnel or police. A description of the patient's condition when first found is essential and should be recorded.

If the patient is conscious, question him about any areas of particular pain. If his condition deteriorates, this information may be valuable later.

Remember to find out the patient's normal medical condition including any past history (e.g. diabetes, myocardial ischaemia or previous chest injury), any current medication such as insulin or steroids and allergies.

On examination

The examination must be a thorough head to toe assessment and include all systems. The findings should be accurately recorded, ideally at the time the examination is being carried out.

Examine the patient methodically, starting with the head and neck and trunk and working down both arms and both legs, looking for possible injuries. This is especially important in an unconscious patient.

Use what is known of the mechanism of the accident to predict sites of injury, e.g. a person hit by a car bumper while standing may have ligament injuries to the knee. A passenger in a car hit on the left side may have a ruptured spleen or kidney.

Start with the head, looking for lacerations, bruising, haematoma or deformity. Check the pupil reaction and size. Measure the conscious level using the GCS (see p. 637).

Next examine the neck, including a careful palpation of the cervical spine for localized tenderness or deformity. Then feel the thoracic and lumbar spine for any possible fracture. If there is any likelihood of an unstable spinal fracture, this must be stabilized before the patient is moved (see p. 662).

Examine the upper limbs next, including the clavicle, joints, bones and soft tissues down to the individual fingers.

Re-examine the chest for rib, lung or mediastinal injury and then feel the abdomen. Palpate methodically around the various organs observing the patient's reaction for any sign of a localized site of tenderness.

Finally, examine the pelvis and the lower limbs.

X-ray

1 The following are routine in all cases of major trauma:
   (a) cervical spine
   (b) chest
   (c) pelvis.
2 Include the following, depending on injuries observed:
   (a) thoracic spine
   (b) lumbar spine
   (c) limbs
   (d) skull X-rays, facial views.
3 Specialist imaging, such as CT, ultrasound or contrast radiology.

Special Investigations

Send off blood to the laboratory for haemoglobin, cross-matching, urea and electrolytes, blood sugar, amylase.

Decide on priorities for management

Decide on the priorities for management. This can be done whilst the patient is being X-rayed. It may well be difficult.

The order should be as follows:

1 Conditions threatening life
2 Conditions which are at present stable but could threaten life if they deteriorate
3 Major injury, no threat to life
4 Minor injury.

Treatment

The management of injuries will be considered under the following headings.

1 Head injury (pp. 634–645).
2 Chest trauma (pp. 646–655)
3 Abdominal trauma (pp. 655–661)
4 Spinal injury (pp. 662–667)
5 Injuries to the pelvis (pp. 664–667)
6 Trauma to the skin and limbs (pp. 668–677)
7 Burns (pp. 677–683).

15.2   Head Injuries

A head injury may present in isolation or in association with other major injuries.

Brain survival depends on adequate perfusion with oxygenated blood. This is governed by the intracranial pressure (ICP), the mean blood pressure and respiratory function. The brain compartment in the skull is of constant volume, with limited room for expansion either by brain swelling or haematoma. As additional volume is added, cerebrospinal fluid (CSF) shifts into the spinal compartment, the venous sinuses are compressed and there may be some vasoconstriction. There is thus little initial change in ICP. Once this leeway is taken up, the ICP starts to rise, until eventually a small increase in volume causes a dramatic rise.

The brain perfusion pressure (BPP) is the sum of the mean blood pressure minus the ICP. A minimum of 60 mmHg is required for adequate brain function. Less than this causes first electrical and then structural damage. In a major injury with head involvement the ICP may rise and the mean blood pressure may fall, resulting in inadequate brain perfusion.

Pathology of brain injury (Fig. 124)
Brain damage is divided into primary damage sustained at the moment of injury, and secondary damage sustained following the injury.

Primary brain damage
Primary brain damage occurs by distortion and sudden movement within the dura and skull. Damage may be focal (e.g. after assault injury), the rest of the brain being relatively normal, or may be a combination of focal and diffuse injury typical of a high-momentum impact. There are three categories of primary injury.

1 Concussion. This is a generalized injury resulting in diffuse loss of nerve function. It is an electrical injury which is reversible.

2 Contusion. This is more localized and consists of bruising of the cortex.

3 Laceration of the cerebral cortex. This is always associated with bleeding into the subdural space. This is structural dam-

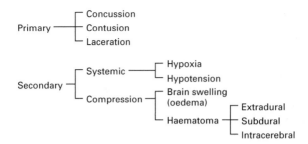

Fig. 124. Pathology of head injury.

age, and thus is irreversible. Diffuse axonal injury is included in this category and is seen after high-momentum rotational injuries.

Secondary brain damage

Secondary brain damage is caused by the following.

1 Systemic factors including:
 (a) hypotension
 (b) hypoxia.
2 Compression, either by brain swelling or by haematoma.

If brain compression is asymmetrical, focal shift occurs between the various brain compartments. The most important of these are as follows:

1 The medial temporal lobe herniating beneath the falx and pressing on the third nerve.

2 The temporal lobe, herniating through the tentorial hiatus and compressing the midbrain.

3 The cerebellar tonsils herniating through the foramen magnum ('coning').

The assessment and management of head injury is governed by the need to prevent, detect and treat this secondary injury. Systemic and local factors responsible for secondary brain damage are correctable. The prevention of hypoxia and hypotension is crucial to the outcome of brain damage and is most important in the first few hours after head injury.

Head injuries can be divided into major head injuries where the patient is unconscious on arrival, and minor head injuries where the patient is conscious.

Major head injury

Assessment

The initial assessment is combined with resuscitation. The following steps are performed:

1 Is the airway patent? If not an airway must be inserted or the patient intubated.

2 Is the patient breathing effectively? There may be active breathing movements but respiratory effort is wasted due to a flail chest.

3 Is ventilation adequate? Central cyanosis indicates inadequate gaseous exchange, which may be due to pulmonary contusion. Blood gases should be performed as soon as possible. Hypercapnia is a potent cause of cerebral vasodilatation and therefore increased ICP.

4 Chest X-ray. An early chest X-ray is mandatory to exclude pneumothorax or haemothorax.

5 Pulse and blood pressure. Is there a pulse and is it strong? Is there evidence of any external bleeding? If so, this must be controlled. Remember that isolated head injury does not cause hypotension so look elsewhere for blood loss.

6 Carotid perfusion. Are there carotid pulses?

7 Cervical spine. A patient with a major head injury must be assumed to have a cervical spine injury until this is excluded. Until this is done, and the patient is seen by an orthopaedic surgeon, a cervical collar should be put on to protect the neck.

Emergency management is performed to achieve cardio-respiratory stability. This may include blood transfusion, insertion of a chest drain for a pneumothorax or haemothorax or even laparotomy for ruptured spleen.

The history

Establish full details of the injury especially from the ambulance personnel. Include the position in which the patient was lying (an unconscious patient lying on his back may have aspirated), the time of the injury, any changes in conscious level, any history of fitting and whether the patient was ever cyanosed or unable to breathe.

Find out about any medical illnesses or drugs the patient was taking.

At the end of this assessment and resuscitation, the mean blood pressure should be restored such that cerebral perfusion is improved even though the ICP may still be elevated.

Once the blood pressure and ventilation are satisfactory carry out a neurological examination.

Table 26 Glasgow coma scale. (From Jennett B. & Teasdale G. (1977) Aspects of coma after severe head injury. *Lancet*, 23 April, 878–81.).

Function	Type of response	Points
Eyes	Open	
	spontaneously	4
	to verbal command	3
	to pain	2
	No response	1
Best motor response	To verbal command	
	obeys	6
	To painful stimulus*	
	localizes pain	5
	flexion — withdrawal from pain[†]	4
	flexion — abnormal (decorticate rigidity)	3
	Extension (decerebrate rigidity)	2
	No response	1
Best verbal response[‡]	Orientated and converses	5
	Disorientated and converses	4
	Inappropriate words	3
	Incomprehensible sounds	2
	No response	1
Total		3–15

*Apply the thumb to the underside of the supraorbital ridge and press up, observing the arms. To localize pain a hand must come above the chin.
[†]Elicit pain by squeezing a finger-nail bed.
[‡]Arouse patient with painful stimulus if necessary.

Neurological examination

Start a chart of the pulse rate, blood pressure, respiratory rate and body temperature as a basis for future observations.

Assess the conscious level. Make a note of the eye signs, motor responses and verbal responses. The Glasgow coma scale is the standard method of recording the level of consciousness and facilitates comparisons later on (Table 26).

Examine the head for scalp lacerations or bruising. Localized tenderness and a boggy swelling due to haematoma may be felt over a fracture site. You may feel a depression in the outline of the skull if the fracture is displaced. Look in the nose and ears for blood or CSF leakage, which may indicate that the nasal sinuses, nasal cavity or middle ear are fractured.

Anterior fossa fractures, as well as causing traumatic rhinorrhoea, may extend into the orbit and cause an effusion of blood, leading to unilateral exophthalmos, disturbance of eye movements and subconjunctival haemorrhage. The posterior border of this haemorrhage cannot be seen. The cranial nerves may also be affected. Bruising behind the ear (Battle's sign), with or without facial nerve palsy, indicates a fracture through the petrous temporal bone.

Examine the eyes noting the pupil size, equality and reaction to light. Try to assess eye movement. Examine the limb movements, noting the tone and testing the reflexes.

The continual assessment of conscious level is a dynamic process, the main purpose of which is to detect the trend indicating rising ICP. This is described further on p. 640.

Management

Early management is governed by the stability or otherwise of the patient's conscious level.

If the unconscious patient is stable, investigations can proceed in an orderly fashion. These should include the following:

1 Repeat blood gases to check respiratory function
2 Haemoglobin
3 Urea and electrolytes
4 Blood sugar
5 Liver function tests
6 Skull X-ray. Look for evidence of a skull fracture. The radiological features of a skull fracture are described on p. 645. If the pineal gland is calcified, it should be central. A shift of the pineal gland is a significant sign of raised ICP on one side.
7 CT scanning. The indications for CT scanning include the following:

(a) a patient who is in coma (Glasgow coma score 7 or less) after resuscitation

(b) any patient with a skull fracture that is associated with confusion, neurological signs or a fit

(c) a falling level of consciousness, (more than 2 on the GCS).

(d) depressed skull fracture or clinical evidence of skull base fracture

(e) a history of penetrating injury such as stabbing or gun shot.

These patients should be discussed with the regional neurosurgical centre.

General care of the unconscious patient

The priorities are to minimize brain swelling, maintain oxygenation and blood pressure and monitor regularly for evidence of deteriorating conscious level.

Nurse the patient with the head elevated 30°. In some centres ICP monitoring is performed. There is no place for steroids in acute head injury.

Respiration

If respiration is not adequate, the patient will need to be ventilated. This enables better control of blood gases. Hyperventilation to lower the P_{CO_2} (partial pressure of carbon dioxide) to 30 mmHg is not now routine since it can cause vasoconstriction so that brain ischaemia may result. Sedation and analgesia (using benzodiazepines and opiates) are necessary during this period if the patient is restless or in pain.

If ventilation is required for longer than 7 days, a tracheostomy may be required.

The daily assessment of the chest should include:

1 Examination
2 Chest X-ray
3 Blood gases.

Chest physiotherapy should be carried out regularly and if possible coincide with turning the patient. Tracheobronchial suction or bronchoscopy may be required.

Cardiovascular system

Ensure cerebral perfusion, avoid hypertension. If the blood pressure increases, exclude raised ICP, pain, hypoxia or a distended bladder and then treat either with a sedative (e.g. chlorpromazine 5 mg i.v.) or hydralazine (5–10 mg i.v.).

Nutrition

This may be given either through a nasogastric tube or by an intravenous route. If the nasogastric route is used, it is important to watch for regurgitation. Also remember that patients with multiple injuries may have an ileus.

Bladder

This should be catheterized. Retention of urine is a common cause of restlessness.

Bowels

They should be controlled by enemas.

Fluid balance

A strict watch should be kept on the patient's fluid balance together with measurements of urea and electrolytes and blood sugar, particularly if mannitol is being given. If anything, the patient should be run with a slight fluid deficit to prevent cerebral oedema.

General body care

The pressure points on the skin should be looked after by regular turning and putting the patient on a sheepskin and/or a ripple mattress. The eyes should be cleaned and kept closed to prevent corneal ulceration. The mouth should be regularly cleansed and kept moist to prevent parotitis or stomatitis. Regular limb physiotherapy is needed to prevent contractures developing.

Epilepsy

Fits following head injury are common, particularly after conditions such as depressed skull fracture with dural penetration and brain damage. Epilepsy requires treatment with anticonvulsants, such as phenytoin or carbamazepine. In an emergency intravenous diazepam is a safer drug to use. There is now no indication for prophylactic anticonvulsants.

Deterioration in conscious level

Deterioration may be seen in casualty or after a period of observation in hospital. The faster the deterioration occurs, the faster must be the response if one is to save the patient's brain. Deterioration is due to secondary brain damage, often a developing haematoma.

The signs of deterioration are as follows:

1 A decreasing level of consciousness
2 Bradycardia
3 Hypertension
4 Deep breathing.

Changes in the pupillary reactions and focal neurological signs such as arm or leg weakness indicate the probable site of such a lesion, as discussed on p. 643.

Carry out a computed tomography (CT) scan provided the patient's cardiorespiratory system is stable. This is to differentiate between generalized brain swelling, brain contusions and haematoma.

Contact the neurosurgical centre. Transfer of the patient may be discussed. Transfer of patients is potentially dangerous. Ensure the patient is well intubated, ventilated and stable prior to moving off.

Active measures can be taken to reduce cerebral oedema. Mannitol (20% 250–500 ml i.v. over 20–30 min) may be given. Frusemide in small doses is also useful. In some centres direct measurement of the ICP is made through a burr hole.

Haematoma

A haematoma causing cerebral compression must be removed. This may be done at the referring hospital, or by a neurosurgeon. Usually transfer is advised, following the resuscitation described above. The management of haematoma is described further on p. 643.

This concludes the final step in successful head injury treatment — namely to reduce the elevated ICP.

Minor head injury

Assessment

This is defined as a head injury where there has been no loss, or only transient loss, of consciousness, with or without loss of memory. The patient is conscious when seen.

Recognizing the pattern

A careful enquiry as to the nature of the injuries is undertaken. Establish whether the patient remembers the whole event clearly or if there is any retrograde or post-traumatic amnesia. Are there any disturbances of smell or hearing which may indicate a fracture causing damage to the olfactory or auditory nerves? Are there disturbances of vision, photophobia, nausea, vomiting or headache? Has the patient had a fit?

On examination the examination is performed as for a major head injury, but in this case with the cooperation of the patient.

The indications for skull X-ray include the following:

1 Loss of consciousness or amnesia at any time
2 Neurological symptoms and signs
3 Leakage of CSF from nose or ear
4 History of penetrating injury or scalp bruising and swelling.

Management

The main decision is whether to admit the patient to hospital or to send him home. The indications for admission to hospital are as follows:

Continued on p. 642

Continued.

1 A history of transient loss of consciousness, with post-traumatic amnesia of more than 5 min.

2 Confusion or other impairment of conscious level at the time of examination.

3 Evidence of a skull fracture.

4 Vomiting or headache, or other neurological symptoms or signs.

5 No witness to the accident or an unreliable history (usually due to drunkenness).

6 Lack of adequate supervision at home.

If the patient can go home, then an instruction sheet may be given, which includes the address and telephone number of the hospital, the date, and advice that the patient should return to hospital immediately if he develops symptoms of nausea, vomiting, headache, drowsiness, photophobia or weakness.

Patients who are admitted should have the following observations quarter- or half-hourly (in order to look for signs of raised ICP):

1 Conscious level, which should be described as in the Glasgow coma scale (p. 637).

2 Pulse, blood pressure, respiratory rate and body temperature.

3 Pupil size, equality and reaction.

4 Limb tone and movement.

Observations should ideally be continued for 24 h, after which the stable patient can be discharged. Children generally should stay longer because this age group can suddenly develop raised ICP within the first 48 h despite being stable.

Intracranial haematoma

Haematomas may be extradural, subdural or intracerebral.

Extradural haematoma occurs between the bone and the dura and is classically due to rupture of the middle meningeal artery following a fractured overlying temporal bone.

Subdural haematoma occurs between the dura and brain, and is usually associated with severe head injury causing cerebral laceration. It is typically less brisk than an extradural haemorrhage.

Intracerebral haematoma is a collection of blood within the substance of the brain and is associated with major brain damage. Occasionally intracerebral haemorrhage due to aneurysm or hypertension is the primary event which caused the head injury.

Recognizing the pattern

A stable patient develops signs of rising ICP as described above. The other presentation of intracranial haemorrhage is of a patient who is unconscious and begins to show signs of rising pressure.

On examination focal signs may indicate the side of the compression.

1 Pupillary size. There is contraction followed by dilatation of the pupil on the side of the haemorrhage (Hutchinson's pupil). As the pressure further increases, the opposite pupil shows similar signs. Bilateral fixed and dilated pupils may be a sign of brain-stem death, seen as the terminal evidence of coning. Remember, though, the effects of drugs, including alcohol, and of fits.

2 Hemiplegia. This is usually contralateral to the side of the first dilated pupil.

Proving the diagnosis

The diagnosis is made on a CT scan. If the patient is deteriorating rapidly, he should still be scanned, if possible, even if this is one or two slices simply to confirm the diagnosis. Occasionally a patient deteriorates so quickly that even this is not possible.

Management

The management is surgical evacuation provided that the patient's clinical condition warrants it. A patient who is found to have a haematoma but is clinically improving can be managed conservatively. Otherwise a craniotomy needs to be performed.

An acute extradural or subdural intracranial haematoma is solid and therefore has to be removed by craniotomy, usually by a neurosurgeon. Skilled anaesthesia is mandatory. Frusemide or mannitol is given while theatre is being prepared.

In the rare event of a patient being taken to theatre on clinical grounds only, exploratory burr holes are performed to decompress the cranium. In determining which side burr holes should be done, the site of a skull fracture or the side of the first dilated pupil are of more significance than localization by observed limb weakness.

OPERATION: CRANIAL BURR HOLES

The burr hole is situated either next to the fracture or at a point 5 cm up from the mid-point of a line drawn between the external auditory meatus and lateral angle of the eye. A linear incision is made in a direction that can be converted into a scalp flap if a craniotomy is to be performed. The temporalis is divided and a burr hole drilled. If a haematoma is found, it is evacuated. If necessary the burr hole may be enlarged (craniectomy) to find and control the bleeding vessel. This is usually beneath the fracture. It is then acceptable to place a swab in the wound and transfer the patient to the local neurosurgical centre. If the wound is closed, the dura must be stitched up to the pericranium around the craniectomy edge to prevent reaccumulation.

If no haematoma is found, other burr holes may be made as appropriate. If haematoma is excluded on each side, the deterioration must be assumed to be due to brain swelling.

Codes

Blood	2 units
GA/LA	GA
Opn time	1 h
Stay	Variable, depends on other injuries
Drains out	0
Sutures out	7 days
Off work	Variable

Postoperative care

The long-term management of head injuries is multidisciplinary. Complications such as epilepsy, chronic subdural haematoma, external hydrocephalus and infection may occur.

Skull fracture

A skull fracture can be closed (simple) or open (compound). An open fracture is one where there is an associated scalp injury, rendering the fracture site open to the atmosphere, with the secondary risk of meningitis or abscess formation. Fractures that run into the nose or middle ear are also regarded as open.

A fracture may also be undisplaced (a linear or fissured fracture) or depressed. A depressed fracture will cause local injury and loss of function depending on its site. The site and the presence of dural penetration determine the treatment required.

Making the diagnosis

This is made on the X-ray and the appearances can be difficult to interpret. A linear fracture is characteristically thinner and darker and has a more angular course than the vascular markings. It is straighter and more defined than the cranial suture lines. On inspecting the skull X-ray, it is important to look for a depression in the fracture, or any evidence of dural penetration (which appears as spicules of bone at right angles to the plane of the vault of the skull). Look carefully at the region at the base of the skull, as it is easy to miss fractures there. Also inspect the outlines of the orbit carefully and compare the appearance with that on the opposite side. CT scanning is indicated in a patient whose fracture is depressed or who has confusion, neurological signs or a fit.

Management

A closed lineal fracture requires no additional management, other than that already described for head injuries. The patient is admitted and regular observations are carried out.

An open linear fracture requires surgical treatment. The wound must be thoroughly cleaned and the fracture inspected. If hair is present, it must be removed, if necessary by craniectomy. Broad-spectrum antibiotics are given (e.g. Cefuroxime 1.5 g i.v.). If there is CSF leakage, the patient remains in hospital until it stops. If the leak persists more then 1 week, surgical repair of the defect may be necessary.

A closed depressed fracture is managed conservatively unless there is evidence of dural penetration or the fracture is overlying an important area of function, e.g. the speech or motor cortex. In this case surgery is indicated. The depressed fracture is elevated and any fragments of bone or damaged brain removed.

An open depressed fracture requires urgent operation to clean the area and remove any dirty bone, fragmented dura or damaged brain. The wound can be closed and skull reconstruction may be carried out at a later date. Antibiotics are required as above.

15.3   Chest and Abdominal Injury

Chest trauma

With any chest injury there is a danger that respiration may be compromised. You should also consider whether there has been associated injury to the underlying pleura, lungs or mediastinal structures including the heart.

Injuries to the chest involve one or more of the following.

1 Chest wall:
(a) fractured ribs (p. 646)
(b) flail chest (p. 647)
(c) fractured sternum (p. 648).
2 Pleura:
(a) pneumothorax (p. 649)
(b) tension pneumothorax (p. 650)
(c) traumatic haemothorax (p. 650).
3 Lung:
(a) pulmonary contusion (p. 651)
(b) pulmonary laceration (p. 651).
4 Mediastinal structures:
(a) ruptured thoracic aorta (p. 652)
(b) ruptured bronchus (p. 652)
(c) ruptured diaphragm (p. 652)
(d) blunt injury to the heart (p. 653)
(e) haematopericardium (p. 654).
5 Penetrating injuries: bullet and stab wounds to the chest (p. 654).

Fractured ribs

Ribs are usually fractured as a result of a direct blow to the chest or a crushing injury. The fractures may be single or multiple and simple or compound. Pneumothorax may occur either due to a compound fracture with air entering through the wound or due to perforation of the underlying lung by a fractured rib.

Recognizing the pattern

The patient complains of severe, localized, pleuritic pain and difficulty in breathing. The latter may either be due to inability to take a deep breath because of pain, or secondary to a pneumothorax.

On examination the characteristic sign is of extreme tenderness at one point along the rib. There may also be bruising or laceration at the site of the injury. Remember to look for signs of an associated pneumothorax.

Proving the diagnosis

The diagnosis is clinical. The fracture may not be seen on a chest X-ray. You must exclude a pneumothorax.

Management

Analgesia

Analgesia must be adequate to allow effective respiration. This is especially important in the elderly and debilitated who are likely to develop an underlying hypostatic pneumonia. Intercostal Marcain nerve blocks are very useful but need to be repeated every 6 h or so. Non-steroidal anti-inflammatory agents such as diclofenac are particularly useful as they do not cause respiratory depression.

Breathing

The patient is given breathing exercises and physiotherapy.

Strapping

Opinions differ about the value of strapping. This is effective in relieving the pain but it does also further restrict normal chest expansion.

Flail chest

A flail chest develops when the chest wall has lost its mechanical rigidity due to multiple fractures. One segment of the rib cage becomes separated from its surroundings and can move paradoxically (i.e. inwards on inspiration, outwards on expiration). This results in inadequate ventilation of the lung and retention of pulmonary secretions. There is associated pulmonary contusion. A dangerous vicious circle ensues in which the lung becomes increasingly oedematous, the patient more and more anoxic and respiratory movements increasingly active. This further exacerbates the paradoxical movement, and progressive anoxia ensues.

Recognizing the pattern

The patient has signs of fractured ribs. Initially respiration may be satisfactory but after 24–48 h there is increasing dyspnoea and the patient becomes more and more distressed. On inspection the flail segment will be seen to move paradoxically.

Proving the diagnosis

The diagnosis is confirmed on chest X-ray. Blood gas estimations are of value and show a low PO_2 (partial pressure of oxygen) and an elevated PCO_2.

Management

The patient should be sat up and given oxygen. As a temporary measure the flail segment can be supported with strapping. Strong analgesia will be required in all cases and is best given either as intercostal blocks or as a thoracic epidural anaesthetic. The patient is observed carefully and, if the respiratory rate begins to climb, further action may be required. Serial blood gas estimations are also used to monitor progress. In severe cases intermittent positive pressure ventilation is needed. A tracheostomy reduces the dead space and facilitates good tracheobronchial toilet. If the flail segment is depressed (stove-in chest), it will require elevation.

Fractured sternum

This is a rare injury. It commonly follows road traffic accidents where there is a forceful impact against the seat belt, steering wheel or dashboard.

Recognizing the pattern

The patient complains of pain over the sternum and is usually breathless. The pattern of bruising from the seat belt may be seen. On examination the sternum is very tender and there may be a palpable step or deformity. Pulmonary complications are rare, but there may be associated damage to the trachea, great vessels or heart. Do a chest X-ray and ECG.

Management

The patient is treated with strong analgesia (e.g. pethidine) to allow chest expansion. If there is severe displacement with a reduction in the anteroposterior diameter of the chest, the depressed segment is pulled forward at open operation and fixed with wires. Cardiac monitoring is vital.

Traumatic pneumothorax

Air may get into the pleura either through a deep wound or through damage to the lung following a penetrating wound or rib fracture. There is frequently an associated haemothorax. If the air leak is valvular, a tension pneumothorax develops (see below).

Recognizing the pattern

Apart from the pain of the original injury, the patient complains of breathlessness and pleuritic pain. On examination the affected side of the chest is not moving and the percussion note is hyper-resonant. The breath sounds are decreased on that side and there may be tracheal displacement towards the uninjured lung if tension is developing.

Proving the diagnosis

This is confirmed on chest X-ray. The absence of lung markings in the periphery of the pleural space is noted, as is the edge of the lung.

Management

Because of the risk of tension, a traumatic pneumothorax must be drained with a large intercostal drain attached to an underwater seal. The insertion and management of a chest drain is described on pp. 253–257.

If the lung has failed to re-expand, suction should be applied to the drain (75–100 mmHg). When the lung has re-expanded (as shown by lack of bubbling from the chest drain on coughing, and confirmed by chest X-ray), the tube is clamped for 12–24 h. Once the lung has remained inflated, the tube may be withdrawn. If the tube continues to bubble even after the lung has re-expanded, there is probably a tear in the lung. This usually seals off after a few days but, if the tear is major or involves the bronchus, a thoracotomy may eventually be necessary. A small pneumothorax may go unnoticed and only become apparent when it rapidly develops into a tension pneumothorax when the patient is ventilated.

Tension pneumothorax

A tension pneumothorax develops when there is a one-way valvular leak of air into the pleural cavity. Air rapidly accumulates, compressing the lung, and urgent treatment is required. Severe respiratory embarrassment develops and death can ensue due to kinking of the great veins secondary to mediastinal displacement.

Recognizing the pattern

A breathless patient with the clinical features of a pneumothorax becomes progressively worse with increasing dyspnoea and evidence of increasing mediastinal shift. Tracheal displacement only occurs if tension is developing. The patient is very distressed. There may be associated surgical emphysema of the chest wall, neck and face. It is the steady deterioration in symptoms which suggests the diagnosis. Impaired venous return causes a tachycardia and hypotension. The deterioration can occur very rapidly.

Proving the diagnosis and management

The presence of tension is confirmed by inserting a chest drain as below. No time should be wasted in wondering whether there is tension pneumothorax or not. If this is a possibility, a chest drain should be inserted urgently. In difficult circumstances, a simple needle straight into the pleural cavity will suffice. The rush of air under pressure confirms the diagnosis. Once the tension has been released, normal chest drainage connected to an underwater seal can be established. The presence of a pneumothorax and the position of the drain is confirmed by urgent portable chest X-ray.

Traumatic haemothorax

An accumulation of blood in the pleural cavity can occur from injury to the muscles in the chest wall, lung, heart or great vessels. There may also be a pneumothorax.

Recognizing the pattern

The presence of blood is irritant and causes pleuritic pain and breathlessness. The patient may be shocked. On examination there are signs of a pleural effusion with lack of breath sounds and a dull percussion note at the lung base.

Proving the diagnosis

The blood in the pleural cavity is seen on chest X-ray and confirmed on tapping the chest.

Management

After resuscitation and cross-match immediate drainage is required. An underwater seal is used and the level of the water in the bottle is marked so that the blood loss can be measured. Further management is usually conservative until the bleeding stops. However, if more than 1500 mLs is removed or if the rate of bleeding is more than 200 mL/h, a thoracotomy may be required.

Pulmonary contusion or laceration

This is bruising, and oedema of the lung beneath chest wall trauma. There may or may not be an associated rib fracture. The injury to the lung has a severe effect on respiration. There may also be an associated pulmonary laceration with blood or air in the pleural cavity.

Recognizing the pattern

The patient is breathless, apprehensive and cyanosed and coughing produces sputum tinged with blood.

Proving the diagnosis

A chest X-ray shows a progression from a patchy diffuse opacity in the lung fields (12–24 h after injury) to a complete 'white out'. Blood gases show hypoxia and hypercapnia.

Management

It is important to keep the patient relatively dehydrated and diuretics may be helpful. Intravenous fluid therapy must be carefully regulated to avoid overtransfusion. Oxygen, adequate analgesia and physiotherapy will help, but the patient may eventually need ventilating.

Closed chest injury

Closed chest injuries are often caused by shearing forces generated during extreme deceleration. The following will be considered:

1 Rupture of the thoracic aorta
2 Rupture of the bronchi
3 Rupture of the diaphragm.

Rupture of the thoracic aorta

Rupture of the ascending thoracic aorta is usually fatal. Rupture of the descending aorta usually involves the intima and media only, resulting in a large periaortic haematoma.

Recognizing the pattern

The patient complains of severe central chest pain. The diagnosis is made by noting widening of the mediastinum on a chest X-ray and it is important to be aware of this potentially lethal condition. Where there is doubt a repeat chest X-ray may show progressive widening.

Management
After control of blood pressure, urgent operation is required. Under cardiopulmonary bypass repair or replacement of the aorta by a Dacron graft is undertaken.

Rupture of the bronchi

This commonly occurs distal to the carina as the bronchus leaves the support of the mediastinum. There is a large escape of air causing bilateral pneumothoraces and mediastinal emphysema. There may be haemoptysis.

Recognizing the pattern

The patient is acutely dyspnoeic and shocked, and surgical emphysema may be felt in the neck.

Proving the diagnosis

This is confirmed on chest X-ray and on bronchoscopy.

Management
Immediate operative repair is required which will restore lung function. Any significant delay will result in infection around the bronchial wound and later stricture formation.

Rupture of the diaphragm

This occurs after a crush injury to the abdomen. The diaphragm usually tears on the dome from front to back adjacent to the pericardium. There may be herniation of the stomach or other organs through the rent. The stomach may distend, collapsing the lung and shifting the mediastinum. Occasionally it becomes strangulated.

Recognizing the pattern

The patient presents with increasing respiratory difficulty following an abdominal injury.

Proving the diagnosis

The chest X-ray may show a raised hemi-diaphragm and, if the left side is involved, a stomach bubble may be visible in the chest. If a nasogastric tube has been passed, it will be seen to lie in the chest. A decubitus film will also show a horizontal fluid level in the chest. A barium swallow is useful.

Management

Following resuscitation and passage of a nasogastric tube, surgical repair is required urgently. If there is no other thoracic injury requiring operation, the diaphragm may be exposed from below through the abdomen. This decreases the incidence of pulmonary complications postoperatively and allows the surgeon to check that the spleen is not damaged.

Blunt injury to the heart

Blunt injury to the heart may cause contusion of the myocardium with necrosis of muscle fibres. Dysrhythmia or heart failure may follow. Occasionally there may be rupture of the papillary muscles or interventricular septum. The thin walls of the atria and right ventricle may burst, causing cardiac tamponade (see below). Cardiac concussion is a condition where there may be dysrhythmia in the absence of myocardial necrosis.

Recognizing the pattern

The patient may present with a dysrhythmia, heart failure or cardiac tamponade following a blow on the chest. There may be a pericardial friction rub on examination.

Proving the diagnosis

The electrocardiogram (ECG) may show changes typical of infarction if there is a large area of cardiac contusion. Cardiac-specific enzymes (e.g. the cardiac isoenzyme of creatinine phosphokinase) are elevated.

Management

It is most important to be aware of the possibility of a cardiac injury. The patients most at risk from complications are those with ECG changes, particularly if other major injuries are present.

The patient must be put on an ECG monitor. Care must be taken during intravenous infusion not to overload the circulation. Measurement of the central venous pressure or intracardiac pressure may be useful. The patient should be examined frequently with particular care taken to auscultate the heart. A cardiothoracic surgeon should be warned about the case if it is severe and transfer considered.

Haemopericardium

The pericardial cavity fills with blood following a penetrating injury to the heart (e.g. stab wound) or following blunt trauma with rupture of the walls of the atria or right ventricle. The outer fibrous pericardium limits distension of the pericardial sac, and blood in the cavity therefore prevents ventricular filling, resulting in cardiac tamponade with decreased cardiac output, hypotension, cyanosis and elevated jugular venous pressure. The heart sounds are quiet on auscultation.

Proving the diagnosis

This is a life-threatening condition. Aspiration of the pericardial cavity with a needle inserted just under the seventh costal cartilage and to the left of the xiphoid process proves the diagnosis and provides temporary relief.

Management

The pericardial cavity is opened through either an anterolateral thoracotomy or a sternotomy, and the defect repaired.

Bullet and stab wounds to the chest

Any penetrating injury to the chest may cause serious complications but the most dangerous are those that occur within the mid-clavicular lines and between the jaw and xiphisternum. These need careful surgical exploration because of the risk to internal organs. The pleura, subcostal vessels, lung, heart, great vessels and main airways may all be involved. Remember that a low or angulated penetrating wound in the chest may have perforated the diaphragm and injured abdominal viscera, especially the liver, stomach and spleen.

Management

Preoperatively a chest and abdominal X-ray must be taken to look for any missiles. Six to 10 units of blood are cross-matched but the laboratory is warned that more may be needed urgently later. If a cardiothoracic surgeon is available, his help should be obtained. Set up at least two good intravenous infusion lines, a central venous pressure line to prevent overtransfusion and chest drainage if necessary.

OPERATION: EXPLORATORY THORACOTOMY
FOR PENETRATING CHEST INJURY
The wound is excised and all dirt, rib fragments and debris are removed either through the same wound or through a separate thoracotomy. The pleural cavity is explored and any pulmonary lacerations repaired. Any other damage is treated as necessary.

Codes

Blood	6–10 units
GA/LA	GA
Opn time	2–3 h
Stay	About 7 days but variable
Drains out	Chest drain 3–4 days
Sutures out	7–10 days
Off work	Variable

Postoperative care
The postoperative care following thoracotomy is described in section 6.1.

Abdominal trauma

Abdominal trauma may be due to penetrating or blunt injuries. Different problems arise in these two categories.

Penetrating injuries to the abdomen

These include the following:

1 Stab wounds
2 Gunshot wounds
3 Penetration by other foreign bodies.

The patient complains of abdominal pain and may be shocked with signs of peritonism.

Management
All penetrating injuries of the abdomen should be explored after the patient has been resuscitated. The laparotomy is undertaken to exclude damage to any hollow viscus which may result in fluid leakage and peritonitis, and also to stop any haemorrhage. The entrance wound is excised and a full laparotomy is performed.

Blunt injury to the abdomen

The external visible damage may be minimal but the internal injuries serious. There may also be delay between a causative injury and the appearance of signs of damage. Finally, the internal injury may be at a different site from the site of the original trauma. The internal injuries to be considered are the following:

1 Ruptured liver
2 Ruptured spleen
3 Traumatic bowel injury
4 Pancreatic injury
5 Renal injury.

Ruptured liver

In blunt abdominal trauma the liver is usually injured by rapid compression and decompression. This tends to produce a ragged tear in its substance. The condition must be suspected in any case of multiple trauma or abdominal injury. This is especially true if there are external marks on the abdomen or if the patient is shocked with no obvious sign of blood loss.

Recognizing the pattern

The conscious patient may complain of abdominal pain situated in the right upper quadrant. The pain is worse on breathing. On examination he will be shocked (pale, sweaty, anxious, with a tachycardia and sighing respiration). The abdomen may exhibit localized tenderness and rigidity in the right upper quadrant. There may also be more generalized tenderness due to a haemoperitoneum. The abdomen is distended.

Proving the diagnosis

Peritoneal lavage will show blood in the peritoneal cavity. The urinary bladder is emptied by a catheter. This also allows the urine output to be monitored. A cannula is then introduced into the peritoneal cavity and saline injected. This is moved around by gently rolling the patient and then reaspirated.

Management

The patient is resuscitated. There is some controversy as to the best course to pursue in this dangerous condition. Some favour initial conservative management in which the patient's condition is very carefully monitored in the hope that, as pressure rises within the abdominal cavity internal tamponade may occur and the bleeding cease. If such management its pursued and the patient's condition continues to deteriorate, urgent laparotomy is required.

Others proceed more rapidly to laparotomy. Fatalities can occur, however, as the patient is anaesthetized and especially when the abdomen is opened and the tamponading pressure is released.

OPERATION: LAPAROTOMY FOR RUPTURED LIVER

The abdomen is opened and the abdominal viscera inspected. If a hepatic tear is confirmed, one of the following procedures is carried out:

1 The tear is sutured
2 The affected part of the liver is excised (partial hepatectomy; see p. 352)
3 The liver is packed to control bleeding. Such packs can be left in place for a few days and then removed at a second laparotomy.

The danger of wide exploration of hepatic tears is that they may extend into the cava. If such a tear is explored at open laparotomy, death from air embolus is common. Elevation of the legs and positive-pressure ventilation can help direct such air embolism into the lower body.

Codes

Blood	10 units
GA/LA	GA
Opn time	Variable, 2–3 h
Stay	14 days but depends on other injuries
Drains out	2–7 days
Sutures out	7 days
Off work	2–3 months

Postoperative care

If the hepatic wound has been successfully sutured or if a partial hepatectomy is performed, the postoperative course

Continued on p. 658

Continued.

should be reasonably straightforward, depending on the other injuries.

If a pack has been inserted, this will need to be removed after about 48 h. In the interim the urea and electrolytes, platelets and clotting screen must be measured frequently.

If there is a large haematoma within the liver substance, the progress of this haematoma can be monitored using repeat radioisotope liver scans.

Ruptured spleen

Splenic rupture may occur as part of an abdominal compression injury or due to a localized blow over the left lower ribs. Rupture may follow trivial injury if the spleen is already enlarged, e.g. due to malaria. Occasionally an injury is sufficient to bruise the spleen but not to rupture the capsule. The haematoma thus formed may rupture after 7–10 days (delayed rupture of the spleen).

Recognizing the pattern

There is pain in the left upper quadrant together with localized tenderness and guarding. The tenderness may be more marked on inspiration. Not infrequently there is an associated fracture of the left lower ribs. The patient also complains of pain in the left shoulder tip (Kehr's sign) and both flanks may be dull to percussion with the right flank exhibiting shifting dullness (Ballance's sign).

Proving the diagnosis

The diagnosis of intraperitoneal bleeding can be confirmed by peritoneal lavage. A straight X-ray of the abdomen may show an elevation of the left hemi-diaphragm and a diffuse splenic shadow with displacement of the gastric air bubble. An ultrasound or CT scan can be very helpful in detecting a splenic haematoma.

Management

The patient is resuscitated. Continued pain, shock and abdominal distension will indicate the urgent need for laparotomy.

OPERATION: LAPAROTOMY FOR SPLENIC INJURY

The abdomen is opened and blood evacuated. If possible the damaged spleen should be repaired but it is often safer to proceed to splenectomy. The spleen may be repaired by one of the following methods:

1 Direct suture of a laceration over a haemostatic material such as Surgicel.

2 Partial splenectomy. The feeding vessels of the damaged area are ligated, the damaged area excised and the cut organ repaired.

If these procedures are not possible, a splenectomy is performed. The bleeding is controlled by grasping the splenic pedicle between the fingers of one hand. The splenic artery, splenic vein and short gastric arteries are ligated and the spleen is removed. Care is taken not to damage the tail of the pancreas, the fundus of the stomach or the splenic flexure of the colon. A drain is left in the splenic bed.

Codes

Blood	6 units
GA/LA	GA
Opn time	60–90 min
Stay	7–10 days
Drains out	3–7 days
Sutures out	7 days
Off work	About 1 month

These figures will be prolonged by associated injury.

Postoperative care
See under splenectomy (p. 369).

Traumatic bowel injury

The bowel may be damaged either by direct injury or indirectly due to damage of its feeding vessels. In the latter case there is risk of rupture some days after the initial injury. Such injuries occur in road traffic accidents when the bowel is crushed against the spine by a seat belt.

Recognizing the pattern

The patient with a bowel injury may have minimal signs at first and the condition may not be suspected in view of other injuries. If the patient deteriorates with increasing abdominal pain and distension after 2–3 days, think of this possibility.

Proving the diagnosis

The diagnosis is confirmed by an X-ray which shows free peritoneal gas. Aspiration of the abdomen produces bile-stained bowel contents.

Management

Ideally this is by early laparotomy and repair or resection of the damaged area together with careful exploration to exclude other abdominal trauma. In cases of multiple trauma it is permissible to leave the bowel injury for 24 h or so while life-threatening injuries are dealt with.

OPERATION: SMALL BOWEL RESECTION
The damaged bowel is resected and an end-to-end anastomosis performed.

Codes

Blood	2 units or more depending on extent of injuries
GA/LA	GA
Opn time	90–120 min
Stay	7 days
Drains out	Wound 48 h; intra-abdominal 2–3 days
Sutures out	7 days
Off work	4–6 weeks

Postoperative care
A nasogastric tube is aspirated regularly and the patient is kept on minimal oral fluids until flatus is passed. Anastomotic problems are rare.

Pancreatic injury

The pancreas may also be damaged by a crushing injury from a seat belt or steering wheel. There is a high amylase content in the peritoneal aspirate and the serum amylase may also be elevated. The diagnosis must be excluded by laparotomy.

Management

The pancreas is explored and sutured or partially resected. The lesser sac and pancreatic bed are drained.

Renal injury

The kidneys may be damaged by blunt injury to the loins or by compression from the front. The injury may then be extraperitoneal although in children the peritoneum is more likely to be breached as there is little perinephric fat. The renal damage may be anything from a subcapsular haematoma to a complete tear. Occasionally the renal vessels are avulsed.

Recognizing the pattern

The patient is shocked and there is tenderness in the loin. Haematuria occurs but may be delayed. There may also be clot colic. On examination fullness in the loin may indicate a perinephric haematoma.

Proving the diagnosis

An IVP should be done urgently to demonstrate whether the damaged kidney is functioning or not and whether there is a normal kidney on the other side. CT with contrast will also show this and demonstrate a haematoma. Renal artery angiography is occasionally useful.

Management

Having excluded other abdominal trauma, the initial treatment is conservative, comprising bed rest and analgesia. If there has been extravasation of urine, antibiotics such as ampicillin (500 mg 6-hourly) or co-trimoxazole (2 tablets 12-hourly) may be given. Laparotomy is indicated if there is continued uncontrolled bleeding.

OPERATION: LAPAROTOMY FOR RENAL INJURY

If possible, the damaged kidney is repaired, although a partial or complete nephrectomy is often required. A full laparotomy is undertaken to exclude other intra-abdominal injury.

Codes

Blood .... 6 units
GA/LA .... GA
Opn time .... 1–2 h
Stay .... Depends on other injuries
Drains out .... 3 days, kidney bed
Sutures out .... 7–10 days
Off work .... Depends on other injuries

Postoperative care

A severe ileus may occur which may need treatment with a nasogastric tube and intravenous fluids. The long-term follow-up should include a repeat IVP after 3 months to check on renal function.

15.4   Spinal and Pelvic Injuries

Fractured spine

The importance of spinal injury lies in the danger of associated trauma to the spinal cord or nerve roots. Injury is more common in the cervical or lumbar region because the vertebrae are relatively unsupported.

A stable spinal fracture will not displace further and there is no continuing danger to the spinal cord. With an unstable fracture abnormal movement can encroach on the vertebral canal with resulting spinal cord damage.

At the scene of the accident, before the patient is moved, a cervical collar should be applied and any movement of the spine kept to an absolute minimum with the patient placed on a spinal board.

Do not move the patient except 'as a log' until an unstable fracture has been excluded.

Recognizing the pattern

Always consider the possibility of spinal injury when a patient has suffered severe trauma.

The patient complains of severe localized pain at the site of the fracture, which may radiate along the distribution of the relevant nerve roots. The patient lies still and the pain is worse on any movement. Ask if there is any numbness, tingling or weakness in the limbs.

On examination there may be visible deformity of the spine. Palpation of the vertebral spine may reveal discontinuity or displacement, and localized tenderness.

Tenderness on one side of the midline suggests muscular or ligamentous injury or damaged transverse processes.

If the cord has been damaged, you may find abnormalities in sensation, movement and reflexes in the limbs. In cervical injuries there may be abnormalities in the pulse, blood pressure and respiration.

Proving the diagnosis

Spinal X-rays must be done in any case of possible spinal injury. Anteroposterior and lateral views are usually taken. There are other specialist views for the odontoid peg or lumbar pedicles. A qualified doctor should be present to supervise the movement of the patient.

When inspecting X-rays check for the following:

1 Ensure that all seven cervical vertebrae can be seen and in addition the C7–T1 junction is clearly seen. Sometimes special views are necessary to demonstrate this.

2 Symmetry between the two sides.

3 Any incongruities in the width of the vertebral bodies.

4 Any incongruities of the joint spaces.

5 On the lateral view look for a step in the posterior or anterior longitudinal ligament disclosing displacement of a vertebra. Loss of this alignment and widening of the gap between the spines are typical of an unstable fracture.

6 Look carefully for evidence of injury to the bones themselves.

CT scanning now provides an alternative to straight X-rays for radiologically inaccessible parts of the vertebral column (e.g. C7–T1 junction, thoracic vertebrae, etc.).

Management

The patient can be rolled but the head, trunk and pelvis are supported so that there is no relative movement of one vertebra on another. Support the patient between sandbags. In a case of a suspected cervical fracture, the head must be held still in slight extension and kept in a straight line with the body axis.

With muscular bruising or a fractured transverse process, the patient may be allowed home, given analgesics and advised to rest on a firm mattress for 7–10 days. Admission may be required if the pain is severe or movement severely restricted.

If there is a stable vertebral fracture, the patient is admitted, given analgesics and put on a bed with a rigid base. The patient is X-rayed again 2 or 3 weeks later and then mobilized slowly.

In the case of an unstable fracture consider transferring the patient to a spinal centre. External support is needed, and active reduction may be required. Skeletal traction with skull calipers is used for unstable cervical fractures. Alternatively, vertebrae may be reduced and fused by open operation.

When there is damage to the spinal cord, attention must be paid to the paralysed limbs to prevent contractures or pressure sores. There may be an ileus for 3 or 4 days. A cervical cord injury may mask symptoms due to other abdominal trauma. Bladder and bowel function may need assistance.

Fractured pelvis

A fractured pelvis must always be considered and excluded after multiple trauma. External evidence of pelvic fracture may be slight but the blood loss can be considerable (e.g. 2 L) and there is a possibility of associated visceral injury to the urethra, bladder or rectum.

Recognizing the pattern

The patient may complain of back pain, particularly if the sacroiliac joints are involved. Movements are painful. On examination there is pain on compressing the pelvis and deformity may be visible.

Proving the diagnosis

The fracture is seen on pelvic X-ray.

Management

A careful examination should be made of both legs, particularly of the arterial and nerve supply. A rectal examination should be performed. Ask about bleeding from the urethra or micturition problems, which may indicate associated visceral damage.

The patient may be shocked and require initial transfusion. At least 4 units of blood should be cross-matched and a good intravenous infusion line set up.

A stable pelvic fracture can be treated conservatively with bed rest, analgesia and lower limb exercises. The patient is mobilized as the improvement in pain permits.

A pelvis fractured in more than two places results in disruption of the pelvic ring and an unstable pelvic fracture. An unstable pelvic fracture may result in severe blood loss and is a potentially life-threatening condition. Such fractures are usually treated initially by external fixation and consideration is given later to planned internal fixation.

Other pelvic injuries

Damage to the urethra

The urethra may be partially or completely torn. The two sites commonly affected are the membranous urethra at the apex of the prostate (following bilateral fracture of the pubic rami) or the bulbous urethra (following a blow in the perineum).

Recognizing the pattern

There is a history of inability to pass urine, meatal bleeding and a distended bladder. A high-riding, mobile prostate on rectal examination suggests a complete membranous urethral tear. When the bulbous urethra is ruptured, a tense perineal haematoma or a swollen, bruised penis and scrotum are seen. Urethral injury should always be suspected following pelvic fracture.

Proving the diagnosis

If the patient is conscious and can spontaneously pass urine, this is tested for the presence of blood. If the patient is unconscious or cannot pass urine a urethrogram is performed before a cautious attempt to pass a small catheter is attempted. An intravenous urogram should also be performed.

Management

1 Resuscitation of the patient is the first priority. The urethral repair can wait 12–24 h if necessary.
2 Antibiotics must be started.
3 If catheterization was not attempted, or was unsuccessful, urine is drained through a suprapubic cystostomy.
4 A ruptured membranous urethra is usually repaired around a catheter which is used as a splint. A ruptured bulbous urethra can be repaired or may be treated conservatively, in which case it should be reassessed at 10–14 days.

If there is associated rectal damage, the definitive repair is delayed until any infection has been treated.

Any collection in the retropubic space, such as extravasated blood or urine, is drained.

Stricture is a common sequel to any urethral trauma, and a follow-up urethrogram or urethroscopy is required. The treatment of stricture is described on p. 483.

Trauma to the bladder

There are two mechanisms of bladder injury. A direct blow to the lower abdomen, when the bladder is distended, causes the viscus to burst with leakage of urine into the peritoneum. A fractured or dislocated symphysis pubis may also pierce the bladder causing extraperitoneal leakage.

When there is extraperitoneal leakage, the patient may have a strong desire to void urine but is unable to do so. Intraperitoneal leakage causes very few symptoms other than anuria, and the diagnosis may be missed, particularly in a trauma victim, where the anuria may be attributed to shock.

Proving the diagnosis
The diagnosis is proved by an intravenous urogram or urethrogram. This should be done if there is any suspicion of bladder injury.

Management
Antibiotics should be commenced. Urgent laparotomy and repair are required. The urethra is catheterized at operation and the peritoneal and extraperitoneal spaces are drained.

A follow-up urethroscopy must be done. Twenty per cent of patients have accompanying urethral damage and there is a risk of stricture formation.

Injuries to the rectum
These are rare. The damage is usually caused by a crushing or burst injury to the pelvis.

Recognizing the pattern
The patient may have bleeding from the anus and shows signs of a pelvic peritonitis. Rectal examination shows blood.

Management
The treatment is laparotomy, a defunctioning colostomy and washout of the bowel. The tear is repaired at a later date.

Damage to blood vessels

Management
The internal or external iliac artery can be damaged but more commonly there is damage to the pelvic venous plexus. These injuries are associated with profuse blood loss and are a surgical emergency. They should be treated by blood transfusion (cross-match 6–10 units), and stabilization of the pelvis by external fixation to encourage tamponade. If these measures fail embolization of the affected vessels may be required.

Nervous injury

The sciatic nerve may be damaged by a traction force or posterior dislocation of the hip. This is usually neuropraxia or axonotmesis (see p. 675) with eventual recovery. Severe disruption of the sacroiliac joints can cause a nerve root injury where the damage is permanent.

Recognizing the pattern

The presenting sign is of foot drop. There is a partial or complete loss of sensation down the leg, apart from the medial surface which is supplied by the long saphenous nerve (a branch of the femoral nerve).

Management

Neuropraxia or axonotmesis should eventually recover. Meanwhile, physiotherapy to the limb maintains the mobility and prevents any contracture deformity. The nerve must be explored if it is thought likely that it is severed, but this is unusual.

Injury to the hip joint

Fractures involving disruption of the acetabulum may later result in osteoarthritis. This risk is lessened if an accurate reduction of the fracture is achieved.

15.5 Trauma to the Skin and Limbs

Management of wounds

The management of skin wounds depends on whether they are clean or contaminated and whether the skin edges are intact (incisional wound) or damaged (crushed or torn wound). There may also be skin loss. The aim is to heal the wound as perfectly as possible and prevent secondary infection by pyogenic bacteria or organisms causing gas gangrene and tetanus.

Assessment

Ask the patient how it happened and how long ago. Is it known to be clean or dirty? Could there be any foreign body in the wound? Ask if the patient has been immunized against tetanus, and if so when the last injection of tetanus toxoid was given. (Tetanus prophylaxis is dealt with on p. 670.) Examine the wound edges and look for evidence of contamination or infection. Examine closely for any injury to underlying arteries, nerves or tendons, especially in the hand.

Management

All wounds are carefully cleaned and debrided, removing dead tissue and foreign matter. Haemostasis is secured. Further management depends on the age of the wound and whether it is contaminated or not.

History of less than 8 h

A clean or lightly contaminated wound is then closed in layers by primary suture. If the skin defect cannot be closed, the area may be covered by a split-skin graft (see below). Antibiotics (amoxycillin and flucloxacillin) are given if the wound is lightly contaminated rather than clean.

A heavily contaminated wound is then left open and dressed. Antibiotics are given as above. It is then re-examined in 3–5 days and if no infection is present the edges are cleaned and the wound closed by delayed primary suture.

History of more than 8 h

A clean wound cannot be closed as it must be assumed that any potential infection has become established. It should be either treated with delayed primary suture, or closed with drainage, and antibiotic cover given.

A heavily contaminated or infected wound is thoroughly debrided and dressed. It is redressed daily after cleaning with further debridement and saline or chlorhexidine irrigation until the inflection has cleared. Then, when the wound is clean, the granulation tissue is removed, the skin edges freshened and the wound closed by secondary suture. Skin defects are closed by split-skin grafts.

OPERATION: SIMPLE SUTURE OF A SKIN WOUND

The skin is cleaned with a suitable agent (e.g. chlorhexidine, cetrimide or povidone iodine). The area is draped off and local anaesthetic is injected around the edges of the wound, using a puncture site outside the wound. The skin edges are debrided of all dead and contaminated tissue. The wound edges are then opposed, using interrupted nylon sutures. In the head and neck multiple small sutures are used so as to minimize 'cross-hatching' in the scar later.

Codes

Blood	0
GA/LA	LA
Opn time	30–60 min
Stay	Variable
Drains out	3–5 days
Sutures out	Head and neck 3–4 days; elsewhere 5–7 days; if the wound is under tension 10–14 days
Off work	Variable

OPERATION: SPLIT-SKIN GRAFT

Donor sites are usually the upper arm or thigh and a graft may be taken using a special knife, under a local or general anaesthetic. It is important to learn how to do this by observing and assisting an experienced surgeon. The donor site is dressed with tulle gras and left for 10 days. The split-skin graft is placed raw face uppermost on tulle gras and then cut to size. Haemostasis in the recipient area is important to prevent blood from lifting the graft. If a mesh graft is used, a larger area can be covered and any haematoma can escape through the holes in the graft. The graft is applied and sutured at the edges with silk, one end of each stitch being left long enough to tie over a sponge or pad soaked in antiseptic lotion.

Codes

Blood 0

GA/LA .... GA or LA

Opn time .... 30 min to 2 h depending on size of graft

Stay .... 7–10 days depending on size of graft

Drains out 0

Sutures out .... 7–10 days

Off work .... Variable

Postoperative care

The top ties are divided and the tulle gras and sponge removed at between 5 and 7 days. The graft can then be inspected and if healing is satisfactory the rest of the sutures are removed.

Tetanus prophylaxis

Tetanus is a disease characterized by muscle spasm caused by the toxin of *Clostridium tetani*, a Gram-positive, anaerobic, sporing bacillus. The spores appear in animal faeces and therefore contaminate earth. Extensive wounds with heavy contamination are typically affected, although tetanus can follow small penetrating injuries. Active immunization with toxoid is now a routine part of the triple vaccine given to children. A booster dose should be given every 10 years. The organism is sensitive to penicillin, metronidazole or tetracycline.

A high-risk wound is one that is heavily contaminated, deep, more than 8 h old and contains dead tissue.

Management

Surgical debridement and toilet must be performed for all wounds.

The type of tetanus prophylaxis given depends on the nature and age of the wound and the immune category of the patient. The measures available include the following:

(a) a booster dose of tetanus toxoid

(b) a complete course of tetanus toxoid

(c) penicillin

(d) antitetanus globulin.

1 Patients with active immunity who have received a dose of toxoid within the last 10 years need no further prophylaxis.

2 Patients who last had toxoid more than 10 years ago require a tetanus toxoid booster and, if the wound is old or deep, or contamination is present, a course of penicillin.

3 Non-immune patients should be given a tetanus toxoid course and a course of penicillin for all but the most minor wounds.

4 Human antitetanus globulin has been produced for passive immunity in patients with high-risk wounds. It is expensive, not readily available and not without risks.

Hand injuries

These are commonly seen in A/E. The importance of careful assessment, particularly of associated injury to artery, tendon or nerve, has been mentioned. The hand should be cleaned, cooled and elevated, and interference kept to a minimum. Severe hand injuries should be referred for a specialist hand surgeon's opinion. Amputated fingertips are commonly seen. If the bone is exposed it is best trimmed back and the wound allowed to granulate. If the wound is less than 1 cm in diameter and particularly in children, re-epithelialization will be satisfactory. If a whole finger has been amputated, reimplantation is possible. The finger should be cooled and the patient referred to a microsurgery unit.

Management of fractures

This section covers the general principles of fracture management as far as these may be required by the general surgical houseman treating a patient with multiple trauma. For the management of specific fractures the reader should refer to a textbook of orthopaedics.

Individual fractures may be either closed, when the skin is intact (simple fracture), or open, when the skin surface over the fracture has been broken to however small an extent (compound fracture). Other terms, which may be applied to fractures, describe the type of break as either transverse, spiral, oblique or comminuted (Fig. 125).

Recognizing the pattern

The patient complains of localized pain at the fracture site and is unable to use the affected limb. The mechanism of injury should be ascertained, as this will give a clue to the type of fracture expected.

On examination. There is swelling, bony deformity and loss of function of the affected limb. Abnormal mobility and crepitus at the fracture site may provide incontrovertible evidence of a fracture.

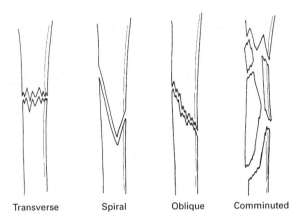

| Transverse | Spiral | Oblique | Comminuted |

Fig. 125 Types of fracture.

Note whether there is a skin wound. If there is, the fracture must be regarded as compound whether or not the bone is visible.

> ### Management
> The precise management depends on the site of the fracture and other associated injuries. In general, however, the steps in management of any fracture are as follows.

Resuscitation and temporary splinting
Fractures of long bones are associated with a significant blood loss, which may require replacement. The pain resulting from a fracture is extreme and analgesic therapy is important. A temporary splint gives relief and protects against further damage whilst the patient is transferred to hospital and X-ray department.

X-ray
Having detected the sites of fractures by clinical methods, an X-ray is essential to define exactly what injury has been sustained. Always ensure that the X-ray includes the joint above and below the fracture.

Repair of skin wounds
If the fracture is compound any skin wound must be carefully explored under general anaesthesia and the bone ends exposed and cleaned. The soft tissue must be cleaned and all dirt and

devitalized tissue must be removed. Associated arterial, nerve and tendon injuries will need to be repaired (see pp. 674–77). The method of wound closure will depend on the time after the injury and the extent of contamination. Clean, recent wounds may be closed immediately, others may have to be closed by delayed primary suture. Antibiotics must be given.

Reduction

If the deformity is putting the overlying skin or neighbouring artery or nerve under pressure, then reduction is urgent. Otherwise it can be delayed whilst more general resuscitative measures are carried out. Reduction may be achieved by closed manipulation under anaesthesia or by open operation.

Fixation

The aim is to maintain the position of the reduced bone ends until they heal together. External immobilization is often achieved with plaster of Paris.

When immobilization is achieved with plaster of Paris, there is a danger of compression of the contents of the limb as the fracture continues to swell. This danger can be avoided by using an initial 'back slab', which can if necessary, be completed later. If a complete plaster has to be applied, it must not be too tight and should contain plenty of padding to allow the fracture to swell. A routine 'plaster check' must be carried out after 24 h and the circulation in the distal limb assessed. If there is any evidence of occlusion, then the plaster must be removed.

Another form of immobilization is the application of traction on each side of the fracture. This may be applied either to the skin or to a pin passed through the skeleton (e.g. a tibial pin for reduction of a fractured femur).

Internal fixation is used when the fracture is reduced by open operation. The bone ends are fixed either by a device placed within the cortex (intramedullary nail, screws or wires) or by a pin and plate placed on the outer cortex.

Rehabilitation

Any prolonged immobilization of the limb will lead to muscle wasting and joint stiffness. Regular physiotherapy is important therefore both during the period of immobilization and once the fracture has healed.

Fat embolism

Fat embolism can complicate major fracture and is more common than generally supposed and occurs when droplets of fat get into the blood stream. The fat may be derived from bone marrow or adipose tissue but may also be of metabolic origin, perhaps by aggregation of chylomicrons. The emboli may lodge in the pulmonary circulation or pass through the lungs and lodge in parts of the systemic circulation such as the brain, skin and kidney.

Recognizing the pattern

The patient is often a young adult with a lower limb fracture, but the condition can also occur in those with severe burns or extensive soft tissue trauma.

There is sudden onset of respiratory distress, drowsiness, restlessness or disorientation 24–48 h following injury.

On examination mild pyrexia and tachycardia are early signs. Petechial haemorrhage due to skin emboli is a helpful sign but may not be present. Cyanosis and right heart failure may occur in severe cases.

Proving the diagnosis

Fat droplets may be found in the sputum and urine. The platelet count is invariably low. An arterial blood gas sample will show hypoxaemia, which is the major cause of death. A chest radiograph shows a 'snow-storm' appearance.

> ### Management
> Oxygen should be given. Other measures which have been advocated include heparinization and intravenous low molecular weight dextran. Severe respiratory distress may require sedation and assisted ventilation.

Arterial damage

Arteries may be damaged by direct trauma transecting the vessel, by external compression (e.g. from a nearby fracture) or by traction which disrupts the intima. Thrombosis and occlusion of the vessel often follow this latter injury, even though the outer wall of the artery is intact.

Recognizing the pattern

Penetrating arterial injury is unmistakable. Bright red pulsatile blood escapes from the wound.

With an acute arterial occlusion the patient complains of pain in the muscles distal to the damaged vessel. The affected tissues are pale and cold and there are paraesthesiae and paralysis. Distal pulses are absent.

Proving the diagnosis

An emergency arteriogram is always indicated when there is a suspicion of arterial injury This is usually performed in the operating theatre by the surgical team.

Management
An occlusion of a main limb artery needs urgent exploration and repair.

OPERATION: EXPLORATION OF TRAUMATIC ARTERIAL OCCLUSION

The artery is exposed and the site of damage identified. If the artery has been transected, the damaged ends are resected and a vein graft used to bridge the gap created. Attention must also be paid to any venous damage.

If the artery is intact, then an occlusion is due either to external compression or to an intimal tear. If any external compression has been relieved and the distal pulses do not return, an arteriotomy is performed and the damaged segment either excised or bypassed.

Codes

Blood	2–4 units
GA/LA	GA
Opn time	1–2 h
Stay	Depends on other injuries
Drains out	Suction drain 48 h
Sutures out	7 days
Off work	Depends on other injuries

Nerve injuries

There are three types of nerve injury.

1 Neuropraxia. This is caused by a blunt injury resulting in concussion of the nerve.

2 Axonotmesis. This is caused by a stretching injury which ruptures the axons but not the nerve sheath. The axons degenerate distal to the injury.

3 Neurotmesis. This is complete severance of the nerve and its sheath.

Recognizing the pattern

The clinical signs of nerve injury are loss of sensation and flaccid paralysis with loss of reflexes. The precise clinical picture depends on the particular nerve which is damaged.

Management

Neuropraxia and axonotmesis

If the injury is a neuropraxia, the treatment is conservative and the nerve usually recovers in 7–10 days. Axonotmesis takes longer because the axons have to grow back down the intact nerve sheath. Physiotherapy is required to prevent contractures and maintenance of normal posture until renervation occurs. The patient needs adequate reassurance and should be told that the nerves grow at the rate of about 1 mm/day (or 1 inch/month). Several weeks may therefore be needed for recovery of an axonotmesis in a limb.

Neurotmesis

When a nerve has been divided, the wound must be carefully explored to identify the nerve ends. These should be freshened and the nerve sheath resutured accurately to restore continuity. If this is done with care, there is a good chance that the axons will regrow down the distal nerve sheath. They also regrow at the rate of 1 mm/day.

Digital nerves

A divided digital nerve can be repaired using a microsurgical technique. Digital nerve injuries particularly in the dominant hand involving the thumb, index or middle finger cause serious disabilities and should always be repaired.

Tendon injuries

Tendons may be partially or completely lacerated. Such tendon injuries are commonly seen after cuts over the dorsum of the fingers, back of the hand or the wrist. Careful repair is essential.

Making the diagnosis

Complete division of a tendon is made obvious by the loss of function of the affected muscle. Where there is a laceration over the anatomical site of a tendon, careful examination of the function of the extensors and flexors should be carried out.

Management

The treatment of partial or complete tendon rupture is surgical repair. The wound should be explored under a general anaesthetic. If necessary the patient can wait 6–8 h until the next morning's operating list, providing there is no associated arterial injury. A partial division of a tendon can be repaired by a continuous suture of fine Prolene or other similar material. A complete division needs end-to-end anastomosis.

Postoperative care

The limb is splinted so as to relax the affected tendon and minimize any tension across the suture line. Physiotherapy is commenced early.

Burns

Major burns are a threat to life. Deterioration can be rapid and the management in the acute stage is critical. There are five types of burns.

1 Dry thermal — flame
2 Wet thermal — scald
3 Chemical
4 Electrical
5 Friction.

The damage is caused by coagulation of proteins with cell death. Burns can be of varying depth and any one burn is rarely uniform.

A mild burn causes vasodilatation and diffuse erythema. Kinins are released which cause pain.

Moderate burns cause some cell death with increased capillary permeability and blister and oedema formation. Sensation remains intact and as these burns are of partial thickness the skin will regrow.

Severe burns cause death of cells involving the dermis and deeper tissues, and appear as white insensitive areas. The full thickness of the skin is damaged and the skin will not regrow as the germinal layers have been destroyed. Such a burn heals by fibrosis with resulting contractures.

The main early danger from major burns is the development of 'burn shock'. Burn shock is due to exudation of protein-rich fluid from the surface of the burn and oedema into the tissues beneath the burn. Both these follow increased capillary permeability. The loss of fluid results in hypovolaemia which can develop rapidly, the extent depending on the size of the burn. A patient with 50% burns, for instance, can lose half his plasma volume within 3–4 h. This fluid loss must be replaced rapidly.

Anaemia can develop due to blood loss, red cell destruction and bone marrow suppression.

Later, the damaged and necrotic tissue, lying in a protein-rich exudate, is an ideal site for infection, which can result in septicaemia.

Assessment

The precise history of the time and cause of the burn must be obtained including the length of time that the causative agent was active. A rapid initial examination is performed to assess the following:

1 Signs of shock — apprehension, restlessness, thirst, pallor, sweating, tachycardia, hypotension and air hunger.

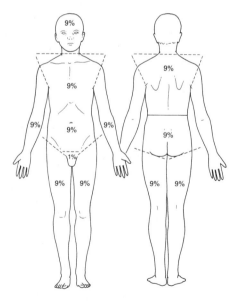

Fig. 126 A method for measuring the extent of burns on the body surface area. 'Wallace's rule of nines' (11 areas of the body, each equal to about 9% of the total surface areas).

2 Whether or not the airway is affected by an inhalation burn — stridor, hoarseness, soot in nostrils, pharyngeal erythema.

3 The size of the burn (Fig. 126). The area of the burn is expressed as a percentage of the total body surface area. It is calculated using 'Wallace's rule of nines' as in Fig. 126. It may be useful to remember that the hand represents 1% of the adult body surface area.

This initial assessment allows burns to be divided into minor or major categories.

Minor burns

These are burns involving less than 10–15% of the adult body surface area (less than 10% in children), with little evidence of systemic upset or disturbance of the airway.

On examination

Draw the size of the burn and map out the areas of definite full thickness, probable full thickness and partial thickness damage. These are judged by the appearance (erythema, blistering or white areas), and the presence or absence of sensation to pin-prick.

Management

Different centres have different regimes. Below is one possible scheme of management.

Local management

1 Superficial burns of the face and superficial scalds are left exposed to the air. They heal in 10–14 days.

2 Partial thickness burns cause erythema and superficial blistering with no break in the skin. They are cleaned with an antiseptic agent and dressed with tulle gras. They are then re-examined in 3–5 days. Check that no areas have become full thickness. The wounds are then redressed and the burns usually heal with little scarring.

3 Deeper burns. Burns with skin loss or those which are dirty must be cleaned with an antiseptic solution and all dirt, large blisters and dead tissue removed. The burn may then be coated liberally with Flamazine cream. This cream contains sulphadiazine and is useful in preventing infection, especially by Gram-negative organisms. It is also useful in treating infected burns. The Flamazine-coated burn is dressed

Continued on p. 680

Continued.

with gauze and ideally is redressed daily. This cream also has a soothing effect. The cream must not be used when a second assessment is required, as it is difficult to examine the burn once it has been applied.

4 Full thickness burns. These heal by fibrosis, causing contractures and scarring, and are best treated by skin grafting. This is done either at 3–5 days or after 3 weeks when the burnt skin is sloughing.

Oral fluids

Those containing sodium are sufficient to counteract any mild hypovolaemia.

Major burns

A burn is described as major when the area involved is more than 15% of the body surface area (10% in children). The regional burns centre should be contacted regarding all major burns.

Management

The main priority is maintenance of the airway and prevention of circulatory collapse. While this is undertaken, the burn is covered with sterile towels.

Airway

If the airway is obstructed or the patient has inhaled soot, pass an airway or endotracheal tube. If severe respiratory damage has occurred, an early tracheostomy may be indicated.

Analgesia

Burns are very painful and adequate analgesia must be given. Intravenous morphine (0.1 mg/kg) gives instant pain relief. Intravenous chlorpromazine (0.5 mg/kg) sedates the patient and acts as an antiemetic.

Fluid replacement

Delay in replacing the fluid lost can lead to rapid deterioration, renal failure and death.

Set up at least one intravenous infusion with a wide-gauge cannula. Avoid using a central venous pressure line if possible, due to the risk of infection. Catheterize the patient to monitor the urine output.

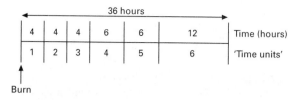

Fig. 127 Six 'time units' after a burn.

During cannulation take blood for haemoglobin, haematocrit, urea and electrolytes, and serum for grouping and cross-matching blood.

Calculation of fluid deficit

There are many formulae to help you do this. The one below (the Mount Vernon formula) is commonly used and estimates the volume of plasma (colloid) required to replace the predicted plasma loss. Different formulae are required if crystalloid is used, as more fluid will then be needed.

The first 36 h after the burn are divided up into six 'time units', as shown in Fig. 127. A similar volume of fluid is given for each 'time unit'. This volume of fluid is calculated from the patient's weight and the area of the burn, as follows:

Plasma volume required for each time unit

$$= \frac{\% \text{ Area} \times \text{weight (kg)}}{2} \text{ cm}^3.$$

For example a 50% burn in a 70-kg man needs 1.75 L of plasma in each time unit.

You will note that the time units immediately after the burn are much shorter than those later on. The first 12 h is the critical period. If therapy is not started until 4 h after a burn, then the fluid deficit must also be replaced. Therefore the calculated volume required for the first 12 h must be given in the remaining 8 h.

One of the problems with a formula that predicts the rate of plasma loss is that, if fluid replacement is not started early, the patient will become hypovolaemic and this in itself will reduce the rate of fluid loss. The above formula will then overestimate the plasma requirements. In this situation the actual (static) plasma deficit may be calculated using the haematocrit, as follows:

Static plasma deficit

$$= \text{blood volume} \ \frac{\text{blood volume} \times \text{normal haematocrit}}{\text{measured haematocrit}}$$

For example, knowing the normal blood volume (5 L) and haematocrit (44) for a 70-kg man, if the above patient's haematocrit was 60, 4 h after the burn, then the actual plasma deficit is 1334 mL. The predicted loss was 1750 mL.

This method gives a prediction of the patient's fluid requirement, and frequent clinical observations must be made to check on the patient's fluid status and urine output. Serial haematocrit estimations are invaluable. As a result of this reassessment, the amount of fluid required in each time unit can be modified accordingly.

Blood requirements

Blood replacement will be required if the burn is deep and more than 10% of the body area. Then, for each 1% burn, give 1% of the patient's total blood volume. The above patient would need 2.5 L of blood. The blood is usually given in the sixth time unit instead of the equivalent amount of plasma. If the burn is 25% or more, it may be given in the second and sixth time units.

An extensive burn causes an ileus and the patient is not therefore able to take oral fluids. In this case the standard body requirements for water and electrolytes must be added to the burn formula regime.

Infection

Systemic antibiotics are usually given in extensive burns prophylactically. Penicillin and flucloxacillin are suitable.

The local management of the burn itself is described on p. 679.

> **Management of burns in special sites**
>
> In deep circumferential burns of the limb or chest, the tight burnt skin may occlude the blood supply to the extremities or affect respiration. The burnt skin must be divided along the length of the limb or in a criss-cross pattern on the chest wall, to release this constricting pressure.
>
> Burns around the eye rapidly result in extensive periorbital oedema. It is therefore essential to examine the eye early before the palpable fissure closes. If the eyelids have been

destroyed, the eye must be bathed with artificial tears and the eyelids restored by plastic surgery at the earliest opportunity to prevent corneal scarring.

Burns of the head and neck with severe facial oedema or evidence of inhalation of soot or hot gases require urgent tracheostomy.

Severe burns to the hands must be cleaned, dressed with tulle gras, and elevated to minimize oedema. The patient should be referred to a plastic surgeon.

List of Operations Index

Index